AF443251

# FILM PROCESSING
## IN
# MEDICAL IMAGING

# FILM PROCESSING IN MEDICAL IMAGING

ARTHUR G. HAUS

*Editor*

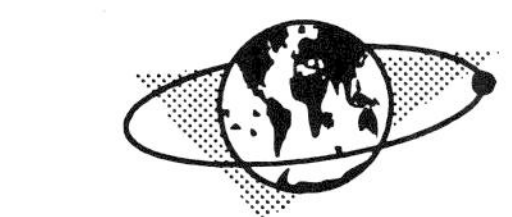

**MEDICAL PHYSICS PUBLISHING**
Madison, Wisconsin

**Published by Medical Physics Publishing**
732 N. Midvale Boulevard
Madison, WI  53705
608-262-4021

ISBN: 0-944838-40-5

Cover design by Becky Chapman-Winter

# Preface

This book is the result of a symposium titled "Film Processing in Medical Imaging: A Practical Update for the 90's", which was held at the Rochester Institute of Technology in March of 1992. The meeting was co-sponsored by the Upstate New York Chapter of the American Association of Physicists in Medicine, the Rochester Institute of Technology Center for Imaging Science and the Health Sciences Division of Eastman Kodak Company.

In medical imaging and particularly in mammography, there is a growing interest and emphasis on film processing and film processor quality control. This book discusses the state of the art of film processing in medical imaging and addresses many areas that have changed over the past decade. Contributions were provided by experts from medical facilitites, including radiologists, medical physicists and radiologic technologists, industrial scientists and engineers, and film processor dealers and service organization representatives. This book should serve as a valuable reference for medical physicists, radiologic technologists, radiologists and equipment engineers.

The contributors to the symposium and to this book have enabled this comprehensive publication and and their efforts are deeply appreciated. The editorial suggestions provided by Mrs. Dawn S. Beck and the symposium coordinating assistance of Mrs. Cheryl R. Siegenthaler and Mrs. Joanna N. Tuzzeo are also greatly appreciated.

Royalties from the sale of this book will be equally divided to support the Robert J. Shalek Graduate Fellowship in Medical Physics program in Clinical Physics at the M.D. Anderson Cancer Center in Houston, Texas and to support students involved in medical imaging at the Center for Imaging Science, Rochester Institute of Technology, Rochester, New York.


Arthur G. Haus

# Contents

# Historical Developments in
# Film Processing in Medical Imaging

**Arthur G. Haus**
Health Sciences Division
Eastman Kodak Company
Rochester, New York

Roentgen's discovery of x-rays in 1895 occurred because a fluorescent screen (barium platinocyanide) emitted light when excited by radiation emerging from a Crookes tube. This radiation also produced an image on a photographic dry plate. After Roentgen discovered x-rays, glass plates, flexible films, and sensitized papers were used to record the radiographic image. Roentgen's original communication discussed the importance of the photographic plate for recording the radiographic image. The first radiograph, Mrs. Roentgen's hand, demonstrated this point.

In the early days of radiology, most radiographs were made by photographers or by physicians whose hobby was photography. Radiography was considered a specialized branch of photography. In fact, it was often referred to as "the new photography." Photographers established "Roentgen studios" and did a lively business in "x-ray sittings." Many of the radiographs were of pieces of art and metallic objects – the precursor of industrial radiography.

The photographer-radiographer used available materials with which they were accustomed to working. Much of the early literature recommended that the operator use the material that was most familiar. An interesting result of the early dependence on the professional photographer was the choice of sizes of sensitized products. In the years just prior to Roentgen's discovery, photographers made life-sized portraits of their clients. The sizes of the plates and film were ideal for radiography. The 1886 price list of one plate and film manufacturer listed popular sizes such as 14 x 17 inches, 11 x 14 inches, 10 x 12 inches, 8 x 10 inches, 6-1/2 x 8-1/2 inches, and 5 x 7 inches. Most radiographs were made on glass plates because glass was considered superior to film and the characteristics of glass were better understood. The consensus was that any fast photographic plate was satisfactory, and good results were achieved.

Many types of developers were used in the days of glass plates; no two were alike. The quantities of chemicals used were not standardized and development was based on the user's experience.

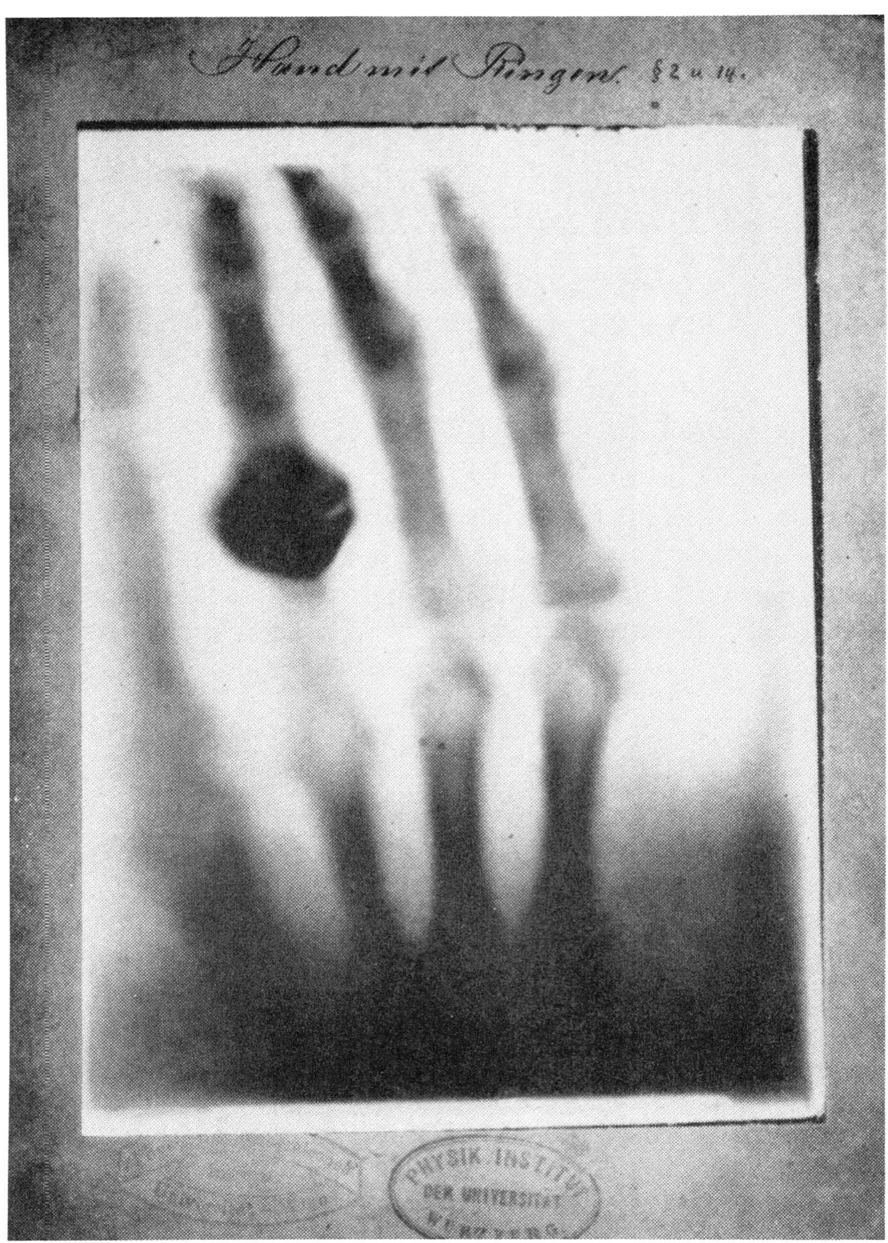

Figure 1. The first medical radiograph. This radiograph of Mrs. Roentgen's hand was made by Roentgen before he announced his discovery of x-rays. On January 1, 1896, Roentgen sent a copy of a separate printing of his first paper on x-rays with examples of his x-ray photographs to several colleagues. Photographic positive prints made from the x-ray plate of his wife's hand and eight other plates formed the collection from which he selected the examples forwarded to his colleagues together with his paper.

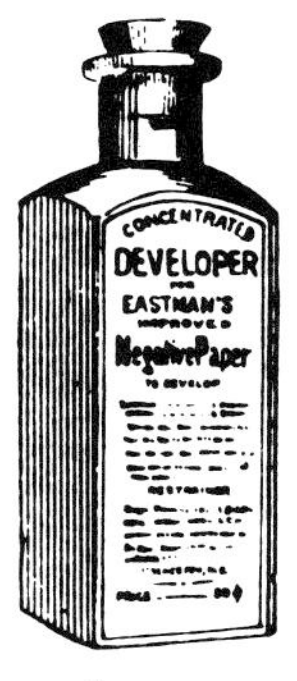

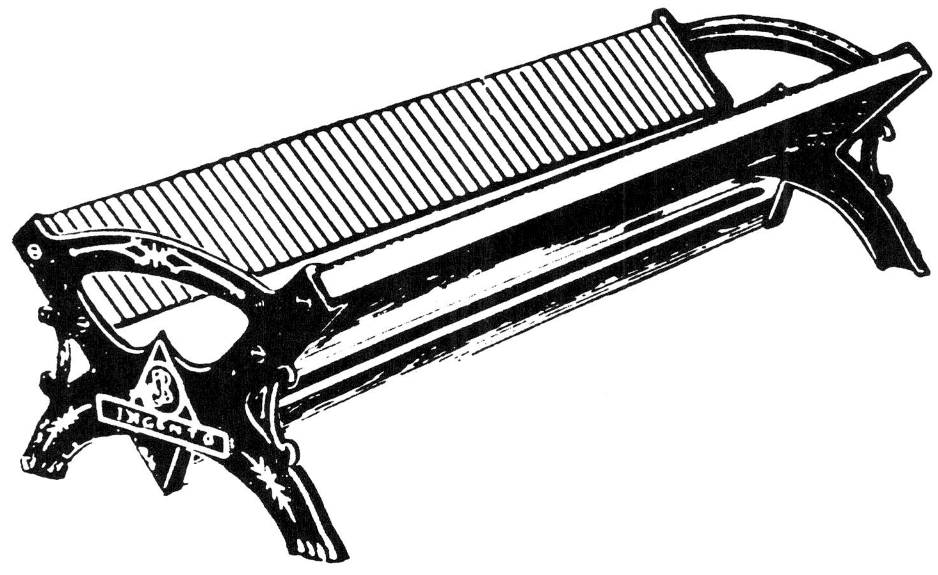


Figure 2. Page of the 1886 price list of the Eastman Dry Plate and Film Company showing the listing for a concentrated solution of developer.

Figure 3. A rack to hold processed glass plates (vertically placed) while drip drying.

A few pioneer radiographers recognized the deficiencies inherent in photographic materials when exposed to x-rays such as low maximum density, lack of contrast and slow speed. In the decade following Roentgen's discovery, experimenters proposed ways to overcome these problems. In December 1896, the first paper designed specifically for x-ray purposes was introduced. This venture failed, however, because the radiographs were difficult to interpret, due to the contrast and the low maximum density of the paper. Several manufacturers began to make special plates for x-ray use with varying degrees of success.

After exposure, the plate was developed to produce a photographic print on sensitized paper rather than a roentgenographic negative. Today, we know that direct interpretation of those plates was almost impossible. Prints were required and interpretations were made from the prints. The early roentgen-ray plate possessed wide latitude with little contrast whereas high quality, distinctive results could be produced in the prints.

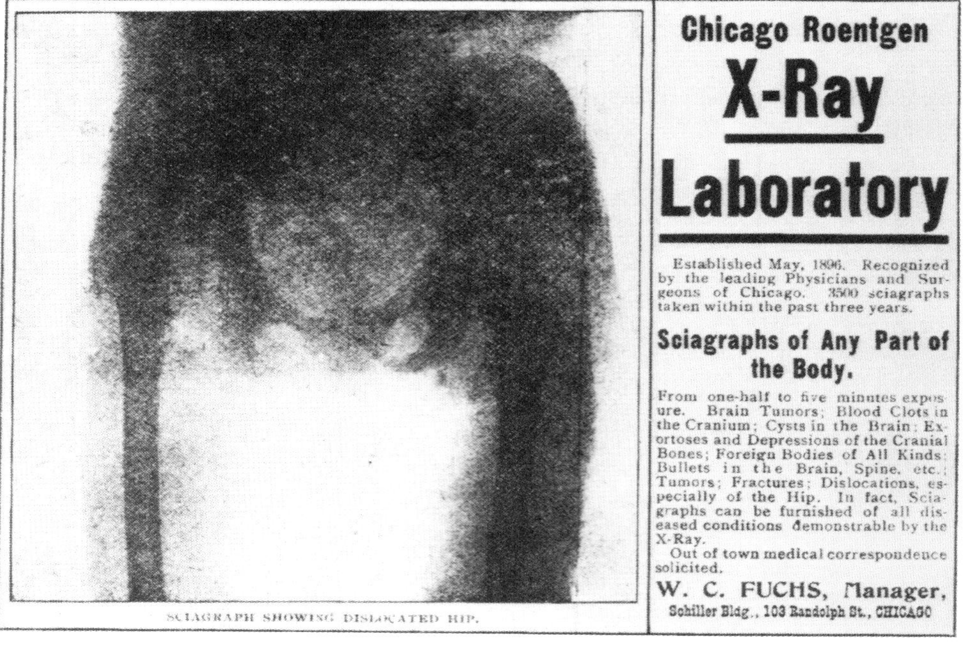


**Figure 4. Early advertisement by Wolfram C. Fuchs. Mr. Fuchs operated his successful and highly regarded laboratory until severe roentgen dermatitis forced his retirement in 1905.**

In the early development of roentgenograms and prints, the roentgenographer developed by means of the old four bottle photographic method, covering the sensitive material first with a solution containing the developing agent, then preservative and accelerator, and then the bromide. As development proceeded, a little more of one solution or another was added in order to "bring out the desired anatomical detail," until development was complete. The roentgenographer or photographer thought that they were able to bring out the desired anatomical detail.

The more successful developers contained pyrogallic acid, metol, or hydroquinone as reducing agents. Various quantities of alkali, sodium sulfite, and potassium bromide were used to accelerate or retard developer activity.

The most prevalent method for increasing the density of the image was after-treatment (intensification) of the negatives; many of the leading roentgen workers of the time resorted to this practice.

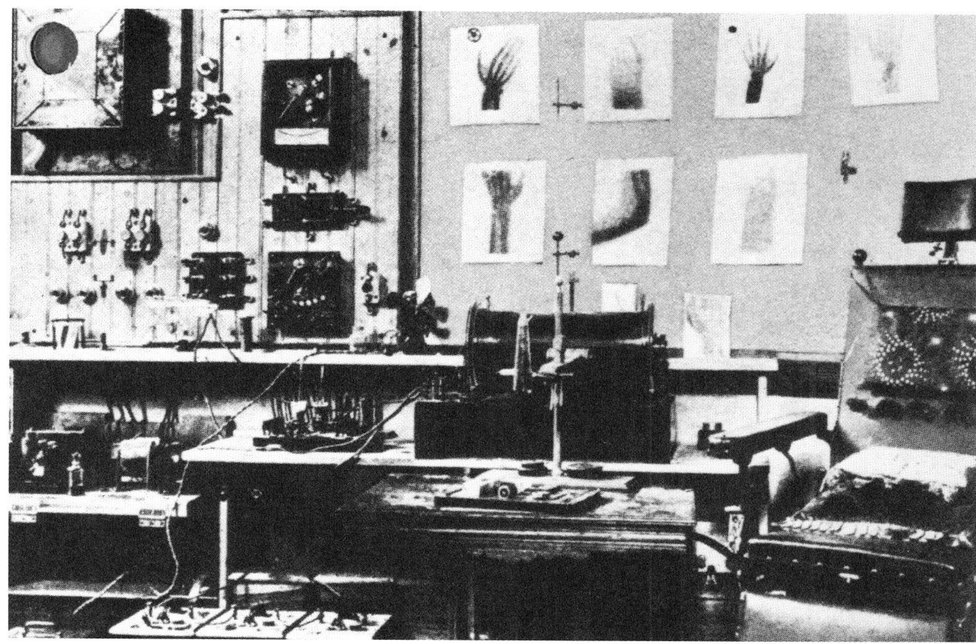

**Figure 5. Laboratory of Wolfram C. Fuchs showing some of the equipment he used along with photographic copies of some of the radiographs he made.**

Before 1900, plates were largely hand-processed in trays. Since each plate required special treatment in development (because the variation of emulsions required unpredictable exposures), close inspection of the developing image was required. Once the speed of plates became somewhat standardized (and the radiation quality and output could be better controlled), it was possible to time the development period more precisely, which varied from about 10 to 25 minutes. During development, the plate had to be agitated constantly to ensure uniform development of the entire image.

As interest in radiography grew, more efficient and quicker processing methods became necessary. By 1906, wooden tanks were made with slotted sides so that plates could be easily inserted in the slots and the development period could be precisely timed. Compartments in the tanks were set apart for the various plate sizes then in use.

By 1910, slotted plate-developing hangers became available which had a crossbar at the top for suspending the plate in the solutions. The hangers could be used to transfer plates to other sections of the tank, thereby eliminating the need for separate compartments for plates of various sizes.

Modified tanks became available which provided for a developing compartment, a rinse area, a fixer compartment, and a large washing area. The first tanks were made of wood or wood lined with lead sheeting; later, they were constructed of soapstone. These tanks produced greater uniformity of results than could be achieved with tray development and also substantially reduced the space required for processing the plates.

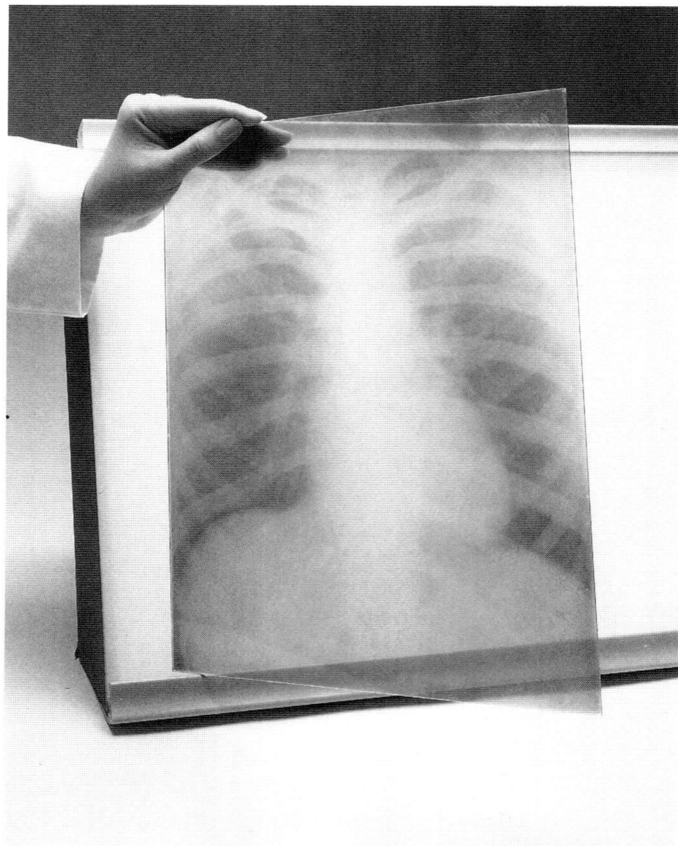

**Figure 6. This chest radiograph was recorded on a single-emulsion glass plate in 1912.**

Many of the problems of using a glass plate as a support for the sensitive emulsion were recognized before Roentgen made his discovery, and roll films for photography developed by Eastman had been marketed as early as 1889. The year 1914 marked the turning point. Most of the glass needed to manufacture photographic plates was produced in Belgium and the start of World War I halted the supply. Simultaneously, the demand for medical radiographs increased and the need for a suitable x-ray film became urgent. In 1913, an x-ray film was introduced that had a cellulose nitrate base coated on one side with an emulsion more sensitive to x-rays than any previously available emulsion. Better radiographs could be produced with less exposure and the new film permitted more extensive use of intensifying screens, with consequent reduction in exposure. Intensive research resulted in an improved product and, in 1916, a non-curling film base was introduced.

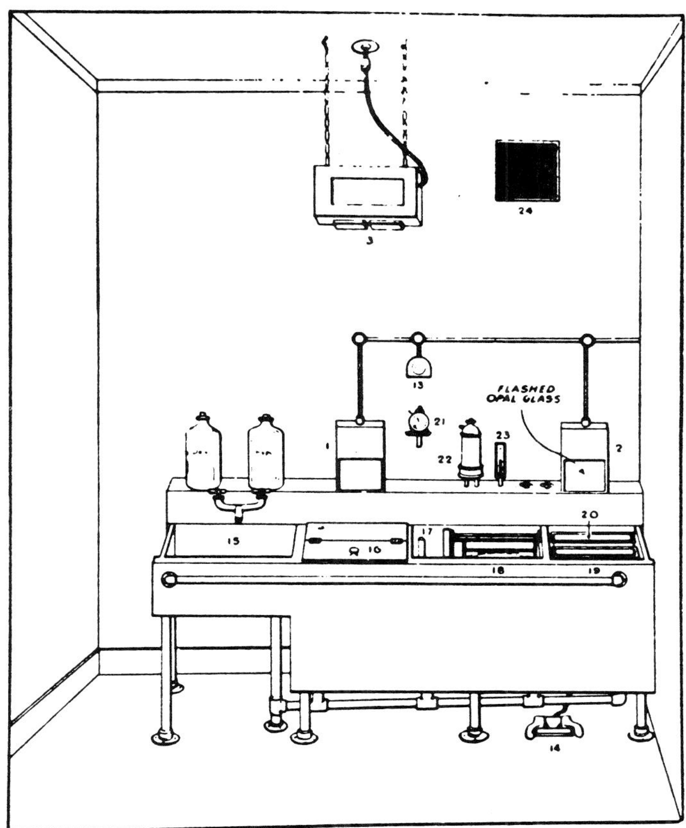



**Figure 7. Darkroom in 1918. Tray processing was satisfactory for plates but not as good for film.**

The year 1918 marked a significant advancement in x-ray film. The first film to have a high-speed emulsion coated on both sides of the support was introduced. It permitted the use of double intensifying screens, which further reduced exposure and exposure times. During the same year, the double-screen technique with "thin" front and "thick" back screens was developed.

Strange as it may seem, it was not easy to convince radiologists and technologists that film offered any appreciable advantage over glass plates. There were years of prejudice to overcome and film could not be processed by familiar techniques. Glass plates and film coated on one side could be processed satisfactorily in trays, but film coated with emulsion on both sides of the support could not be processed satisfactorily in this way. By 1920, however, film hangers and deep tanks for processing were readily available. Fortunately, excellent intensifying screens were also available, and the necessary cassettes and other film holders were soon placed on the market. The reluctance to use film gradually broke down and the popularity of glass plates lessened as continuous improvements were being made in the speed, contrast and emulsion uniformity of x-ray film.

Efforts to quantify the relationship between exposure and the appearance of the resulting image are as old as photography itself. The first real success in this search was the classic work of Hurter and Driffield, published in 1890. Their plot of optical density versus exposure, continues to be useful today and is known as a characteristic curve, or H and D curve (after the originators). The study and measurement of these relationships is known as sensitometry.

In 1917, M. B. Hodgson published a work showing that Hurter and Driffield's methods of evaluation could be used for radiographic as well as photographic materials. In his article, Hodgson noted, "The following factors could be investigated more or less precisely and mathematically: (a) sensitivity or speed, (b) contrast, (c) sensitivity and contrast with wavelengths, (d) development characteristics, and (e) fluorescent screen efficiency characteristics."

Sensitometry was used to evaluate film contrast differences resulting from factors such as development (time and temperature) and recording media (x-ray film and paper). Initially, sensitometry of x-ray materials was performed with exposure to light sources simulating the emission of fluorescent screens. This method was used for many years because calcium tungstate screens predominated, and because a good approximation of their emission had been devised. This method of sensitometry continues to be useful today for quality control of film processing.

A method of standardized tank development was reported in 1929 by Martin, Smith and Hodgson. These investigators recommended the establishment of a constant time of development for a given temperature based on the rate of exhaustion of the developer. This "exhaustion system" assured uniformity of results and made it possible to check exposure time.

In 1947, Crabtree and Henn described the "replenisher system" of development. This technique was designed to maintain the activity of the developer by the addition of developer replenisher solution at a constant rate. It made possible the use of a constant time of development for a given temperature for the life of the solution.

Before the introduction and routine use of automatic film processing in radiology, medical x-ray films had to be hand processed. In hand processing, the exposed radiographic film was loaded onto metal hangers. Then the film was immersed for approximately six minutes in a tank containing developer at 68°F; then immersed in

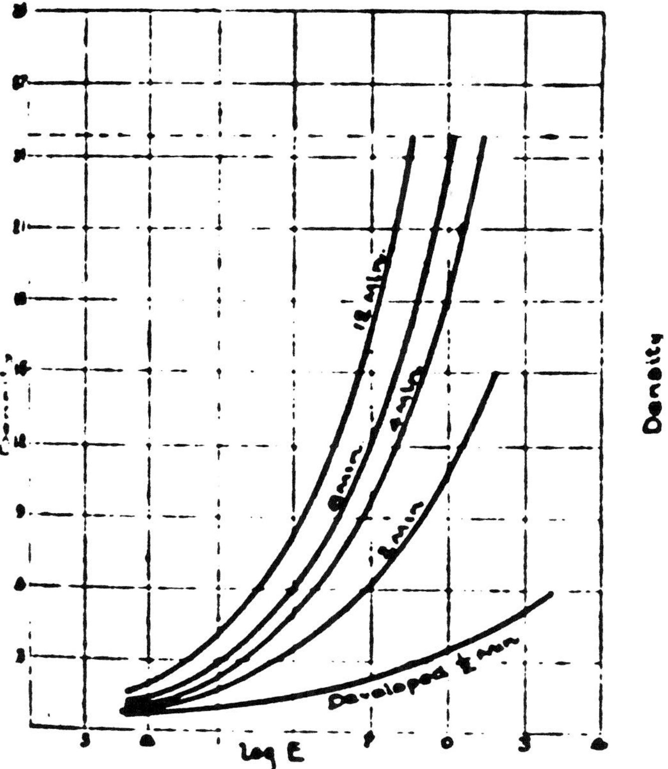


**Figure 8. Characteristic curves, published in 1917 by Hodgson, compared films processed at different developer temperatures.**

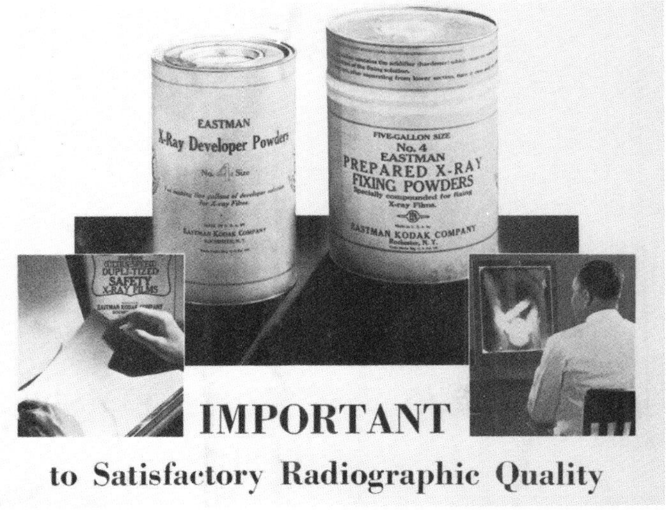


**Figure 9. Advertisement from 1934 isssue of Radiography and Clinical Photography discussing the importance of processing chemicals for radiographic quality.**

a stop bath; followed by immersion in a fixer solution. The film was then washed in running water and hung up to drip dry. It took approximately one hour to obtain a completely dry and ready-to-read radiograph. The number of films processed per hour depended on the size of the processing tanks, dryer capacity, number of darkroom personnel, and so on. Image quality, reproducibility of results, and patient exposure were dependent on the user's control of processing time, solution temperatures and freshness, agitation, and general housekeeping. Frequently, exposure was increased to permit shortened development time for early inspection of the radiograph. This procedure tended to reduce contrast and increase patient radiation exposure.

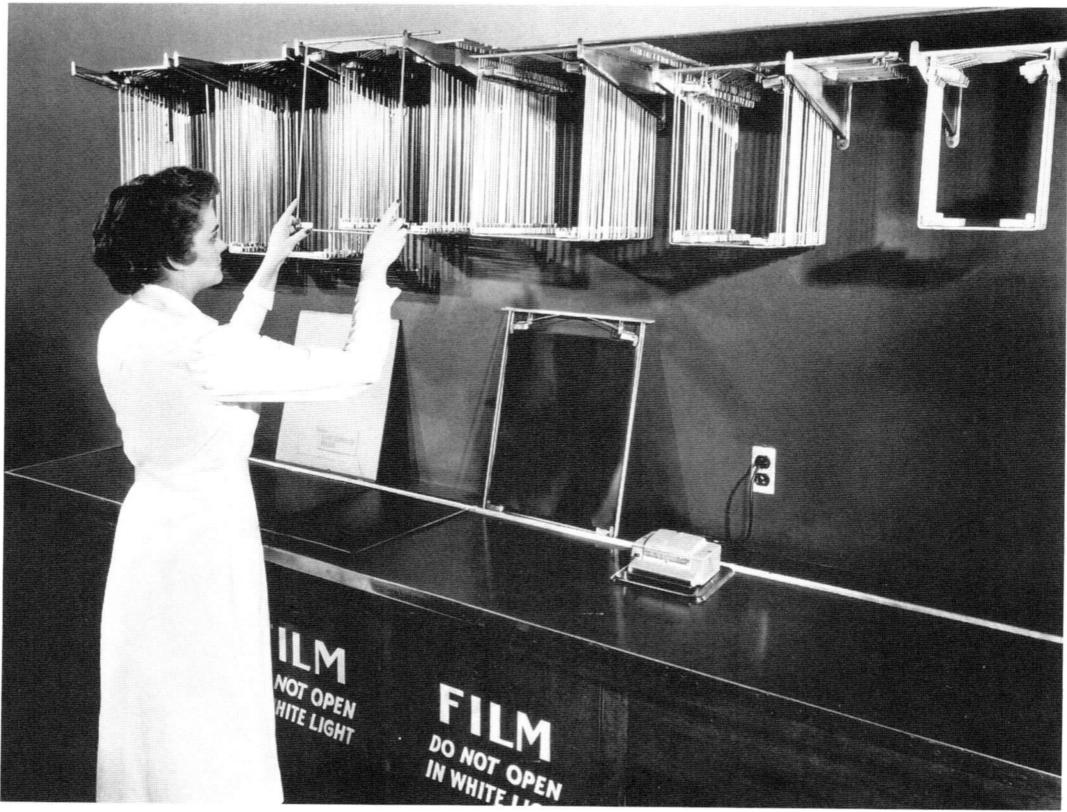


Figure 10. X-ray processing room in the 1940's, showing an x-ray technologist removing metal film hanger from rack.

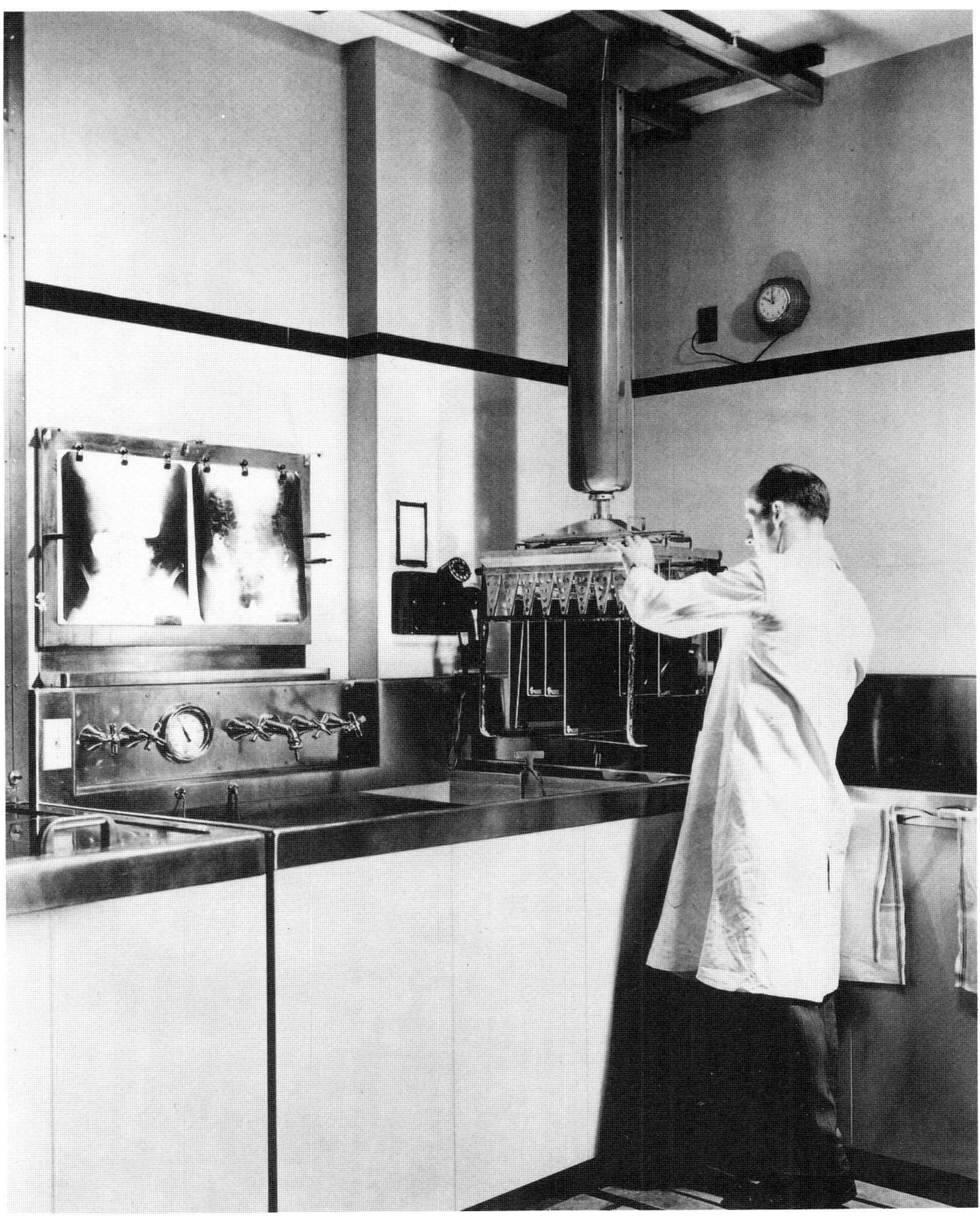

**Figure 11.** X-ray processing room in the 1940's, showing film being removed from processing solutions.

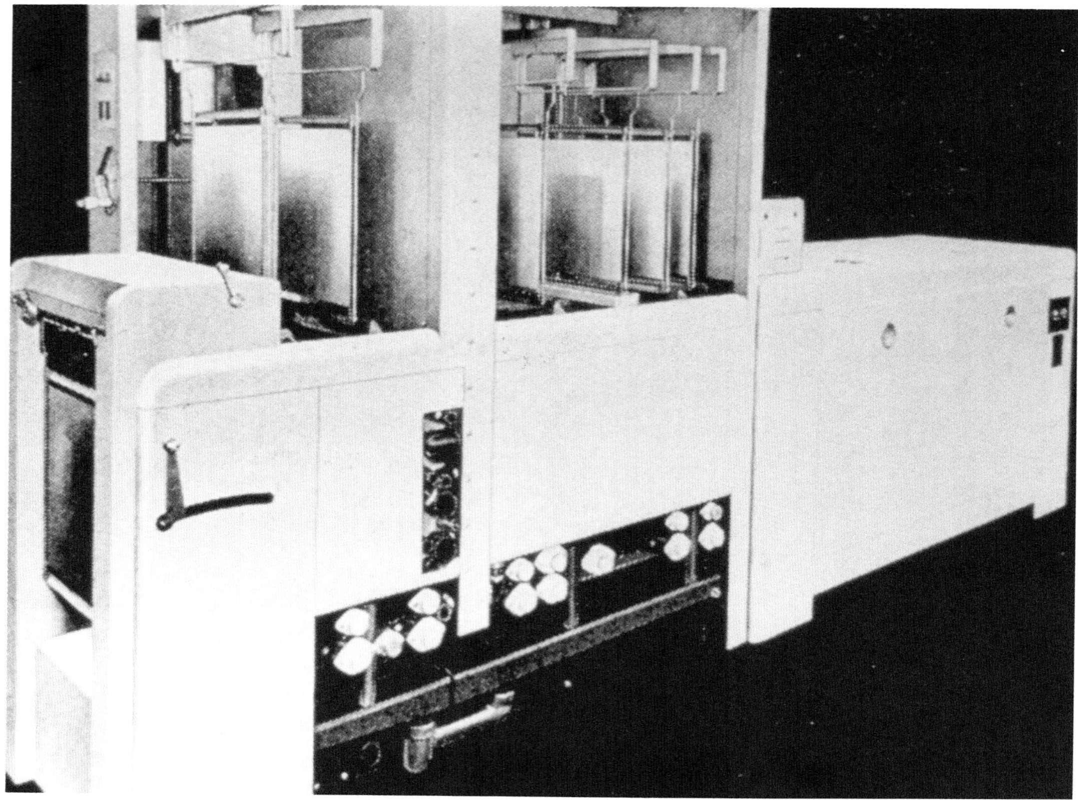

**Figure 12. The first automatic film processor introduced by Pako.**

The first prototype automatic x-ray film processor was introduced by Pako in 1942. The first commercially available model processed 120 films per hour using special film hangers; the total time for processing one film was approximately 40 minutes. A significant improvement in automatic x-ray film processing was made in 1956 when Kodak introduced the first roller transport processor for processing medical radiographs. This processor accommodated all medical x-ay films designed for exposure with intensifying screens. It not only avoided the need for hospitals to change their film inventories, it also avoided the complication of supplying different films to areas without automatic processors such as the emergency room, surgery and urology departments. The processor was about 10 feet long, weighed nearly three quarters of a ton, and sold for approximately $33,000 ($180,000 based on today's dollar).

Automatic processing was a boon to busy departments; finished radiographs became available in 6 minutes and the variability in results caused by the human element was eliminated from processing altogether. Radiologists and radiographers were now able to further standardize techniques in order to reduce the number of retakes as well as the length of time a patient needed to wait for radiographs to be read.

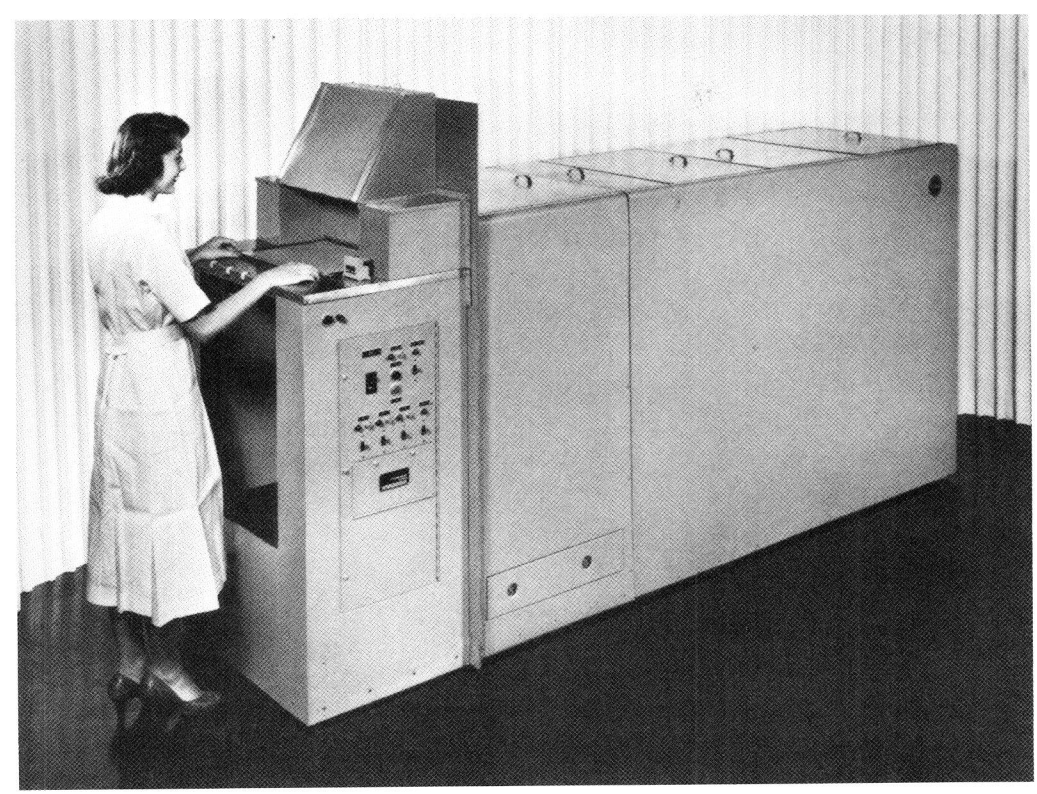

**Figure 13a. Kodak X-Omat processor introduced in 1956. The entire unit, which produced a radiograph in six minutes, occupied about 25 square feet of floor space and measured approximately 10 feet in length. The loading section extended 22 inches into the darkroom.**

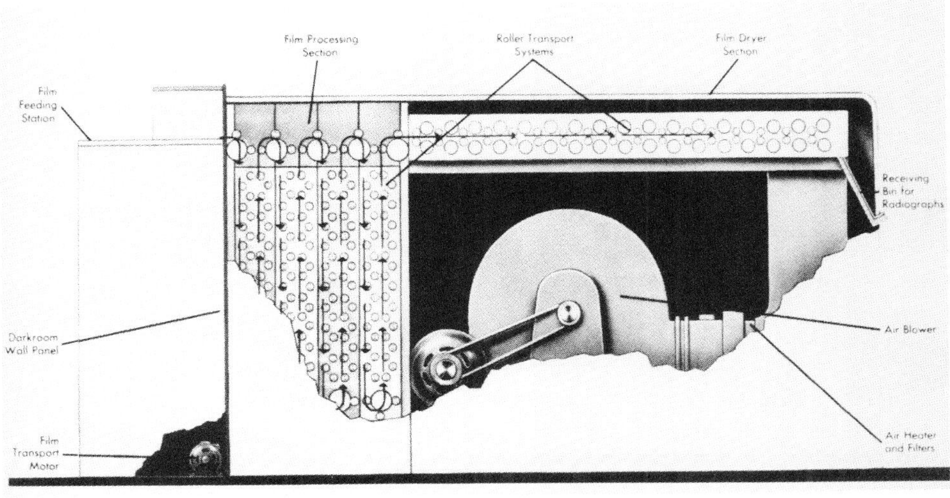


**Figure 13b. Cutaway view of the Kodak X-Omat processor introduced in 1956.**

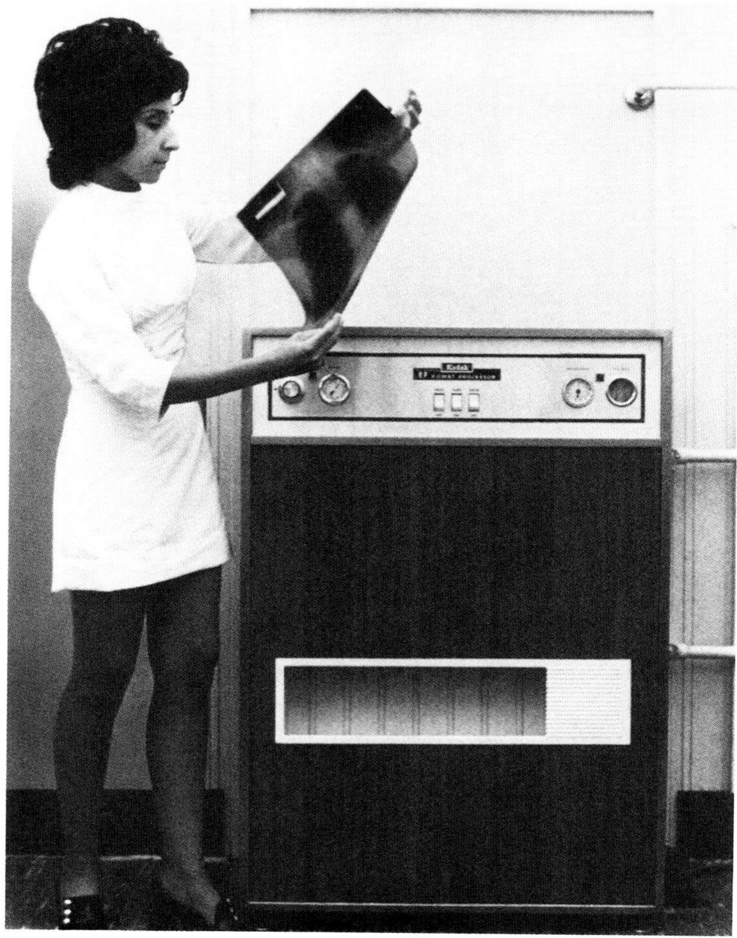

**Figure 14a. This Kodak RP X-Omat processor produces a radiograph in 90 seconds. The entire unit occupies less than five square feet of floor space. The film-feeding station extends only 15 inches into the darkroom; and outside, in the lighted area, the unit requires a space only 22 inches long and 30 inches wide.**

In 1965, another significant breakthrough in the processing of medical x-ray films led to the introduction of 90-second rapid processing by Kodak. This advancement combined new chemistry and new film emulsions, an increased development temperature (95°F), and the use of a polyester film support for better roller transport—all which led to faster drying time. The processor, which was 36 inches long, 30 inches wide, and 42 inches high, processed 215 sheets of film per hour in a dry-to-dry time of 90 seconds per film. This type of automatic processing system remains the industry standard as we know it today. Automatic film processors today range in list price from approximately $6,000 to $28,000.

In 1987, an automatic film processor was introduced by Konica which had a processing cycle of approximately 45 seconds and required special films. In 1990, Kodak introduced an automatic film processor with an approximate 38-second processing cycle; this processor also requires special films and chemicals.

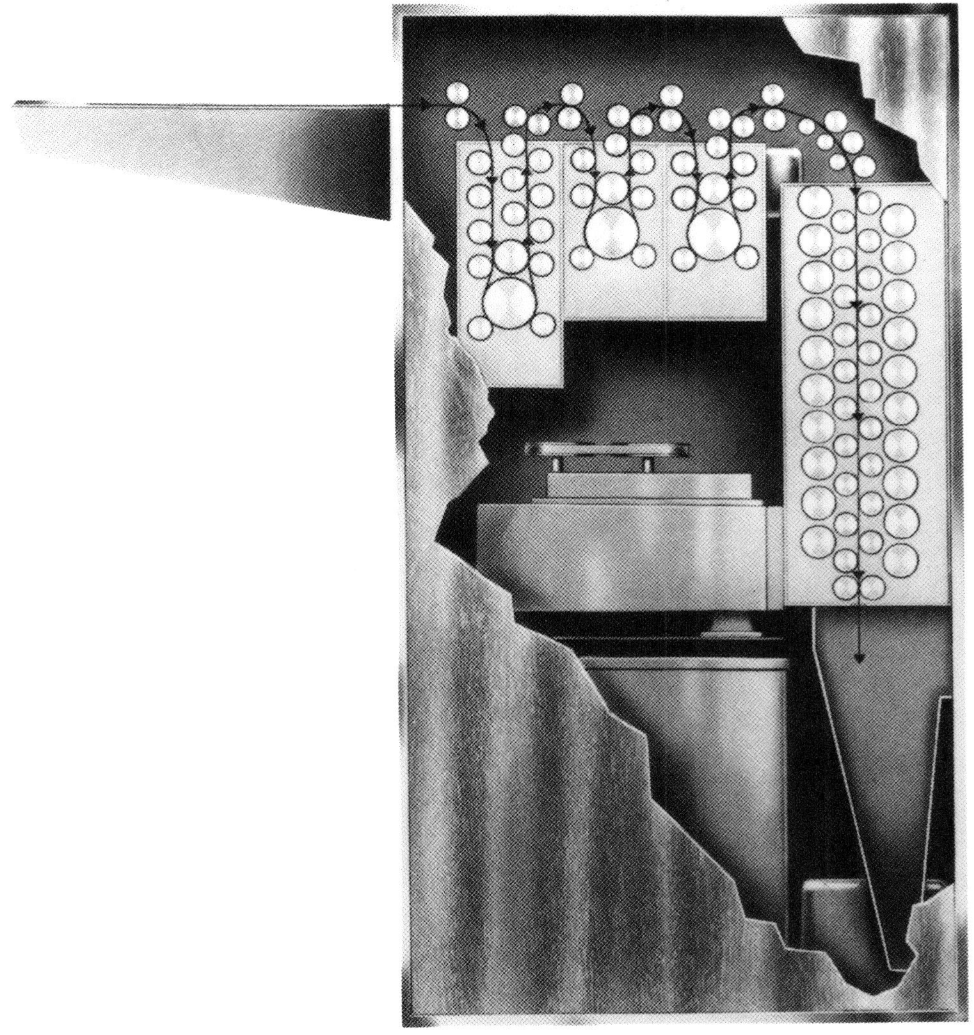

**Figure 14b. Cutaway view of the Kodak RP X-Omat processor. Note the simplification that has taken place since 1956.**

## References


1. Röentgen WC. Ueber eine neue art strahlen. (Vorläufige Mittheilung.) Sitzber, *Physik-Med Ges Würzburg* 1895; 9:132-141.

2. Eisenberg RL. Radiology An Illustrated History. St. Louis, MO. Mosby Year Book Inc.1992.

3. Grigg ERN. The trail of the invisible light. Springfield, IL. Charles C. Thomas, 1965.

4. Martin FC, Fuchs AW. A historical evolution of roentgen ray plates and films. *AJR* 1931; 26:540-548.

5. Kodak and radiography. *Medical Radiography and Photography* 1970; 3:79-106.

6. Haus AG, Cullinan JE. Screen-film processing systems for medical radiography: A historical review. *Radiographics* 1989 9:1203-1224.

7. Hodgson MB. The sensitometry of x-ray materials. *Br J Photogr* 1917; 64:654-657.

8. Martin FC, Smith EE, and Hodgson MB. A new system of standardized tank development. *X-ray Bulletin* 1929 5:6-10.

9. Crabtree JI, Henn RW. Developer solutions for x-ray films. *Medical Radiography and Photography* 1947 23:1-12, 38-46.

# Film Processing: Clinical Requirements

**Perry Sprawls, Jr.**
Emory University
Atlanta, Georgia

## Introduction

The ideal medical-image receptor would be one which produces an immediate image with high diagnostic quality, the lowest possible radiation exposure to the patient, minimum labor requirements, low cost, and no adverse effects on the environment. Today we do not have the ideal receptor. The silver halide film used for most medical imaging applications requires chemical processing to produce the visible image. Chemical processing is a major element which causes film to be less than the ideal receptor component described above. Film processing in the clinical environment can contribute to:

1. Delays in image availability
2. Loss of image quality
3. Unnecessary patient exposure
4. Reduced productivity
5. Increased cost
6. Environmental contamination

The general clinical requirements are to reduce these undesirable effects as much as possible.

## Processing Goals

Several of the clinical requirements listed above relate to the two major operational goals of clinical processing. They are:

1. Processing accuracy
2. Processing consistency

Accurate processing is the level of processing which produces the design sensitivity and contrast characteristics of a film. This is achieved when the processing conditions in the clinical facility produce the same results as the processing used by the film manufacture. Accurate processing conditions are necessary in order to achieve an optimum level of processing.

After accurate processing is established it is necessary to maintain consistent processing over a period of time. This is achieved by means of an ongoing quality control program.

Processing accuracy and consistency are affected by the many variables associated with the processing system. As shown in Figure 1, there are both physical and chemical variables which must be considered.

There are two categories of clinical requirements which must be considered in order to achieve these goals.

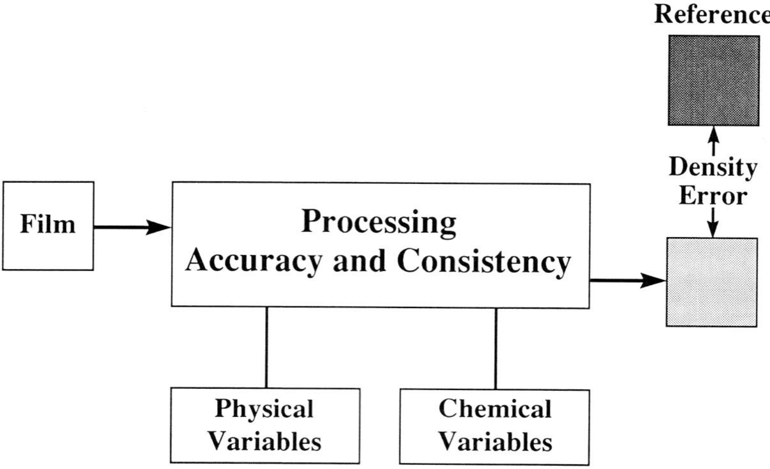


**Figure 1. The two categories of variables that have an effect on processing accuracy and consistency.**

## Requirements of the Clinical Facility

In order to achieve the most desirable processing conditions, there are certain requirements of the clinical facility which must be fulfilled by the industry. These requirements relate to:

1.  Processing equipment design
2.  Chemical formulation
3.  Maintenance and service

## Requirements for Clinical Personnel

The actions performed by clinical personnel which will impact on the quality of film processing include:

1.  Processor equipment selection

2. Chemical selection
3. Processor operation

Clinical personnel must be concerned with both categories of requirements. However, this chapter will give primary emphasis to processor operation, which is most directly under the control of the clinical staff.

## Processing Equipment and Chemicals
A film processor is actually a system consisting of two major components: the equipment and the chemistry.

## Processing Time
The primary design characteristic of a processor which impacts on clinical operation is the time required to process a film. This cycle time is measured from when a film enters the processor until it drops out and is ready for viewing. There are three basic categories of processors with respect to processing time.

### Standard Processing
Most medical film processors are designed for a cycle time of 90 seonds. This time is divided into the four phases:

1. Development
2. Fixing
3. Washing
4. Drying

The immersion time in the developer solution is the primary factor which determines total cycle time. The developer immersion time is in the range of 23 to 32 seconds, depending on the type of film processor. Development temperature and replenishment rates are determined based on the processor cycle time.

### Extended Processing
An extended processing cycle is used in some mammographic applications. Developer immersion time is increased in order to achieve more complete processing of the film and a generally higher contrast for film types which are not fully processed in the standard cycle. A typical developer immersion time for extended processing is 47 seconds with a total cycle time of about 180 seconds. The benefit of extended processing depends on the type of film which is being used. Some film types benefit more from extended processing than others.

## Rapid Access Processing

A general thrust in processor design is to reduce the total cycle time. These are generally known as rapid access processors which have a cycle time of 45 seconds. This faster processing is achieved by using specially formulated chemicals.

Processing time is the principal factor which contributes to:

delays in image availability

reduced productivity

## Processing By-products

Film processing creates several by-products which are potential sources of environmental contamination. The principle by-product in this category is the silver which is removed from the fixer solution and sold because of its significant economic value. However, if the silver recovery process is not completely efficient,  it is possible for the unrecovered silver to pass into the environment through the waste water system.

The completeness of silver recovery and its environmental impact is an important design characteristic of the silver recovery component of the system.

## Film Characteristics

Processing has a major effect on several specific film characteristics. These film characteristics can, in turn, have an impact on image quality and patient exposure.

## Film Sensitivity (Speed)

The sensitivity (speed) of a film determines:

the exposure required to produce an image

the image density resulting from a specific exposure

Each type of medical imaging film is designed with a specific sensitivity value which is appropriate for the film's intended application.

## Unnecessary Patient Exposure

If processing conditions do not produce the intended film sensitivity, it then becomes necessary to increase the radiation exposure in order to obtain an adequately exposed image.

When film sensitivity fluctuates over a period of time, exposure errors will increase. This, in turn, can increase the number of repeated examinations which results in additional and unnecessary exposure to the patient.

### Contrast

The primary function of processing is to produce image contrast. The level of contrast in an image is determined by a combination of the film design characteristics and the level of processing. A specific film can produce the contrast it is designed for only if it is adequately processed.

### Artifacts

The processing operation can produce a variety of image artifacts. The frequency of artifacts is generally related to the physical condition and level of maintenance of the processing equipment.

### Processor Operation

The principle problem with film development is that it is an unstable process which is subject to considerable variability. It is this variability in processing which contributes to:

Reduced image quality.

Unnecessary patient exposure.

The primary requirement in the clinical facility is to control the processing variables in order to achieve and maintain optimum processing conditions.

### Level of Processing

The level or degree to which a film is processed is  a continuum which depends on many of the variable processing parameters. The level of processing for a particular film generally falls within one of the following three ranges. The variables which affect the level of processing will be discussed later.

### <u>underprocessing</u>

An underprocessed film has two undesirable characteristics: a reduced sensitivity (speed) and a loss of contrast. The reduction in sensitivity can result in an "underexposed" film or the need for unnecessarily high exposure to produce an adequate film.

### <u>optimum processing</u>

An optimum level of processing produces film characteristics in the clinical setting which match the design characteristics of the film. Optimum processing is the principal goal in the clinical facility.

### overprocessing

Overprocessing is somewhat more complex than underprocessing. It generally increases the sensitivity (speed) of the film. This might appear to be an advantage in that exposure can be reduced. However, overprocessing can produce overexposed films, especially when the processing is inconsistent. Overprocessing also has an impact on the contrast characteristics of a film. In some cases, a moderate degree of overprocessing decreases contrast because of the added density and fog.

## Processing Variables

There are many individual variable processing parameters which contribute to the overall variability in processing.

## Chemical Variables

Figure 2 shows the major chemical variables which can have an effect on processing accuracy and consistency.

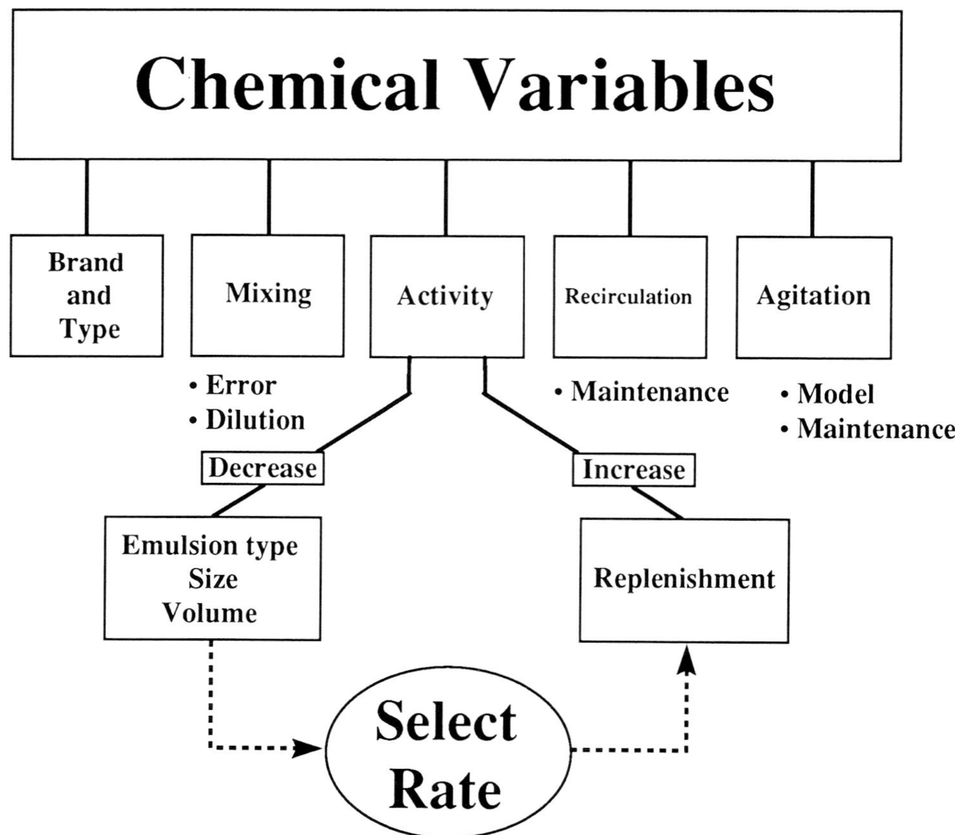


**Figure 2. The Chemical variables which have an effect on processing accuracy and consistency.**

### chemical brand and type

There are some variations in the chemical formulation among the processing chemicals provided by the various manufacturers. Some manufacturers also provide more than one formulation or type of chemistry. While it is not necessary to match chemistry and films on the basis of brand name, it must be demonstrated that a specific chemistry type is capable of producing adequate and accurate processing for each type of film which is being used.

### chemical concentration (mixing)

Processing chemicals are produced in a concentrate form which are then mixed with water and diluted to the appropriate concentration. This mixing is performed either manually or by automatic mixing devices attached to individual processors.

Inadequate chemical concentration can result from mixing errors (manual or automatic) or intentional over-dilution for reasons of economy or profit.

### chemical activity (replenishment)

The activity of the developer chemistry is a dynamic characteristic which must be set and maintained at the appropriate level. The activity is decreased by the development process at a rate determined by the type of emulsion, film size, and the number of films (volume) processed. Automatic replenishment compensates for this decrease in activity. The crucial factor is selecting a replenishment rate which provides the appropriate compensation.

### contamination

The accidental contamination of the developer solution by other chemicals, such as the fixer, can significantly alter the chemical activity and the resulting level of processing.

### recirculation

A relatively stable chemical activity requires the constant recirculation of the solution. A defect in the recirculation system is a potential cause of changes in the level of processing.

### agitation

The level of processing can be affected by the degree of mixing and agitation at the film surface where the chemical interactions actually occur. This can vary from one type of processor to another and might be affected by the level of maintenance.

### Physical Variables

Figure 3 shows the two major physical variables which have an impact on the level of processing.

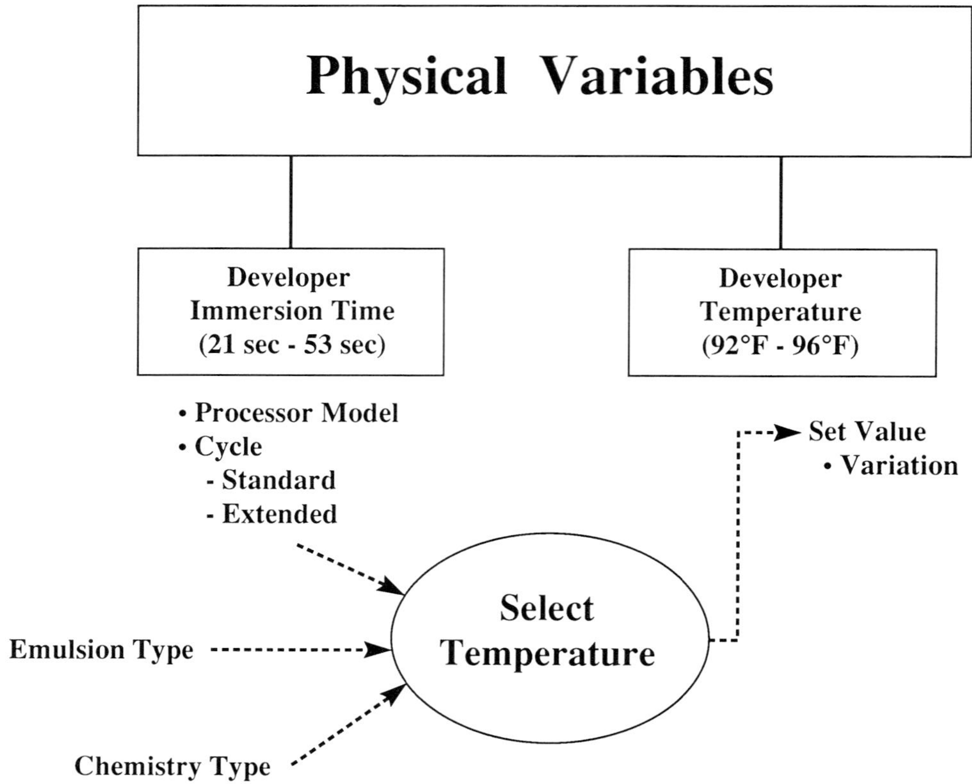


Figure 3. The major physical variables which have an effect on processing accuracy and consistency.

## immersion time

The immersion time is determined by processor design and the specific processing cycle which has been selected.

## temperature

Developer temperature has a major effect on the level of development. The appropriate temperature for a specific emulsion type depends on the type of chemistry being used and the processing cycle. The film and chemical manufacturers recommendations should be consulted for the appropriate temperature value which will achieve accurate processing. Variation in temperature should be minimized for the purpose of achieving consistent processing.

To obtain the goal of optimum processing, two steps are required. The first is to establish accurate processing conditions, the second is to maintain consistent processing conditions.

## Accurate Processing Conditions

Figure 4 illustrates the concept of accurate clinical processing. Accurate processing is achieved when the clinical processing conditions produce film characteristics (density and contrast) which are consistent with the characteristics obtained with the manufacturer's recommended processing. As a general rule the density and contrast values should not vary from the film manufacturer's recommendations by more than 15%. Figure 4 shows the several sources of potential error.

There are two basic steps to achieving accurate processing.

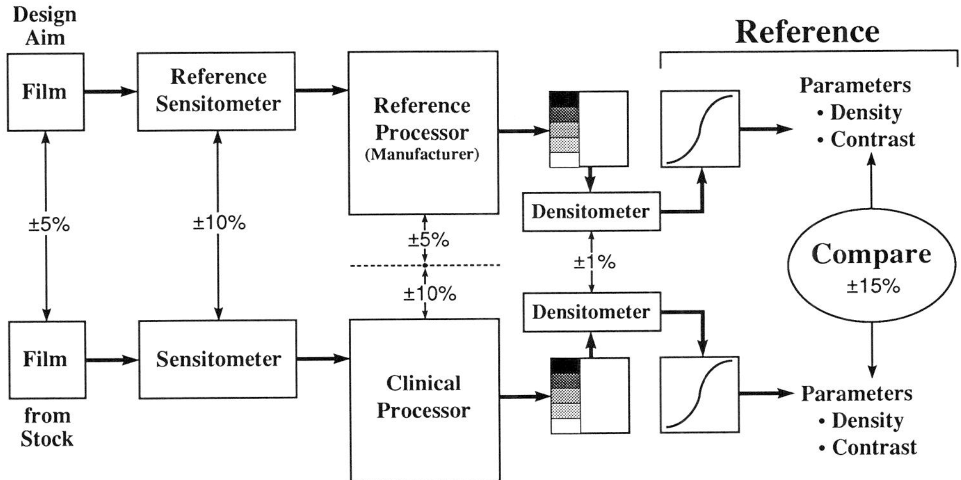


**Figure 4. The concept of clinical processing accuracy as compared to the film manufacturer's recommendations.**

## <u>manufacturer's recommendations</u>

The first step to ensure that film will be processed to produce its desirable design characteristics is to consult the film manufacturer's recommendations with respect to factors such as:

>Type of chemistry.
>
>Developer temperature.
>
>Replenishment rate.

Recommendations on type of chemistry can produce potential problems. It is expected that a film manufacturer will recommend processing in their compatible brand of chemistry. However, it is a widespread practice of clinical facilities to use chemistry manufactured by companies other than the film providers. It then becomes necessary for the chemistry manufacturer to provide recommendations for proper film processing.

The appropriate replenishment rate depends on the type and quantity of films being processed. The developer temperature which will produce optimum processing depends on the type of film and chemistry and the developer immersion time which is a design characteristic of the processor.

### verification

The second step is verification that film contrast, speed (sensitivity), and base plus fog values are being obtained as intended by the film manufacturer. Because of the complexity of processing, just setting all conditions according to the manufacturer's recommendations does not ensure accurate processing. The level of processing should be verified by comparing the characteristics of a test film to a standard reference provided by the film manufacturer.

### Consistent Processing Conditions

There are three basic actions in a QC program for maintaining consistent processing.

### testing

The first step is to periodically test the processing. This is done by processing a film which has been exposed with a sensitometer and then measuring the resulting density values with a densitometer. The density values of specific exposure steps, and the contrast between steps, will vary with the level of processing.

### charting and analysis

Selected density and contrast values are plotted on a control chart so that they can be compared on a day-to-day basis. The control charts must also have established limits showing the maximum acceptable range of variability for each factor. There are two conditions which will indicate a need for corrective actions. A continuing change in a density or contrast value in the same direction generally indicates an unstable processing condition which will often continue and eventually exceed the established limits. This type of gradual trend is typically associated with changes in the chemical activity. Abrupt changes in density or contrast can result from factors such as a shift in temperature, some form of contamination, or an error when replacing chemicals. This requires more immediate corrective action.

### corrective action

This requires a person who is knowledgeable in the technical aspects of processing. This person can be on the staff of the clinical facility or the company providing the processor maintenance and service.

# Results of Federal and State Studies on Film Processing

**Orhan H. Suleiman**
Food and Drug Administration
Center for Devices and Radiological Health
Rockville, Maryand

## Introduction

The Office of Training and Assistance of the Food and Drug Administration's Center for Devices and Radiological Health is an educational arm of the Center. Its role is primarily educational. The first step in solving a problem is identification of the problem. Professional problems are usually ones of ignorance; therefore, once a problem is identified and industry or the user is educated about the problem – an important step towards solving the problem has been taken.

This discussion focuses on a series of studies conducted over a period of 15 years. Many of these studies are still very relevant today.

## The X-ray Generator and Film Processing

Although processing is the subject of this proceedings, it is important to understand the relationship between radiation output and film response. X-ray equipment is not designed by photographic scientists or engineers. If you have ever looked at the control panel of an x-ray generator, you will notice that the milliampere (mA) stations are linear, i.e., there will probably be a 100, 200, 300, and 400 mA technique factor available for selection. This is also true for the exposure time stations, where you will observe 0.1-, 0.2-, 0.3-second exposure times. The x-ray engineers should have first consulted with their counterparts in photography! Many of you have 35 mm photographic cameras. Have you noticed what the exposure time settings are? They are 1/1000, 1/500, 1/250, 1/50 seconds, not a linear progression but geometric! Why? Film does not respond linearly; it responds in a logarithmic manner. Understanding this relationship between exposure and film denity is essential to appreciate the consequences of poor film processing on radiation exposure.

## Darkroom Fog

Film processing cannot be discussed without first discussing the darkroom. Although these data were published 10 years ago,[1] it is still timely.

Darkroom fog has a detrimental effect on image quality. If the effect is dramatic enough it will result in a clinical film which may have to be repeated – resulting in increased radiation exposure to the patient and increased costs. If the examination is not repeated, the fog will affect the diagnostic quality of the resulting radiograph by increasing the overall density of the clinical image and reducing the contrast level of the radiograph. This degradation in image quality is not desirable. In addition to causing some repeat exposures and degradation in image quality (increased density, reduced contrast), darkroom fog also introduces an intermittent variable that really needs to be controlled because it may introduce density fluctuations into the daily sensitometry routine which may not be that easy to identify. You should never have to rely on a sensitometry test to identify excessive darkroom fog. The test for measuring darkroom fog is simple and easy to perform.

In order to measure fog, a uniform exposure must first be given to the test film. This usually results in a density in the 0.8 to 2.0 region. Film is most sensitive in this region, and the effect of fog will be greatest on the resulting clinical image. Anecdotal stories continue to be told about people measuring fog with unexposed film! This is wrong! Unexposed film is very insensitive to fog. What may manifest itself on a clinical image will not always be detected on unexposed film. The only consolation to using unexposed film is that if you do measure fog, you can be confident that you have a very serious problem.

## Darkroom Fog Tests

There are several different ways that have been recommended for measuring fog. We recommend exposing a fresh film which is routinely used clinically, loaded in a cassette, and using an aluminum step wedge. The resulting step wedge image results in a range of different densities (associated with each of the steps), one of which will provide the requisite clinical density. The advantage of this test is that one exposure will usually yield an adequate test film. This test is especially recommended for the surveyor going into different facilities who does not know what radiographic technique will yield a mid-density radiograph.

All of these methods generate a test film with a mid-range density. The film is then partially shielded in the darkroom, usually by bisecting half of the film with opaque material. Any increase in density accompanied by a visible border corresponding to the border between the shielded and unshielded portion of the film is attributable to poor ambient light conditions in the darkroom and is defined as darkroom fog.

The time of exposure for the test film should ideally represent the typical film handling time in the darkroom. You may conduct the test using 30-second, 1-minute, 2-minute, or 4-minute time intervals. We recommend a 2-minute interval, a period of time sufficiently sensitive to detect significant fog levels, but short enough to be practical. Another method, recommended by Kodak, involves exposing the film, loaded in a cassette, in order to obtain a film with a uniform density which corresponds to a mid-range value. The disadvantage of this test is that it may take several exposures and several sheets of film to obtain an appropriate density. The advantage is that different portions of the single sheet of film can be exposed to different time periods in the darkroom, permitting measurement of fog levels associated with these time intervals. This test can be easily performed in-house, assuming one knows the necessary radiographic technique to obtain a mid-range optical density.

The darkroom fog test film for the 1992 mammography NEXT survey uses the image of the mammography phantom, which has the required mid-range density.

The American College of Radiology (ACR) fog measurement protocol involves using a strip exposed by light from a sensitometer, rather than a film exposed in a cassette, to obtain the mid-range density. The advantage of this test over the other tests is that it eliminates the need for a radiographic exposure. A drawback is that to bisect a light sensitometric strip requires more skill than to cover half of an entire x-ray film.

In the 1982 study, fog levels were measured in approximately 900 darkrooms for 1-, 2-, and 4-minute time intervals. The 2-minute time interval seemed to be the most practical. In that study, fog was detected in 73% of the tested facilities when using levels greater than 0.05 density for a 4-minute time interval. Sixty-three percent of the tested darkrooms exceeded this value for a 2-minute exposure, and 53% for a 1-minute exposure. Today, darkrooms having fog levels 0.10 density units or greater for a 2-minute time interval are considered unsatisfactory and require corrective action.

When performing the fog test, if you do not obtain a visible border, the increase in density may simply be due to inherent non-uniformity of the x-ray beam due to the heel effect, scatter, or geometry. A typical, "uniformly exposed" radiograph may have density differences as high as 0.2 density units across the films; therefore, the magnitude of the difference alone is not sufficient to define a film as fogged. This is one of the reasons why we use an action level of 0.10 density.

To put this quantity into perspective, you must appreciate the fact that a 2-minute exposure yielding a fog level of 0.10 would correspond to a fog level of 0.025 for a 30-second exposure, a fog level of 0.05 for a 1-minute exposure, or a fog level of 0.20 for a 4-minute exposure. If films are handled for very long periods of time in your darkroom, you should use a longer time interval when performing the test.

The main point to be emphasized is that darkroom fog is prevalent and needs to be measured properly. Don't use unexposed film. The test film should be the same type as the film used clinically, the increase in density attributable to the fog level should be measured in the mid-density region, and a visible border must be present.

There are two major sources of darkroom fog – safelights and light leaks. Fog caused by safelights may be due to inappropriate safelight filters for the film; aged, cracked or scratched filters; too many safelights; and safelights located too close to the film-handling area. Light leaks may come from a multitude of sources, including seams between doors and walls, electrical outlets, and even air-conditioning conduits. The wide array of electronic products has also proliferated a wide array of indicator lights which sometimes find their way into the darkroom. These may be on telephones, intercoms, and even on the processors themselves. Darkroom fog was recently discovered to be caused by a warning light that was only on when one of the two interlocked darkroom doors was open.

We have developed a fog folder for measuring fog. The novel thing about it is that the letters "FOG" appear on the test film if detectable fog is present.

## The Relationship Between Exposure and Density

Before discussing processing, it is important to review the relationship between density and exposure (Figure 1). This relationship is described by the characteristic curve of the film, or density-log relative exposure curve, originally described by Hurter and Driffield a century ago, and sometimes referred to as the H & D curve.

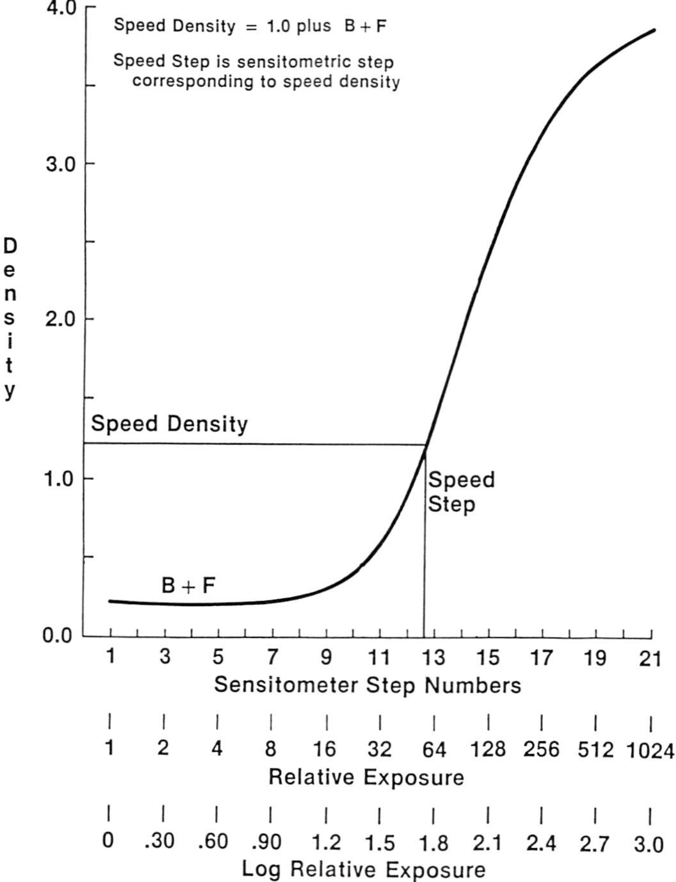


Figure 1

For a film with a gamma of 4.0, a density difference of 0.10 corresponds to an exposure difference of 5.9%, but for a film with a gamma of 3.0, this same density difference corresponds to an exposure difference of 8.0%. Restated, you would have to increase the radiation output by 8.0% to increase the density by 0.10 density for a film with a gamma of 3.0. Gamma is the slope of the line, and it changes as a function of density.

$$\text{Gamma} = \frac{(\Delta \text{ Optical Density })}{(\Delta \text{ log relative E })}$$

Most commercial sensitometers have a stated precision of $\pm 0.02$ log relative exposure ($\pm 4.7\%$). This corresponds to a $\pm 0.06$ density difference for films with a gamma of 3.0, and $\pm 0.08$ density difference for films with a gamma of 4.0.

### Sensitometry: Steps, Relative Exposure, Log Relative Exposure

When we evaluate processing, the film density that is tracked is the speed density, the density that corresponds to a base plus fog (B+F) density plus 1.00, or a net density of 1.00. After the speed density is determined, the sensitometer step number corresponding to the speed density is determined. This is referred to as the speed step.

If we have a sensitometer that gives us a density of 1.20 on step 11, and the B+F on your film happens to be 0.20, that means that step 11 is your speed step – the sensitometric step that corresponds to speed density.

The sensitometers we use have step increments that increase the exposure of each consecutive step by $\sqrt{2}$, 1.41, or 41% (Table 1). What this means is that if step 11 provides a relative exposure of 1.0, then step 12 yields a relative exposure of 1.41 of step 11; step 13 will yield 1.41 of step 12, or double ($\sqrt{2} \times \sqrt{2} = 2$) the relative exposure of step 11.

### Table 1. Sensitometer Step Number versus exposure

| Step Number | Relative Exposure | log Relative Exposure |
| --- | --- | --- |
| 10 | 0.71 | -0.15 |
| 11 | 1.00 | 0.00 |
| 12 | 1.41 | 0.15 |
| 13 | 2.00 | 0.30 |

Photographic or imaging scientists do not use sensitometric step numbers and does not customarily use relative exposure. Instead, they deal with the log of the relative exposure. The log relative exposure difference between step 11 and 12 is 0.15. Exposure differences which are relative differences of 41% will be reported as a log relative E of 0.15.

To develop this concept further, start interpolating between step 11 and step 12 (Table 2). A 5% (1.05) relative increase in light exposure corresponds to a log relative exposure difference of 0.02. This happens to be the stated precision of most commercially available sensitometers. Stated another way, these sensitometers' exposure precision, or reproducibility, is therefore ± 5%. The sensitometer step number that would yield this exposure would correspond to a theoretical step of 11.13. A 12% (1.12) relative increase in exposure would correspond to a log relative exposure difference of 0.05.

**Table 2. Sensitometer Step Number versus exposure**

| Step Number | Relative Exposure | log Relative Exposure |
|---|---|---|
| 10.67 | 0.89 | -0.05 |
| 11.00 | 1.00 | 0.00 |
| 11.13 | 1.05 | 0.02 |
| 11.33 | 1.12 | 0.05 |
| 12.00 | 1.41 | 0.15 |

## Processing Speed and Relative Exposure are inversely related.

Relative Exposure = K x (1 / Processing Speed)
where K is a constant relating units of exposure with speed.

If we assume that the standard sensitometer step number which yields the speed density – when the film is developed according to the film manufacturer's recommended processing specifications – is assigned a relative exposure value of 1.0 (Table 3), we then assign this "Standard" processing system a speed value of 100.

**Table 3. Sensitometer Step Number versus exposure**

| Step Number | Relative Exposure | Speed (1/rel E) x 100 |
|---|---|---|
| 10.67 | 0.89 | 112 |
| 11.00 | 1.00 | 100 |
| 11.13 | 1.05 | 95 |
| 11.33 | 1.12 | 89 |
| 12.00 | 1.41 | 71 |

For example, a processing system which develops a film with a resulting sensitometric speed step of 12.00 requires one additional sensitometric step of exposure than the properly developed film (which had a speed step of 11.0). This film, therefore, required a higher relative exposure of 1.41, and has a speed of 71.

What does this difference mean in terms of density? Table 4 shows the density differences due to differences in exposure, along with the relative speed. Please note that these density differences are calculated for a film with a gamma of 3.0, which is typical of conventional medical x-ray film. The density differences can manifest themselves in two ways. Assuming that the "appropriate" clinical density is associated with a system having a speed of 100, the processor with a speed of 112 (Table 4) will now generate a film with an increase in density of 0.15; a processor with a speed of 71 will generate a film with a decrease in density of 0.45. These differences in density may be acceptable and, therefore, no change in radiographic technique may be made. What is more likely, however, is that the radiographic technique will be adjusted to compensate for the increase or decrease in density. In this example for the system with a speed of 112 the exposure will have to be reduced by 11% (1.00 - 0.89 = 0.11). Radiation exposure will have to be increased by 41% (1.41) for the processor with a speed of 71.

### Table 4. Sensitometer Step Number versus exposure

| Step Number | Relative Exposure | Speed (1/rel E) x 100 | Density Difference Gamma = 3.0 |
|---|---|---|---|
| 10.67 | 0.89 | 112 | -0.15 |
| 11.00 | 1.00 | 100 | 0.00 |
| 11.13 | 1.05 | 95 | 0.06 |
| 11.33 | 1.12 | 89 | 0.15 |
| 12.00 | 1.41 | 71 | 0.45 |

In Table 5, density differences have been calculated for films having gammas of 2.0, 3.0, and 4.0. Films that are being underdeveloped will have gammas approaching 2.0, while high-contrast films, being properly developed, such as those used in mammography, will have a gamma greater than 4.0.

The overall implication of this is that, initially, a processing system which is underprocessing, i.e., with a speed less than 100, will produce films with lower density. Conversely, a system which is overprocessing, i.e., having a speed greater than 100, will produce a film with higher density. If the clinician is satisfied with the images, there will be no compensating radiographic adjustment. Eventually the lighter or darker than normal clinical films will have to be adjusted. What probably happens is that as the processing deviates from normal conditions, adjustments for the changes in processing will be made by adjustments to the radiographic technique, not in the processing. A film processed in a system with a speed of 60 will initially be 0.44 density units light (for a film with gamma = 2.0). In order to recapture this lost density, the radiographic exposure will have to be increased by 67%.

### Table 5. Density Adjustment vs Processing Speed

| Speed | Radiation Exposure | Gamma = 2.0 | Gamma = 3.0 | Gamma = 4.0 |
|---|---|---|---|---|
| 60 | 67% higher | + 0.44 | + 0.66 | + 0.88 |
| 80 | 25% higher | + 0.20 | + 0.40 | + 0.60 |
| 100 | "Normal" | 0 | 0 | 0 |
| 120 | 17% lower | - 0.16 | - 0.24 | - 0.32 |
| 140 | 29% lower | - 0.30 | - 0.45 | - 0.60 |

We consider anything with a speed ranging from 80 to 120 as "normal", or in compliance with film manufacturers' recommended processing specifications. This really is a very liberal standard. It corresponds approximately to a $\pm 2°C$ ($\pm 4°F$) developer temperature difference.

## The New Jersey Processor Study

Almost 500 automatic film processors were evaluated during the New Jersey Sensitometry study in 1977.[2] During the analysis phase of the study, we realized that reporting processor performance as a range of densities associated with a single sensitometer step was not correct. As pointed out earlier, the magnitude of the density difference is highly dependent on processing conditions. During the intermediary phase of the analysis, sensitometer step number was being used along the x-axis, a surrogate for log relative exposure. Prior to publishing these data we still felt uncomfortable with how the data were being presented. Density differences or sensitometer step numbers did not convey the real effect of what was being observed. Once processing speed was used instead of sensitometer step number or density, we felt that the data were more clearly presented, and the problem, therefore, more clearly defined.

The important thing about the New Jersey study was that it documented a wide range of processing performance. This observation was neither original nor unanticipated, since others had previously reported similar observations.[3]

## Sensitometric Technique for the Evaluation of Processing (STEP)

As a direct result of the New Jersey study an empirical test method for evaluating processing was developed. This survey technique is known as the Sensitometric Technique for the Evaluation of Processing, (STEP).[4,5,6,7] The test measures processing speed, a term analogous to photographic film speed. Speed, as used here, should not be confused with processor cycle time.

The measurement of processing speed with the STEP method has been an integral part of the Nationwide Evaluation of X-ray Trends (NEXT) survey program since 1984. The data to be presented have been collected as part of the NEXT program.

The NEXT survey program is conducted collaboratively by FDA with the Conference of Radiation Control Program Directors (CRCPD), the umbrella organization for state and local radiation control agencies. The main objective of NEXT is to measure the radiation doses associated with selected diagnostic examinations. Since 1984 we have measured the dose to the typical patient for examinations such as chest radiography (1984, 1986), mammography (1985, 1988, and 1992), and abdominal radiography, specifically the lumbosacral spine and abdomen (1987, 1989). Our most recent studies addressed computed tomography (1990), the upper gastrointestinal fluoroscopic examination (1991), and mammography (1992).

The NEXT surveys are comprehensive, measuring not only the radiation intensity associated with these examinations, but also relevant technical information such as x-ray beam quality, geometric factors, screen and film manufacturer and type, and processing speed. The data to be presented later will be strictly limited to the processing.

## The Effects of Different Film Chemistry Systems on Processing

In 1980, one of the questions prior to developing STEP was how different are standard processing conditions from one manufacturer to another. We discovered, much to our surprise, that only Kodak and Dupont provided standard processing recommendations.[8] We also learned in that study that most films will respond to different chemistries and changes in processing in subtle and different ways. The more important lesson was that, although we could observe subtle differences in processing between films, the differences were less than the experimental uncertainty associated with the sensitometers and densitometers we were using.

We repeated this study about two years ago.[9] Again, we used common, off-the-shelf chemistries, and the most frequently observed films from the NEXT surveys. Essentially this study revalidated what we had observed 10 years earlier – that different films respond differently, although in a subtle manner, to different processing conditions. We also were able to verify that flat-grain films are less sensitive to changes in processing than conventional films. Despite this, all tested films increased in speed as developer temperature increased. Poor processing will affect all films, although the magnitude of the effect will be highly dependent on the type of film.

We also tested the films in extended processing,[10] a technique where the processor's developer immersion time is doubled. This technique has been promoted to increase contrast for some mammography films.

An interesting observation was that one of the tested orthochromatic mammography films, the contrast as measured using the blue emission of the light sensitometer reached a maximum at the developer temperature recommended by the film manufacturer. The same film's contrast, as measured using the green emission from the same light sensitometer, reached a maximum during the extended cycle. This apparent difference in where contrast reaches a maximum is apparently related to the differences between the blue and green emissions of the light sensitometer and their interactions with the film emulsion layer. The implication is that the evaluation of film contrast should probably not be performed with a light sensitometer. It seems prudent to use light from an intensifying screen when evaluating two films with respect to contrast, rather than a light sensitometer.

## Pre-exposed Sensitometric Film Versus Freshly Exposed Sensitometric Film

Another question that is raised very frequently is, "What about pre-exposed sensitometric strips?" The answer is a qualified no; do not use pre-exposed sensitometric films for quality assurance testing.

In a study published in 1985,[11] the feasibility of eliminating the sensitometers for use in STEP by using pre-exposed films was evaluated. Several batches of film were divided into a pre-exposed group and a freshly exposed group. The pre-exposed films were all exposed to a light sensitometer and packaged in a light-tight box at the beginning of the study. The films to be freshly exposed were stored along with the pre-exposed films; they were exposed to the same light sensitometer immediately before developing the films.

The two groups were also divided into a properly stored film set, i.e., films were stored within the darkroom at conventional room temperatures, and an improperly stored film set. The improperly stored film set was stored in a light-tight box located in the trunk of a car during the summer months.

The results proved so interesting that the study was repeated the following summer with an expanded number of films. Films were observed for periods as long as 70 days.

Density differences between freshly exposed and pre-exposed films were observed as early as 2 minutes for some films; these differences became very dramatic as the pre-exposed time period increased. Density differences as great as 0.72 density units were observed between the pre-exposed and freshly exposed films.

Other observations included films where the density increased with storage time, decreased with storage time, or did not change with storage time. The proper term for such changes to the latent image is latent image instability, since some films had latent image fading, while other films actually had latent image enhancement, i.e., the density increased with time.

Sensitivity differences were studied between the pre-exposed films and the freshly exposed films to detect changes in processing: as processing deteriorated it was sometimes impossible to detect these changes using pre-exposed films. In one case the properly stored pre-exposed film actually increased in density, while the improperly stored pre-exposed film and the freshly exposed film decreased in density.

The differences that were observed in density were not surprising, but the magnitude of the differences was. Another surprising observation was that the freshly exposed film that had been improperly stored performed the same as the properly stored film!

So, should pre-exposed film be used for sensitometry? Generally, no. The latent image is highly susceptible to changes attributable to time and storage conditions; there is also a strong possibility that the pre-exposed film may not be representative of the film routinely used in the facility.

In special cases pre-exposed film can be used successfully. But these typically involve a large batch of pre-exposed film which is used within a very short time period by skilled individuals. Film companies have done this on occasion. The advantage is that it eliminates the need to have a large number of calibrated sensitometers. The use of pre-exposed sensitometric strips is not recommended when either the individuals conducting the test or the elapsed time and storage conditions are not controlled. The differences one may observe will just as likely be attributable to latent image changes, and not differences in processing.

## Processing in Clinical Facilities

Having discussed some of the reasons why pre-exposed film should not be used to evaluate processing, and why processing speed is measured instead of density, let's turn to some data in clinical facilities which have been observed over the years. It is important to remember that "normal" processing is a very liberal standard, i.e., 100 $\pm 20\%$; underprocessing facilities, therefore, are very likely underestimated.

Please appreciate that the consequence of underprocessing is a higher radiation exposure and degradation in film contrast. Ironically, the underprocessing condition which requires a higher radiation exposure may also have the beneficial effect of reducing noise by reducing quantum mottle, although this is probably not being done intentionally.

In 1984, as part of the NEXT survey, hospitals conducting chest radiography were surveyed. The important fact is that processing in hospitals was observed. In 1986, another NEXT survey was conducted on chest radiography, but this time the survey was limited to private offices. In 1987, a survey was conducted on hospitals conducting the lumbo-sacral spine and abdomen radiographic examinations. Forty-two percent of films in private offices are underprocessed. This compares with 18% for hospitals in 1986, and 33% of hospitals in 1987. No matter how you look at the data, hospitals are doing a better job than private facilities.

The trend toward poorer processing in hospitals (Figure 2) between 1984 and 1987 is somewhat disturbing. When these data were presented at the Radiological Society of North America Meeting in 1990,[12] most radiologists suggested that it was the effect of cost containment efforts because it was the QA technologist position which was usually the first to be eliminated. Although the underprocessing component for hospitals increased from 18% in 1984 to 33% in 1987, it was still better than the 42% underprocessing observed in private offices.

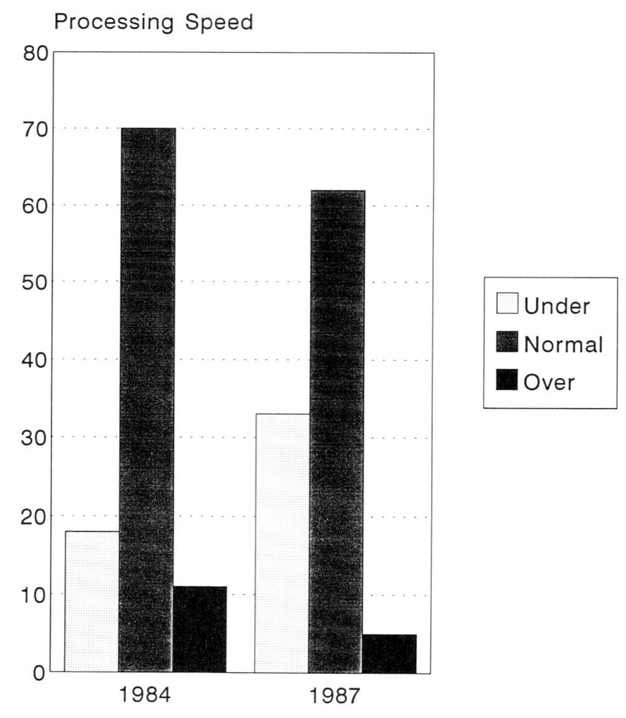


Under (<80), Normal (80 - 120), Over (>120)

**Figure 2**

In 1989 when abdominal radiography was undergoing evaluation (Figure 3), 63% of surveyed radiologists in private offices, 60% of non-radiologists (excluding chiropractors), and only 40% of chiropractors were developing their films normally. The more important observation is the proportion underprocessing, 48% of surveyed chiropractors in 1989 were underdeveloping their films, compared with 33% of non-radiologists, and 25% of radiologists.

# Processing Speed
## Private Practice 1989 (Abdomen/LS Spine Examination)

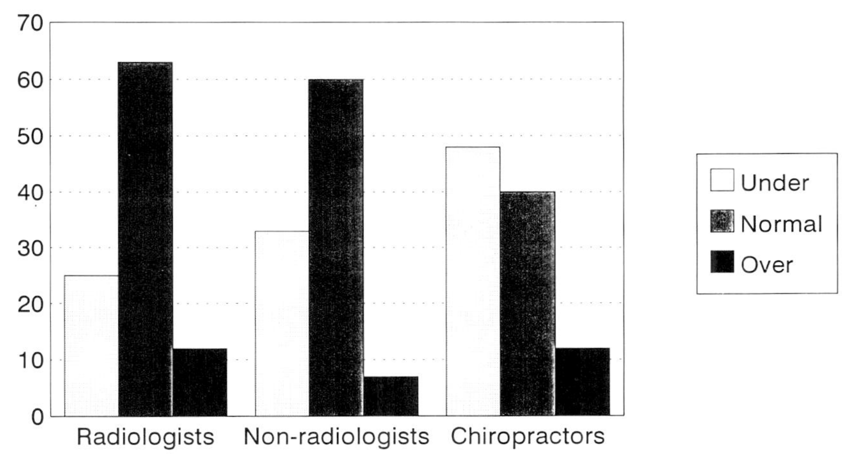


Under (<80), Normal (80 - 120), Over (>120)

**Figure 3**

On the other hand, 18% of mammography facilities (Figure 4) were underprocessing in 1985, which was comparable to the 18% observed in the 1984 hospital survey. By 1988, however, the mammography facilities improved from 1985's 18% underprocessing to 7%, an improvement in the quality of processing contrary to the hospital trend.

It is obvious that except for mammography facilities, film processing is in generally poor shape. Why are mammography facilities processing their films better than other facilities? When a number of us started promoting Quality Assurance years ago, the question was asked, "Are you going to regulate QA?" My answer was that QA problems were ones of ignorance. QA is a win-win situation. Doses are reduced, either by reduced repeat films or lower radiation doses per film. QA is beneficial; there were numerous studies demonstrating the cost / benefit in terms of saved film, chemistry, x-ray tube life, and equipment downtime. Most important of all, it improved image quality. It improved the quality of the clinical examination. How could any professional ignore these factors.

# Mammography
## 1985 vs 1988

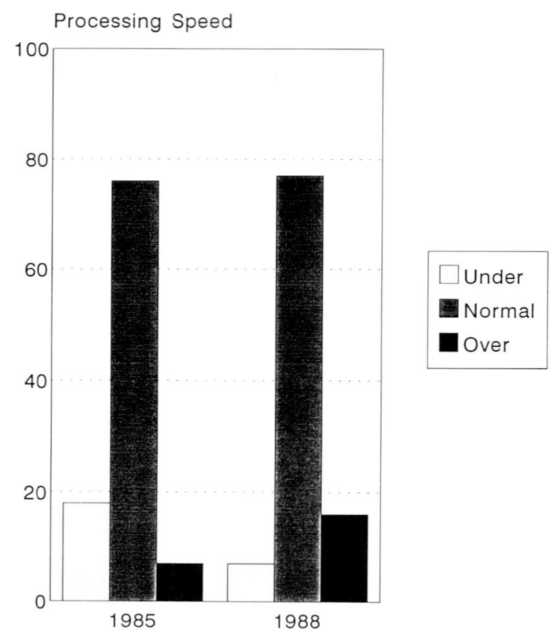


Under (<80), Normal (80 - 120), Over (>120)

**Figure 4**

Unfortunately, there are apparently limits to voluntary education. Our office is educationally oriented. We feel that if we identify the problems, the appropriate professional groups will respond to the challenge.

What bothers me professionally, because it appears that we have failed professionally, is that the threat of the stick has had more impact than the professional incentives. The stick, in this case, is the failure to be reimbursed by the Health Care Finance Administration (HCFA) for mammography services, and the "peer pressure" to be accredited by the ACR in mammography. I wonder how many facilities would be attempting to obtain ACR accreditation in mammography if there was no reimbursement requirement?

Processing affects image quality for all films in a diagnostic radiology department, including hard copy films from non-x-ray imaging modalities. Yet because of the attention mammography and QA are getting, only mammography facilities appear to be aware of the importance of good film processing

## Summary

1. Evaluate the darkroom, a very simple thing, but people often overlook it.

2. Ensure that the processing is optimal, or more specifically, that the film manufacturer's recommendations are followed.

In 1980, when we started evaluating film processing, only two film manufacturers were providing such guidance, Kodak and Dupont. Fortunately, more film manufacturers provide such information today. A lot of times you'll hear the statement that the film manufacturer's technical representatives in the field will make the necessary adjustments. I think that's a way of sidestepping the issue. I suspect that what actually happens is that the technical representative matches film processing to existing departmental technique charts to avoid the risk that all the departmental films may start coming out dark. What they should do is optimize the processor, either empirically or by setting up the processor according to proper specifications. This should only be done with the support of the x-ray service personnel, ready to make adjustments immediately to phototimers and automatic exposure detectors in the radiographic rooms serviced by these processors.

3. Do not make decisions regarding contrast based only on light sensitometry studies.

The evaluation of contrast is complex and will be dependent not only upon the characteristics of the film, but also on the quality of the light from the intensifying screen exposing the film. Spectral characteristics of light sensitometers will not accurately match those of intensifying screens.

4. Do not use pre-exposed sensitometric film for QA testing unless you are knowledgeable enough to know its limitations, in which case you should be knowledgeable enough to avoid using them in the first place.

I do not want to condemn pre-exposed sensitometric strips completely. There are some very limited applications where they can be useful, but I am not aware of any useful role for them for an in-house QA program!

## References

1. Suleiman OH, Showalter CK, Gross RE, and RE Bunge. Radiographic film fog in the darkroom. *Radiology* Vol. 151:237-238, April, 1984.

2. Suleiman OH, Showalter CK, Koustenis G., Hotte E.: Sensitometric evaluation

of film-chemistry-processor systems in the state of New Jersey. HHS publication FDA 82-8189, April 1982.

3. Cleare, HM and Trumbauer. An analysis of variability in radiographic image recording. Second Image Receptor Conference: Radiographic Film Processing. IN: Proceedings of a Conference held in Washington D.C., March 31-April 2, 1977. HEW Publication (FDA) 77-8036, pp 11-23 (August 1977).

4. Suleiman OH and CK Showalter. Sensitometric Technique for the Evaluation of Processing. Scientific exhibit presented at the Conference of Radiation Control Program Directors, Portland, Maine, May 1982.

5. Suleiman OH and CK Showalter. Sensitometric Technique for the Evaluation of Processing. Scientific exhibit presented at the Annual Health Physics Society Meeting, Las Vegas, Nevada, 1982.

6. Suleiman OH. S.T.E.P. – Sensitometric Technique for the Evaluation of Processing of Medical X-ray Film. Videotape (33:25 minutes), National Center for Devices and Radiological Health, FDA, VT2061, September 1982.

7. Suleiman OH, Conway BJ, Rueter FG,  and Slayton RJ. Automatic Film Processing Analysis of 9 Years of Observations. *Radiology* 1992; 185: 25-28.

8. Patterson JF, Suleiman OH, and D McKenna. Comparison of processing variations on different film/chemistry combinations. In: Proceedings of the Health Physics Society Fourteenth Mid-Year Topical Symposium, pp:355-364, December, 1980.

9. Suleiman OH, Slayton RJ, Conway B, Rueter FG: Effects of temperature, chemistry, and developer immersion time on x-ray film. Scientific Exhibit and paper presented at Radiological Society of North America Meeting, Dec, 1990. *Radiology* 1990; 177:132.

10. Tabar L, Haus AG. Processing mammographic films: Technical and Clinical Considerations. *Radiology* 1989; 173: 65-69.

11. Suleiman OH and AW Thomas. A comparison of freshly exposed and pre-exposed control film in the evaluation of processing. In: Proceedings of Medical Imaging and Instrumentation (*SPIE* Volume 555, pp:96-102) April, 1985.

12. Conway BJ, McCrohan JL, Rueter FG, Slayton RJ, Suleiman OH: Processing trends: Observations from 8 years of national automatic film processing data (1982-1989). Presented at 1990 Radiological Society of North America Meeting in Chicago, *Radiology* Vol 177 (P): 173.

# American College of Radiology Mammography Accreditation Program and Legislative Issues Related to Film Processing

**R. Edward Hendrick**

Division of Radiological Sciences
Department of Radiology
University of Colorado Health Sciences Center
Denver, Colorado

It is especially timely to discuss the American College of Radiology (ACR) Mammography Accreditation Program (MAP) and legislative issues in mammography. It is an interesting opportunity to be able to focus on ACR MAP recommendations and legislative requirements on the specific topic of film processing.

To set the stage, a brief review of some of the modern history of mammography is in order. A few of the main developments are summarized in Table 1. As the table indicates, the first dedicated mammography units were commercially available in the mid-1960's, and the first screen-film combinations designed specifically for mammography were introduced in the early 1970's. Since that time, both dedicated x-ray equipment and image receptors for mammography have undergone steady improvement. This has resulted in steadily improved image quality and reduced breast doses in mammography through the last two decades.[1,2]

**Table 1. A Brief Review of the Development of Modern Mammography Equipment**

| | |
|---|---|
| First Dedicated Mammography Unit | 1965 |
| First Screen-Film System Specifically for Mammography | 1970 |
| First Xeromammography Unit | 1971 |
| First Micro-focal Spot (Magnification) Mammography Unit | 1977 |
| First Grid Developed Specifically for Mammography | 1978 |
| Improved Screen-Film Image Receptors for Mammography | 1980 |
| Xeromammography Equipment Sales Discontined | 1989 |

By the mid-1980's, many believed all that was needed to perform high-quality mammography was a dedicated mammography unit and an image receptor designed specifically for mammography. Then, in the second half of the 1980's, it became clear that all was not right with the performance of mammography in the United States. The

Nationwide Evaluation of X-ray Trends conducted in 1985 (NEXT-85) by the Centers for Devices and Radiologic Health in conjunction with State Radiation Control Divisions demonstrated that there were wide variations in image quality and dose among the 232 mammography sites surveyed.[3] A smaller study conducted in the Philadelphia area by Galkin, Feig, and Muir and presented at the 1986 Radiological Society of North America (RSNA) Annual Meeting revealed that breast doses varied by a factor of 10 and that image quality was below optimal standards in 34% of the 29 dedicated screen-film sites surveyed.[4] In addition, this study found that 41% of the sites had poor processor stability over a 15-day period. This was some of the first evidence pointing to the critical role and variability of film processing in mammography.

With the establishment of the ACR MAP in 1987, additional data from across the United States became available on the wide variations of image quality and dose in mammography. Those data demonstrated that no correlation existed between breast dose and image quality parameters; higher breast doses did not result in better images from site to site.[5] An example of those early data, based on the first 1,000 sites tested for ACR accreditation, are presented in Figure 1, showing image quality scores for the visualization of fibers, specks, and masses using the RMI-156 Mammography Phantom as a function of average glandular dose. Each symbol on a graph represents one mammography unit's dose. Each symbol on a graph represents one mammography unit's dose and fiber, speck, or mass score. For example, a fiber score of 4.0 means that an average of the four largest fibers were seen by the three medical physicists who independently reviewed the phantom image. The small correlation coefficients indicate that no statistically significant correlation exists between image quality scores and breast doses.

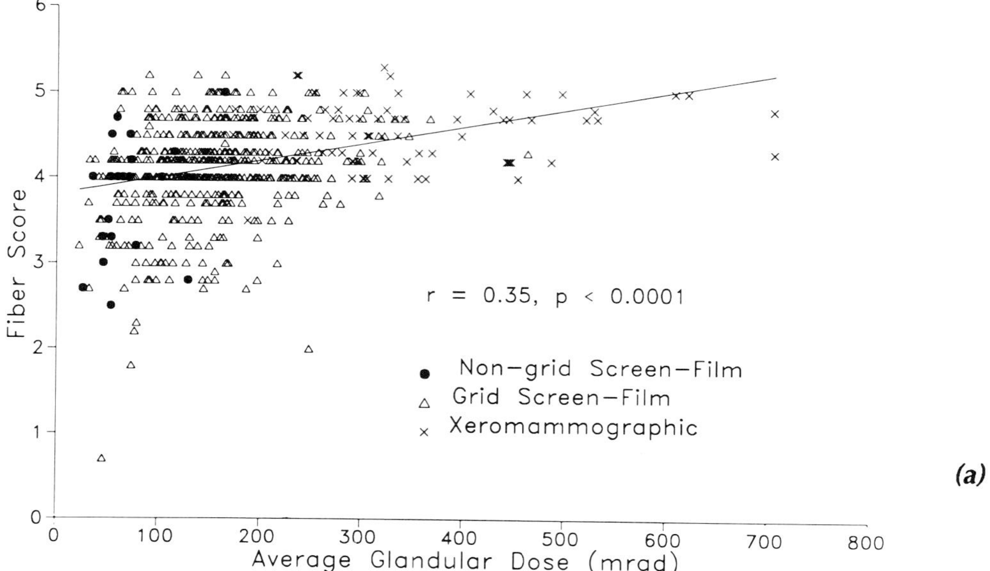

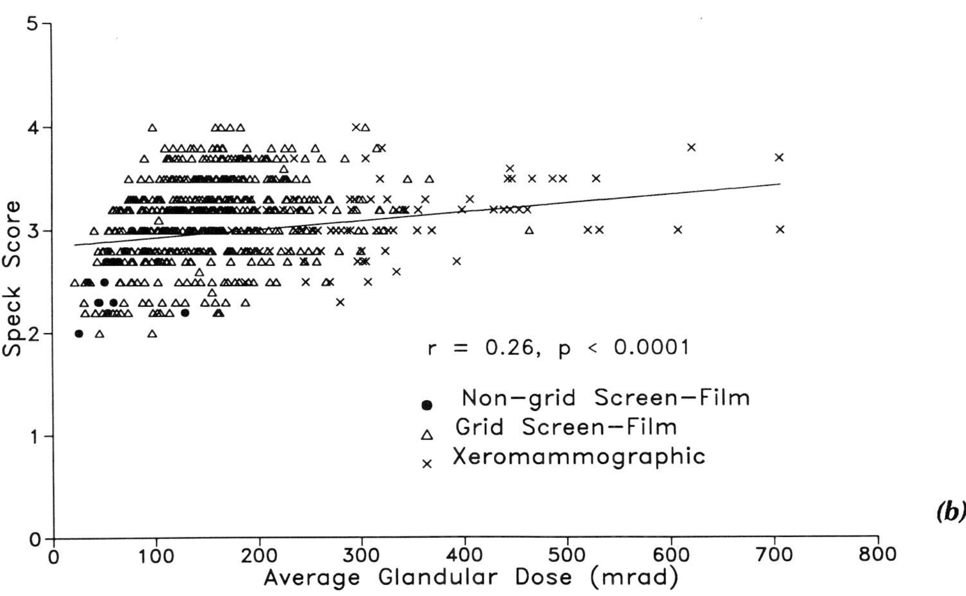

*(b)*

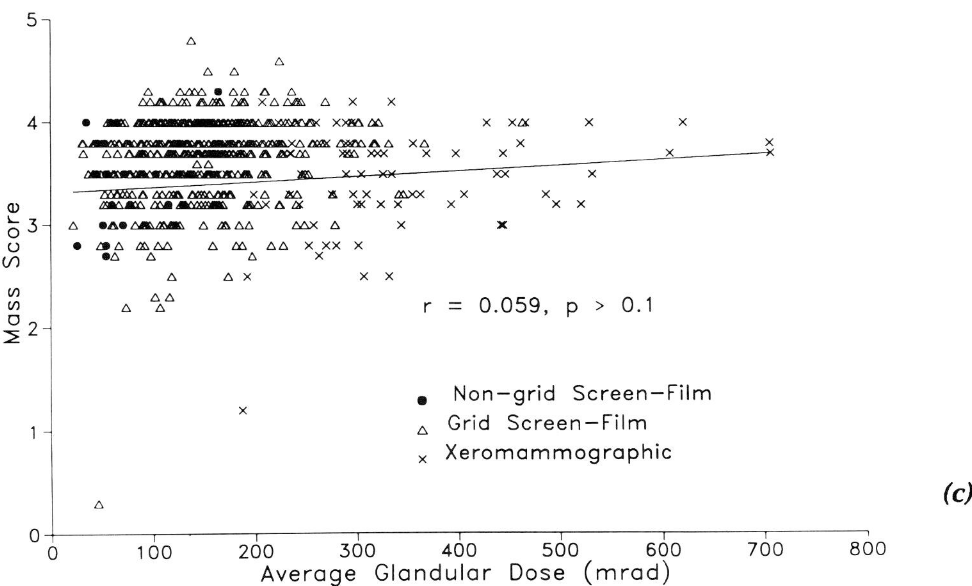

*(c)*

**Figure 1. Distributions of image quality scores and average glandular doses from the first 1000 units tested for ACR mammography accreditation. a) Fiber scores versus average glandular doses. b) Speck scores versus average glandular doses. c) Mass scores versus average glandular doses.**

Since its inception, the ACR MAP has attempted to ensure that mammograms are read by a qualified physician, that the patient is positioned and images are taken by a qualified technologist, that the equipment used is appropriate for mammography, producing excellent image quality at low radiation dose, and that equipment is surveyed at least annually by a qualified medical physicist.[6] Since July 1990, the ACR MAP has also tried to ensure that processing of images is consistent from day to day, requiring submission of a month's processor quality control data. While the period of accreditation is three years, ACR accredited sites are required to submit annually a medical physicist's report, a month's processor QC data, and any changes in equipment or personnel from the site's complete accreditation application.

The site survey form, which is the first phase of ACR MAP application, provides data on quality control practices performed by sites at the time of application to the ACR MAP. Analyzing responses submitted from 5,800 sites during the first four and one-half years of the program, between August 1987 and November 1991, indicates that 64% of applicant sites performed at least daily processor sensitometric testing. Eight percent of sites stated that they performed sensitometry weekly, 7% monthly, and 9% less frequently; 12% stated that they did not perform processor sensitometry at all.[6] In 1990, we performed an independent survey of approximately 100 sites in Colorado and learned that only 38% of sites were performing at least daily processor sensitometry, while 27% of sites were not performing sensitometric testing at all.

Quality control (QC) is defined as those activities that monitor and improve the technical aspects of mammography. The ACR MAP data demonstrated that problems existed in most areas of mammography QC, not just processor QC. Generally speaking, the problems in QC are: 1) mammography technologists are not performing routine QC tests in the manner and at the frequencies needed to be sensitive to imaging system changes; 2) medical physicists often fail to evaluate the most important technical aspect of mammography (the evaluation of image quality and artifacts using a phantom); and 3) radiologists often fail to motivate and support an effective QC program. Such a program requires that a single mammography technologist be chosen to be the QC technologist and that the designated QC technologist be given the training, time, test tools, encouragement and support needed to conduct an effective QC program.

As a result of the identified need for improved QC practices at most mammography sites, in late 1990 the ACR published the ACR Mammography QC Manuals. A revised second edition of these manuals became available in July 1992.[7] The specific QC tests and recommended minimum frequencies of tests from the ACR Mammography QC Manuals are listed in Table 2. In January 1992, the ACR MAP began requiring that accredited sites perform QC tests according to the procedures and minimum frequencies described in the ACR Mammography QC Manuals.

With regard to processor testing, the QC technologist has two direct tests to perform on the processor: daily processor sensitometry and at least quarterly testing of fixer retention in film. Daily processor sensitometry should be performed by setting aside a fresh box of the film most commonly used for mammography. The QC technologist should expose the film in the darkroom using a 21-step sensitometer. A mid-density index should be established by selecting the density step resulting in an optical density closest to 1.20. A density difference index should be established by selecting the upper step as the one resulting in an optical density closest to 2.2, and the lower step as the one resulting in an optical density closest to, but not less than 0.45. The density difference index is recorded as the difference in optical densities of these two steps. Once the particular steps to be used in determining mid-density and density difference levels are selected, they should not be changed. The base plus fog index is the optical density resulting from an unexposed portion of the film. A five day average should be taken to establish the control levels of each of these three processor indices.

The processor is considered to be "in control" if 1) the mid-density index remains within ±0.1 of the mid-density control level, 2) the density difference index remains within ±0.1 of the mid-density control level, and 3) the base plus fog index remains within 0.03 of the base plus fog control level.

Action must be taken if one or more of the following occurs: 1) the mid-density index differs from the mid-density control level by more than ±0.15; 2) the density difference index differs from the density difference control level by more than ±0.15; or 3) the base plus fog index exceeds the base plus fog control level by more than +0.03. An important aspect of quality control is that appropriate action must be taken when processor control levels exceed action limits. It is important to isolate the source of the processor problem (e.g., temperature, chemistry, or replenishment) and correct the problem that has caused processor variation. Too often technologists perform quality control tests, but fail to take appropriate action when processor performance fluctuates widely. Action limits have been defined in the ACR Mammography QC Manuals to indicate the points at which appropriate action should be taken.

The fixer retention test, to be conducted at least quarterly, is a simple test performed with a sheet of mammography film and a fixer retention test kit available from some film manufacturers. A drop of fluid is placed on an unexposed, processed film. After two minutes the density (or color) is assessed by comparing the film to a test chart to determine the amount of fixer solution retained in the film after processing. If fixer retention is excessive, film will discolor over long periods of time (years or tens of years).The two tests described above and described in more detail in the Technologist's Section of the ACR Mammography QC Manuals are the only two direct tests for the processor.

Other QC Tests listed in Table 2 that are processor-related include phantom evaluation of image quality, conducted by both the technologist and the medical physicist, and artifact evaluation, conducted by the medical physicist. These tests assess the entire imaging system chain, including the processor. Other tests indirectly related to the processor include the darkroom cleanliness test and the darkroom fog test.

**Table 2. Quality Control Tests in the ACR Mammography QC Manuals**

| Technologist's Tests | Frequency |
| --- | --- |
| Darkroom Cleanliness | daily |
| Processor Quality Control | daily |
| Screen Cleanliness | weekly |
| Viewboxes and Viewing Conditions | weekly |
| Phantom Images | monthly |
| Visual Checklist | monthly |
| Repeat Analysis | quarterly |
| Analysis of Fixer Retention in Film | quarterly |
| Darkroom Fog | semi-annually |
| Screen-film Contact | semi-annually |
| Compression | semi-annually |

**Medical Physicist's Tests**
**(To be conducted At Least Annually and After Major Equipment Changes)**

Cassette Holder Assembly Evaluation
Collimation Assessment
Focal Spot Size Measurement
kVp Accuracy/Reproducibility
Beam Quality Assessment (HVL Measurement)
Automatic Exposure Control (AEC) System Performance Assessment
Uniformity of Screen
Breast Entrance Exposure and Average Glandular Dose Measurement
Phantom Evaluation of Image Quality
Artifact Evaluation

In addition to the voluntary ACR MAP, there are national requirements on mammography.[8] Table 3 summarizes the past and proposed national legislation on mammography.

## Table 3. National Legislation on Mammography

| Legislation | Outcome |
| --- | --- |
| Catastrophic Health Act of 1988 | Not Passed |
| The Breast and Cervical Cancer Mortality Prevention Act of 1990 | Passed |
| Omnibus Budget Reconciliation Act of 1990 | Passed |
| Breast Cancer Screening Safety Act of 1990 | Not Passed |
| Breast Cancer Screening Safety Act of 1991 | Not Passed |
| Women's Health Equity Act of 1991 | Not Passed |
| Mammography Quality Standards Act of 1992 | Passed |

Two bills enacted by the United States Congress in 1990 contain mammography quality assurance provisions. The Breast and Cervical Cancer Mortality Prevention Act of 1990 (PL 101-354) appropriated $50 million and funded $29.1 million in fiscal year (FY) 1991 for state programs to provide breast and cervical cancer screening to indigent women.[9] Federal funds were provided with requirements of matching funds from applicant states and of quality assurance by all providers. In summary, quality assurance provisions require that sites use only dedicated equipment, that the equipment be checked at least annually by a qualified medical physicist, and that sites meet ACR MAP standards. The legislation provided for additional funding for FY1992 and FY1993 to increase the number of participating states and the number of women screened for breast and cervical cancer.

The 1990 Omnibus Budget Act included funds to reimburse screening mammography for Medicare-eligible women: approximately 17 million women aged 65 and over and 1.5 million disabled women between 35 and 64. Sites voluntarily choose to qualify as Medicare screening sites, but are required to meet quality standards if they choose to qualify. The Interim Final Rules were published on December 31, 1990, as a preliminary version of the Medicare quality standards.[10] These standards include personnel qualifications, equipment standards, safety standards, and quality assurance standards. Responsibility for meeting these quality standards rests with the physician consultant, normally the radiologist reading the mammograms.

Medicare equipment standards require that mammography x-ray equipment and image receptors be specifically designed for mammography. However, there is no requirement that the mammography processor be dedicated only to mammography. The processor developer temperature should be appropriate for the mammography film and chemistry used.

Medicare quality assurance standards require daily processor sensitometric testing, with the same monitoring of mid-density, density difference, and base plus fog levels as required by the ACR. Mid-density and density difference levels should not differ from operating levels by more than ± 0.1 and base plus fog levels should not exceed the base plus fog control level by more than +0.03. Medicare also requires QA checks of darkroom integrity and film storage adequacy, and at least monthly evaluation of image quality using a phantom. At mobile mammography sites, phantom image quality testing must be performed at each new location before the unit is used for patient imaging.

In 1990, national legislation – the Breast Cancer Screening Safety Act – was introduced to require that quality standards be met by every mammography site in the United States. The same legislation was reintroduced in 1991 as the Breast Cancer Screening Safety Act and as one of 22 bills packaged together as the Women's Health Equity Act.[8,11] Neither bill passed in 1991 but the Breast Cancer Screening Safety Act was reintroduced in slightly modified form as the Mammography Quality Standards Act of 1992;[12] it was recently passed by Congress, signed by the President, and is scheduled to take effect on October 1, 1994. The bill requires each mammography site to become certified through a private non-profit accreditation body (such as the ACR MAP) that has been approved by the Secretary of Health and Human Services. The bill requires sites to use dedicated mammography equipment, to have equipment checked annually by a qualified medical physicist, and to establish and maintain an appropriate QC program. The bill does not contain explicit quality standards for processors, but requires sites to meet quality standards comparable to those of the ACR.

While there are a variety of state regulations on mammography, most state regulations do not specify processor equipment or performance requirements. The Conference of Radiation Control Program Directors recently drafted a set of suggested state regulations on mammography that do specify processor performance limits. These suggested regulations stipulate daily processor monitoring of mid-density, density difference and base plus fog levels, with correction required if mid-density or density difference levels vary from control levels by more than ± 0.15, or if base plus fog levels exceed the base plus fog control level by more than +0.03. These levels are identical to the action limits specified in the ACR Mammography QC Manuals.

I would like to conclude with a challenge concerning processor performance: determine a method by which each mammography site may know that their processor is set up properly. While the ACR processor QC protocol can determine consistency, it cannot determine that the processor has been set up properly in the first place. The processor QC protocol may be ensuring that the mammography site is producing consistently poor quality images! What is needed is a procedure using a standized sensitometer and densitometer by which a film manufacturer can specify the sensitometry results that should result if the site's film processing is optimal. Then, routine processor QC testing, as specified in the ACR QC Manuals, can ensure that film processing remains optimal from day to day.


## References

1. Haus AG: Technologic improvements in screen-film mammography. *Radiology* 1990; 174: 628-637.

2. Bassett LW, Gold RH: Evolution of mammography. *Am. J. Roentgenol.* 1988; 150: 493.

3. Conway BJ, McCrohan JL, Rueter FG, *et al*: Mammography in the eighties. *Radiology* 1990; 177: 335-339.

4. Galkin BM, Feig SA, Muir HD: The technical quality of mammography in centers participating in a regional breast cancer awareness program. *Radiographics* 1988; 8: 133-145.

5. Hendrick RE: Standardization of image quality and radiation dose in mammography. *Radiology* 174: 648-656, 1990.

6. McLelland R, Hendrick RE, Zinninger MD, Wilcox PW. The American College of Radiology Mammography Accreditation Program. *Am.J.Roentgenol.* 1991; 157: 473-79.

7. American College of Radiology Mammography Quality Control Manuals. Second Edition, Reston, VA: American College of Radiology, 1992.

8. Hendrick RE. "Quality Assurance in Mammography: Accreditation, Legislation, and Compliance with Quality Assurance Standards" in *Radiologic Clinics of North America*, Breast Imaging: Current Status and Future Directions, LW Bassett, ed., Philadelphia: WB Saunders, Volume 30, Number 1, p. 243-255; January 1992.

9. Public Law 101-354, The Breast and Cervical Cancer Mortality Prevention Act of 1990.

10. *United States Federal Register*, Washington, DC. Volume 55, No. 251, December 31, 1990, p. 53510-53525.

11. S.1777. The Breast Cancer Screening Safety Act of 1991, 102nd Congress, 1st Session.

12. HR.5938. The Mammography Quality Standards Act of 1992, 102nd Congress, 2nd Session, October 1, 1992.

# Film Processing Area Layout Considerations

**Karen LeRoy**

Management Services Division
Eastman Kodak Company
Rochester, New York

Following the six-step planning process, as outlined in this paper, is very important when designing a film processing area. Proper planning will prevent a number of problems at the time of the actual construction and equipment installation. Examples of avoidable problems are: not allowing for adequate space for the equipment, failing to provide the necessary utilities, or installing the equipment incorrectly. Some of these unforeseen problems cannot only be very costly to correct, but may result in frustrating delays in the completion of a very vital part of a radiology department. Thorough planning will also ensure that the floor space is utilized efficiently. This is very important because space is limited in most hospitals. The six steps are:

1) Determining the requirements of the area
2) Evaluating the current area
3) Defining the redesign or design needs
4) Obtaining equipment information
5) Developing a conceptual plan
6) Reviewing plans with an architect

## 1. Determining the Requirements of the Area

The first step is to make the major decisions regarding the requirements for the area. First, consider the functions that will be performed in this space. Next, decide what type of processing area (darkroom or roomlight area) is most appropriate. A significant decision is whether or not a darkroom for processing films is adequate, or if space for viewing, sorting, or any other work, is required. The minimum amount of space that is required for a darkroom with one processor is approximately five feet by eight feet. More space is required for two processors. Additional space might also be required, depending on what functions will be performed in the area.

### Advantages of Roomlight Processing Areas
* Automated film handling
* Easy access to equipment
* Fast turnaround time
* Effective use of people
* Different functions (processing, viewing, work, etc)
  can easily be combined in one area

### Advantages of Darkrooms
* More flexibility in processing certain specialty films
* Lower investment in equipment

One of the major benefits of the roomlight equipment is easy access to the equipment. With roomlight equipment, a technologist can literally walk out of the control area and immediately be at the equipment. This is especially important in trauma rooms or emergency room areas where staying with the patient as much as possible is essential. These rooms are also generally staffed twenty-four hours a day; on the off-shifts, the technologists are probably processing their own films. Convenience is extremely important in this situation.

After a cassette is fed into the roomlight equipment, it is automatically opened and unloaded, the film is transported into the processor, and the cassette is reloaded with new film. With the darkroom, the technologist must enter the darkroom and manually unload and reload the cassette and feed the film into the processor, exit the darkroom, and retrieve the processed films.

The roomlight equipment also offers fast turnaround. The cassette is reloaded and returned in a matter of seconds. Roomlight equipment is also easy to incorporate into an open, multifunction work area. Therefore, the processing, quality control, and sorting functions can easily be combined into one very efficient space. With the darkroom, the space is dedicated only to processing. With the introduction of roomlight equipment, operating costs may be reduced because labor is used more effectively. Of course, this must be weighed against the initial cost of the equipment.

Roomlight areas are not always ideal, however. There are some cases where darkrooms are more appropriate. They are more flexible, especially for certain specialty films, such as orthopedic films. Darkrooms also require a lower investment in equipment. Even with roomlight equipment, a small darkroom is generally needed to load the magazines. Therefore, the darkroom cannot be completely eliminated. It may be possible, however, to share a darkroom with another area.

The next decision concerns equipment needs. The major decision is the number and models of processors that will be required. This is really dictated by the film volume. Determine the expected workload for the rooms that will be using the roomlight equipment and/or darkroom. The equipment manufacturer can provide information on equipment capacities, as well as guidelines for appropriate uses. It is also important to give serious consideration to the need for a backup processor. Replenisher tanks and silver recovery units also need to be selected. Again, the size of these units depends on the film volume.

Centralized systems for replenishment and silver recovery are also an option. The centralized systems remove the chemicals from the immediate vicinity of the processor and offer advantages of scale. Other pieces of equipment to consider include duplicators, identification cameras, passboxes, and film bins.

## 2. Evaluating the Current Area

The second step in the planning process is evaluating the current area. The information is especially useful when renovating an existing space, but most of the points also apply to new construction. The only difference is that new construction offers more flexibility with space. In an existing facility it is common to have limitations on the amount of space that is available. It is important to compare the amount of space that is available against the requirements determined in the first step to determine the changes that need to be made.

When evaluating the current space, be sure to note the location of existing utilities such as power, water, and drains, since they are required for the processors. The processors also require exhaust venting. It is also very important to locate any load-bearing walls or columns, since these cannot be changed.

## 3. Defining the Redesign Needs

The third step in the planning process is to determine the redesign needs. This involves comparing and reconciling the information obtained in steps 1 and 2, and making major decisions such as any walls that may need to be moved or relocated. Examples of very common renovations are: removing walls to open up a darkroom into a large work area, reducing a darkroom in size to accommodate roomlight equipment outside, or adding walls to create a darkroom out of an open space.

Another consideration is determining where utilities need to be provided. Whenever possible, utilize the current utilities, since this is most cost-efficient. When this isn't possible, utilities will need to be brought into the area; this will add to the cost of the redesign. Moving or adding a drain is one of the most difficult changes to make, especially on a ground floor concrete slab.

## 4. Obtaining Equipment Information

The fourth step is to contact the manufacturer to request more detailed equipment information. It is helpful to obtain specific information on all equipment that is under consideration. When contacting the manufacturer, ask for site specifications, which provide detailed information on the equipment dimensions, the required clearances for proper use, utility requirements, and installation information. It is important to get this information early in the process in order to avoid costly changes later.

## 5. Developing a Conceptual Plan

After all of this information has been gathered and most of the fundamental decisions have been made about the processing area, it is time to develop the conceptual design. This may be something as simple as a sketch if the changes are minor, such as removing one processor and replacing it with a new processor. But, it is important to develop a detailed drawing if any major changes are being made. Consider getting assistance from an architect or the equipment manufacturer when creating the drawings, especially if the space that is available is limited. One of the most important considerations in developing a conceptual design is to plan for the optimal placement of the equipment for good work flow. It is very important to allow for the recommended clearances around the equipment for service and ease of use. In many cases, using only the minimal clearances may increase the service time of the equipment or make the equipment less efficient to use. An architect should make construction blueprints if any structural changes are to be made.

There are some specific guidelines to consider when designing a darkroom. The first is determining the appropriate size of the darkroom. The proper size depends on the functions to be performed in the darkroom and who will be utilizing the darkroom. For example, if a darkroom tech will be in the darkroom most of the time to process the films, it can be smaller than if many people will be using the darkroom. Also, if the darkroom will be used for duplicating, space must be planned for that equipment.

Another consideration is whether or not a revolving door is required or if a hinged door is adequate. The revolving door allows access to the darkroom at any time without allowing light to enter, but it has the disadvantages of being more expensive and taking up some floor space. Consideration should also be given to the work counters and storage cabinets to ensure that there is adequate work space.

The work flow must be understood in order to plan properly for roomlight equipment. Observe and ask questions of those working in an existing processing area to understand the work flow. The objective is to place the equipment for easy access and good traffic flow, which result in a very functional area. If possible, place the feed end of the equipment close to the control areas of the x-ray rooms that will be utilizing it. Be sure to allow for space around the equipment for good traffic flow, so that one person standing by the equipment will not block the traffic flow through the area. If the equipment is located off a main corridor, try to set the equipment back a few feet from the corridor so that a person who is using the equipment will not block the traffic flow in the corridor. Providing the recommended clearances around the equipment will result in an efficient work area and easier service. When space is limited, consider requesting assistance from the manufacturer for best utilization of space. Some manufacturers offer assistance with facilities planning involving their equipment.

There are also some general layout considerations that apply to darkrooms and roomlight areas. For instance, it is most convenient to orient the processor's receiving bin toward the viewing counter. Then when the processed films drop into the receiving bin, they can be picked up and reviewed immediately. Consider locating the processing area close to the film assembly, reading, and work areas. As was mentioned before, be sure to plan for the necessary utilities and allow for the proper clearances for service. Utilizing less than the recommended clearances will increase the service time, which results in more downtime. Plans must also be made for cleaning the processor racks. If there is no janitor's closet nearby, try to include a large sink right in the processing area.

The last item to think about is the best location for replenisher tanks and silver recovery units. They need to be in a location that is easy to access and close to the processor. Consider locating them under a hinged or removable counter so they are out of the way, yet close to the equipment. This results in a cleaner processing area.

## 6. Reviewing Plans With the Architect

Once the conceptual design has been developed, it should be reviewed with an architect. This step is absolutely necessary if any structural changes are being made. A conceptual design is not suitable for construction purposes. The architect will make sure that all of the proper construction plans have been made and will develop blueprints.

## Example 1: Typical Layout

Two typical layouts are included to illustrate some of these points. Please refer to drawings 1 and 2. In the first example, the current layout shows four x-ray rooms around a darkroom and viewing area. There is a corridor leading between two of the rooms to provide access to the darkroom. There is access to the darkroom from the other rooms by exiting into the corridor and walking through the main work area and into the darkroom. Passboxes are located in each of the x-ray rooms.

The proposed layout illustrates some of the points that have been discussed regarding roomlight equipment. The current darkroom was eliminated completely. The area was opened up to create a large, open area for work space. Since the control areas for two of the rooms were not convenient to the processing equipment, they were relocated. Now there are four doors leading from the control areas that open up close to the feed-end of the processing equipment. This is a very convenient layout for the user, and service clearances are adequate for easy service. Plenty of work space is provided at the busy feed-end of the equipment.

The processor remains in its current location, which minimizes the cost, since the existing utilities can be utilized. Moving the control areas does result in additional construction costs, however. A small darkroom area has been added in the former

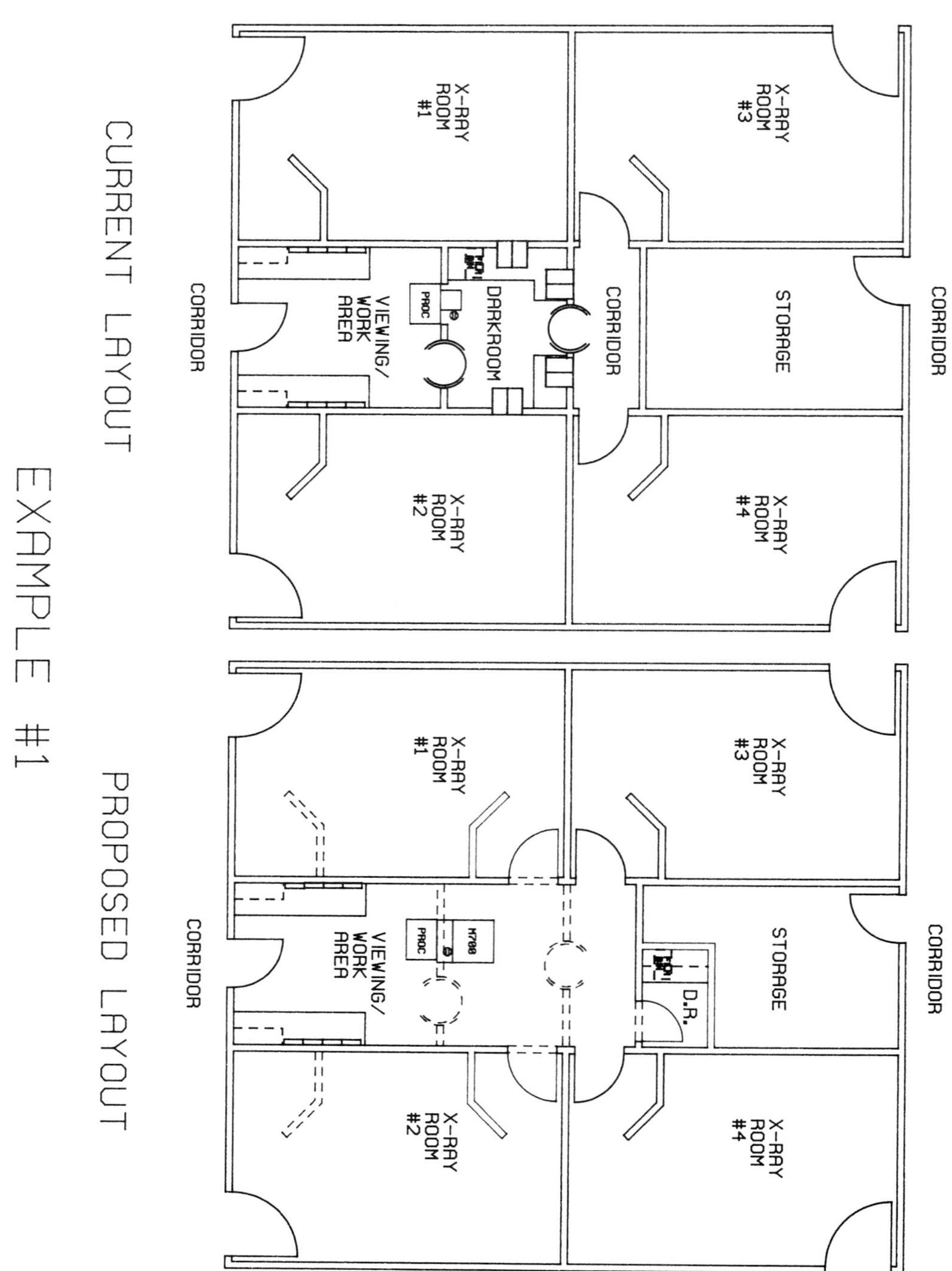
CURRENT LAYOUT
EXAMPLE #1
PROPOSED LAYOUT
X-RAY ROOM #1
X-RAY ROOM #2
X-RAY ROOM #3
X-RAY ROOM #4
CORRIDOR
CORRIDOR
CORRIDOR
STORAGE
DARKROOM
VIEWING/ WORK AREA
PROC
X-RAY ROOM #1
X-RAY ROOM #2
X-RAY ROOM #3
X-RAY ROOM #4
CORRIDOR
CORRIDOR
CORRIDOR
STORAGE
D.R.
VIEWING/ WORK AREA
PROC

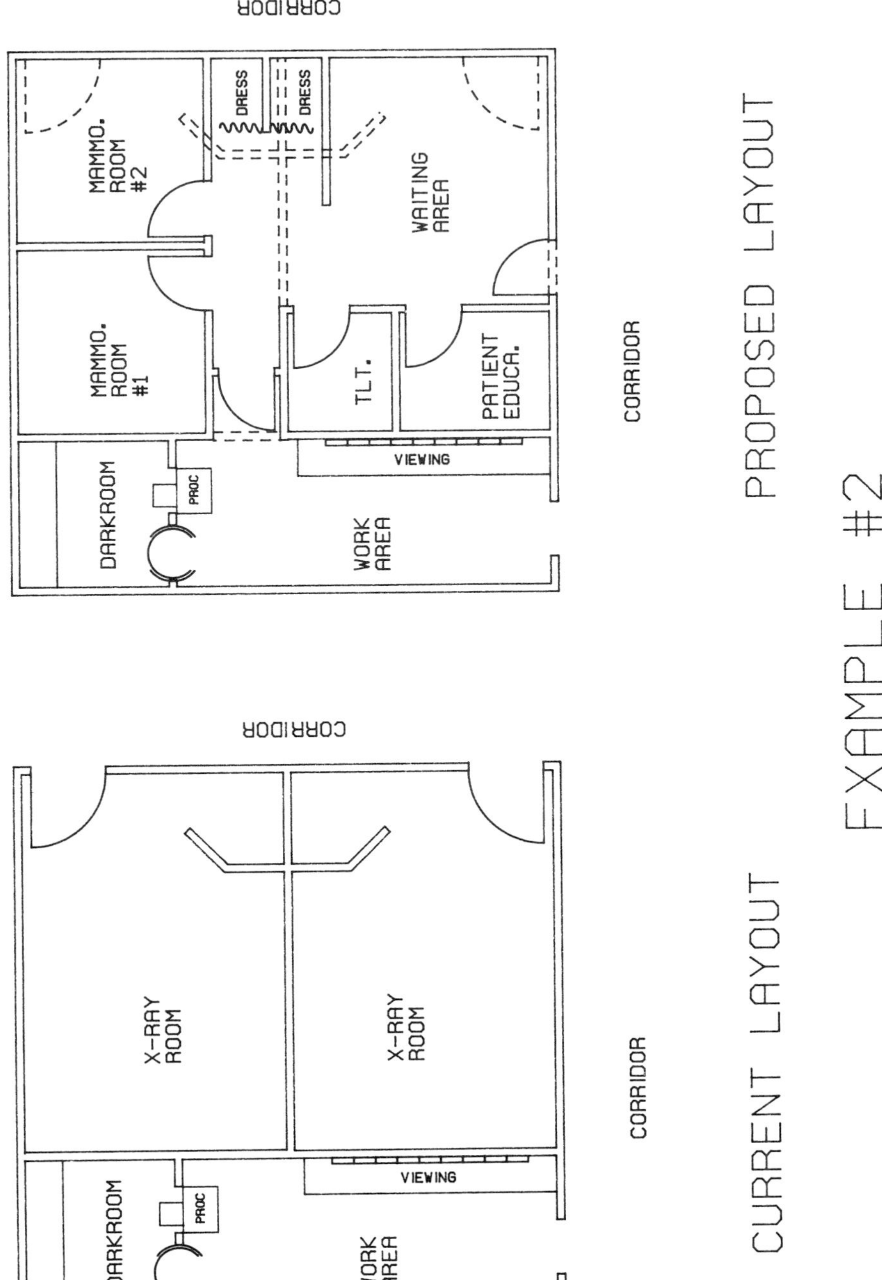
CORRIDOR
MAMMO. ROOM #2
DRESS
DRESS
WAITING AREA
MAMMO. ROOM #1
TLT.
PATIENT EDUCA.
DARKROOM
PROC
WORK AREA
VIEWING
CORRIDOR
PROPOSED LAYOUT
CORRIDOR
X-RAY ROOM
X-RAY ROOM
DARKROOM
PROC
WORK AREA
VIEWING
CORRIDOR
CURRENT LAYOUT
EXAMPLE #2

storage area. If there is no other darkroom relatively close by, consider adding a processor in the darkroom as a backup.

## Example 2: Typical Layout

This example illustrates the renovation of an existing x-ray area into a new mammography suite. The two previous x-ray rooms have been replaced with two new mammography rooms.

The suite has been designed for good traffic flow. A waiting area with a separate room for patient education is located inside the entrance from the corridor. Just beyond the waiting area are the dressing rooms. A toilet is located across from the dressing area. The two mammography rooms are located just beyond the dressing area.

Since the area was already adjacent to a darkroom, it was not necessary to add a new one. Direct access to the processing area has been provided by adding a new walkway from the mammography suite, with a door for privacy. This allows for convenience, but also keeps this area out of the patients' view.

## Conclusion

This six-step planning process illustrates a logical series of activities for the design or redesign of a film processing area. While it may sound like a lot of work - and it does take some effort — it will result in a very functional workspace. Spending a little extra time up front will save a lot of time near the end of the project and will greatly improve the chances of having a problem-free renovation.

# Co-optimization of Film and Process Chemistry for Optimum Results

**Robert E. Dickerson**
Health Sciences Division
Eastman Kodak Company
Rochester, New York

## Introduction

Silver-halide-based medical radiographic films are uniquely suited for their role in medical imaging. Silver halide films fill the role of imaging receptor, display and storage media in one form and in a very cost-effective manner. Film processing is critical for developing this image, and the interaction between film and processing needs to be understood and co-optimized to achieve optimum results. This paper will discuss the role and theory of latent image formation and the conseqences of inefficient processing of light photons, a description of the theory of development and a discussion of a film/chemistry/processor system that was co-optimally designed to achieve very rapid access processing. There will also be discussion of the fate of several key developer components on developer use, and the sensitivity towards variability of these components with two commercially available films. One film contains older conventional 3-dimensional silver halide microcrystals, whereas the second contains tabular silver halide grains.

## Role of Silver Halide Film

Silver halide films fulfill several of the needs of medical imaging in a cost effective and efficient manner. The various roles film plays are as follows:

1. Detection
2. Display
3. Storage

It is in the role of detection that silver halide microcrystals are unparalleled. A discussion of relative differences of systems for information content is difficult to make and many assumptions need to be made. Comparisons of silver-halide-based film to commercially available computed radiography systems show film/screen systems to have 2.6 times the information content of electronic imaging systems. In addition to the role of detection, film displayed on high-quality light boxes have for years been the basis of radiographic viewing and diagnosis. It is recognized that conditions such as light intensity, color temperature of the light bulbs and film masking are important to achieve optimized viewing. Finally, film serves the role of image storage that survives generations with minimal or no degradation in quality. All of these roles are accomplished in a very cost-effective manner.

## Latent Image Formation

The following is a discussion of the stages of latent image formation caused by the processing of light photons generated during X-ray exposure and subsequent emission of an X-ray intensifying screen. It is intended to be an overview and not a comprehensive explanation of latent image theory. More detailed explanation of theory can be found in photographic theory references. The stages of latent image formation include in the following and are illustrated in Figures 1-4.

1. Exposure
2. Nucleation
3. Growth
4. Development

Silver halide emulsions are manufactured with both chemical and optical sensitizers to form sensitivity specks which are efficient receptors for light photons produced during exposure (Figure 1). On exposure the energy produced from an absorbed light photon results in catalysis of a silver bromide molecule into a silver ion, a bromine atom (or photohole as it is sometimes called) and an electron (Figure 2). Migration of the electron and absorption to the sensitivity speck produces a partial negative charge which in turn attracts a positively charged silver ion. This process is called nucleation (Figure 3) and eventually will result in latent image formation. The literature reports that the minimum size of the latent image formation is at least four silver atoms. It is also important to deal with the bromine atom or photohole. If not removed, the photohole can recombine with the nucleated sensitivity speck and destroy the latent image. Failure to deal with the photohole can result in problems such as latent image fading and reciprocity law failure. (Figure 4).

## Amplification of Latent Image

The formation of latent image as a function of exposure does not in itself produce a useful image. It is the amplification of this latent image to a viewable size that forms the basis for medical radiography. This amplification process is called development and can be described in several stages. These include the following:

# *Latent Image Formation*
## *Silver Halide Microcrystal*

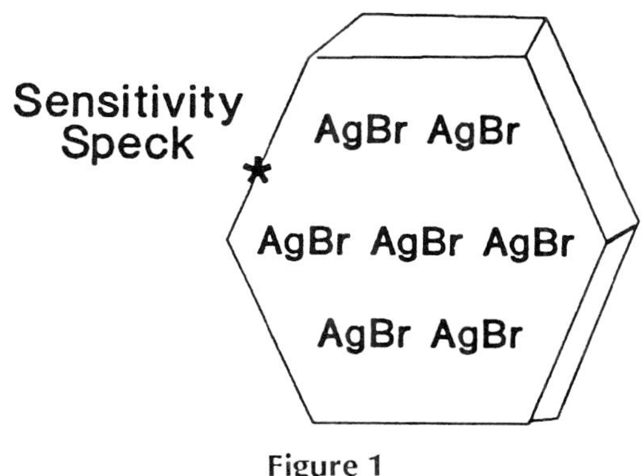


Figure 1

# Latent Image Formation
## *Silver Halide Microcrystal*
### *Exposure*

**Light Photon**

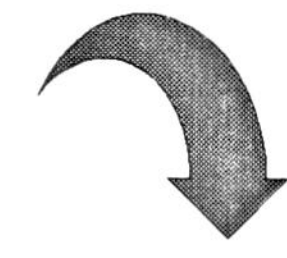

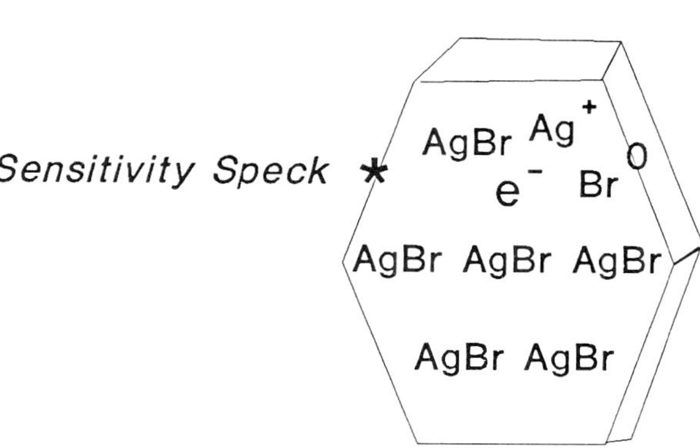


Figure 2

# Latent Image Formation
## *Silver Halide Microcrystal*
## Nucleation

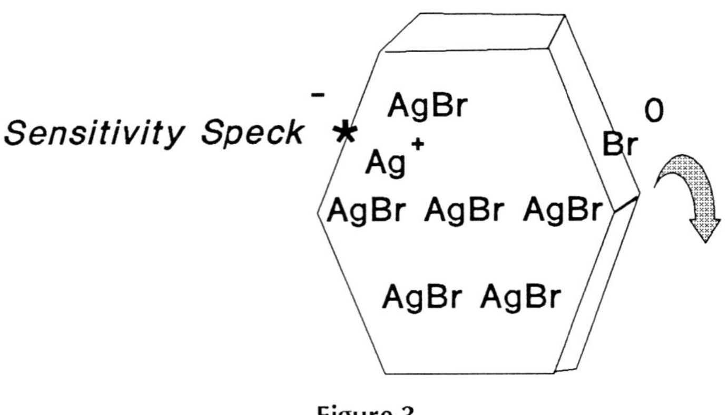



Figure 3

# Latent Image Formation
## *Silver Halide Microcrystal*

## Growth

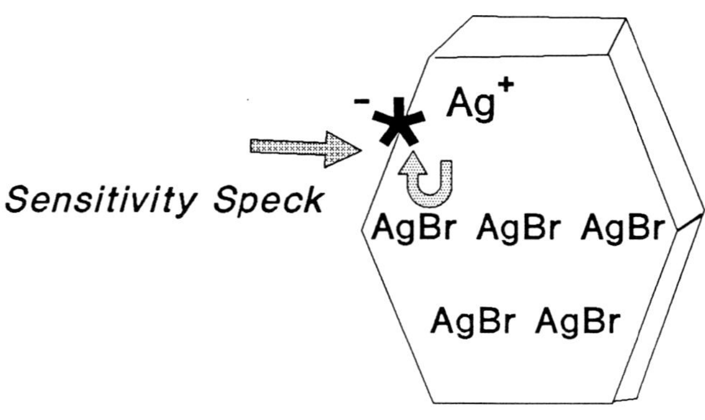



Figure 4

1. Diffusion of developer components
2. Adsorption of developer to latent image centers
3. Transfer of electron to latent image centers by ETA
4. Regeneration of electron transfer agent by hydroquinone (HQ)
5. Reduction of silver halide to metallic silver

## Stages of Development

### 1. Diffusion of Developer

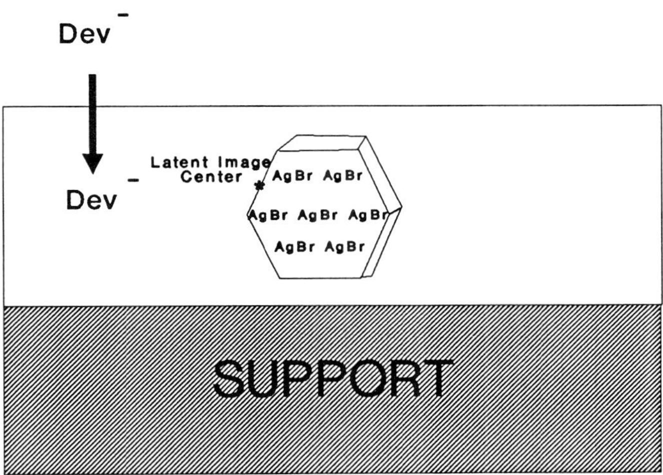


**Figure 5**

Figure 5 illustrates the diffusion of the developer components into the gelatin matrix, which is dispersed silver halide microcrystals containing latent image as a function of exposure. Figure 6 shows the next step that involves adsorption of the developing agents which include both hydroquinone and an electron transfer agent such as Phenidone. On adsorption, the developing agents transfer an electron preferentially to microcrystals containing latent image centers. Subsequent steps (Figure 7) involve regeneration of the electron transfer agent by hydroquinone. This process is called superadditivity; it continues the process of development until the grains containing latent image centers are reduced to metallic silver which forms the viewable image that radiologists have used for diagnosis for many years. The amplification factor that results from latent image to the fully developed grain is a factor of $5 \times 10^9$. Few, if any systems in nature provide this type of system gain or sensitivity. Figure 8 a,b and c show electron micrographs of an undeveloped, partially developed and fully developed grain.

## *Stages of Development*

1. Diffusion of Developer
2. Adsorption of HQ to Latent Image Center (LIC)
3. Transfer of Electron to LIC

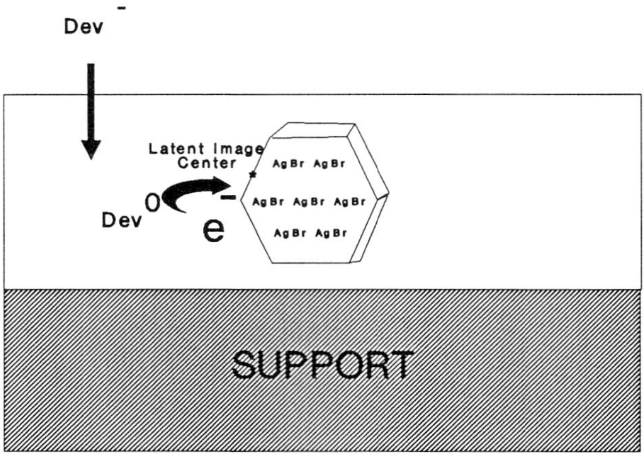


Figure 6

## *Stages of Development*

1. Diffusion of Developer
2. Adsorption of HQ to Latent Image Center (LIC)
3. Transfer of Electron  to LIC
4. Regeneration of HQ by Electron Transfer Agent (ETA)
5. Reduction of Silver Halide to Metallic Silver

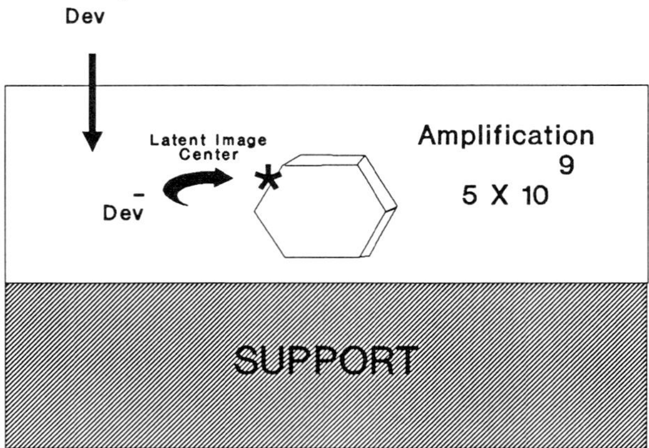


Figure 7

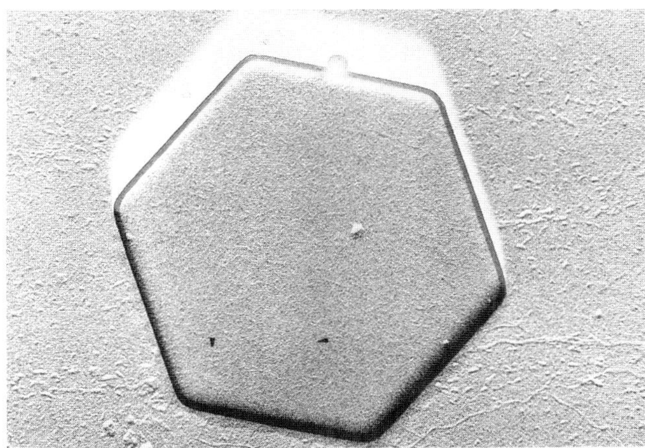

Figure 8a. Undeveloped grain

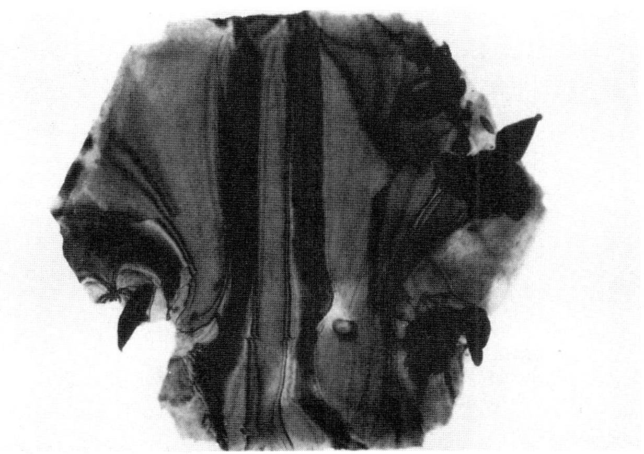

Figure 8b. Partially developed grain

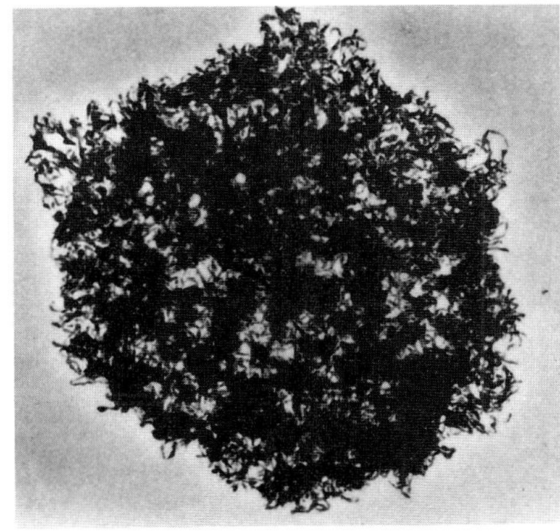

Figure 8c. Fully developed grain

## Factors Affecting Development

Because the amplification factor from latent image formation to viewable image is so large, correct developer composition and proper response of the film to the developer are critical. Table 1 shows a partial list of some of the developer components contained in Kodak RP X-Omat chemistry and their function. There are other components, as well, such as salts to act as pH buffers, metal ion sequesterants and others which are necessary to insure the consistent chemical processing that is needed in medical radiography.

What is the fate of this developer solution that was previously shown to be responsible for the very large $5 \times 10^9$ amplification? Concentration and composition can vary due to several causes. These include the following:

### <u>Factors Affecting Developer</u>

1. Mixing and preparation
2. Depletion through use
3. Oxidation
4. Evaporation

## Table 1. Developer Composition

### KODAK RP X-Omat Developer

| Component | Function |
| --- | --- |
| Hydroquinone | Reducing Agent |
| Phenidone | Electron Transfer Agent |
| Bromide | Restrainer |
| AF3 | Antifoggant |
| AF5 | Antifoggant |
| Glutaraldehyde | Hardener |
| Sulfite | Antioxidant |
| pH | Controls developer activity (typical value is 10.1 with starter) |
| # of parts | 3 |
| Starter | Seasons the fresh chemistry |

## Table 2.  Factors Affecting Activity

| Component | Preparation | Depletion | Evaporation | Oxidation |
|---|---|---|---|---|
| Hydroquinone | ⇓ | ⇓ | ⇑ | ⇓ |
| Antifoggant | ⇓ | ⇓ | ⇑ | |
| Bromide | ⇓ | ⇑ | ⇑ | |
| pH | ⇓ | ⇓ | ⇑ | ⇑ |

Table 2 shows some relative changes in concentration of several developer components as a result of these factors. First, concentration and composition can vary during the preparation and mixing stage. Mistakes in mixing or dilution generally can result in lower than recommended levels of chemistry. Secondly, as a result of use, hydroquinone, antifoggants and pH are reduced but bromide ion increases. Proper replenishment can compensate for this. Thirdly, lack of use can cause increases in concentration because of evaporation. Lastly, oxidation from absorbed oxygen can result in lower hydroquinone levels but higher pH. How these changes affect sensitometry of silver halide films depends on the type of films that are to be processed. Figure 9 shows two films, one containing older, conventional 3-dimensional (3D) or pebble-shaped grains while the second film contains tabular or T-grain microcrystals. The next series of figures show the sensitivity to changes of concentration ($\pm 50\%$) on the sensitometric response of these two films. The Y-axis shows changes in speed (in CR units) or contrast. The X-axis shows concentration $\pm 50\%$ of a developer component centered at the normal level. Figure 10 a and b show the effect of hydroquinone concentration on speed and contrast. As can be seen, the tabular-grain film shows much less sensitivity to changes in hydroquinone concentrations. Figure 11 a and b show a similar trend with changes in pH. Figure 12 a and b show the response for changes in bromide concentration. Here the T-grain film is seen to be slightly more sensitive for speeds although the relative magnitude of change is small. The effect of bromide concentration on contrast is interesting to note; these two films show an opposite trend towards bromide ion concentration although the total magnitude of change is small. Figure 13 a and b show the effect of varying the total developer concentration $\pm 50\%$. Again, the 3-D grain film shows the greater sensitivity, particularly at low concentrations.

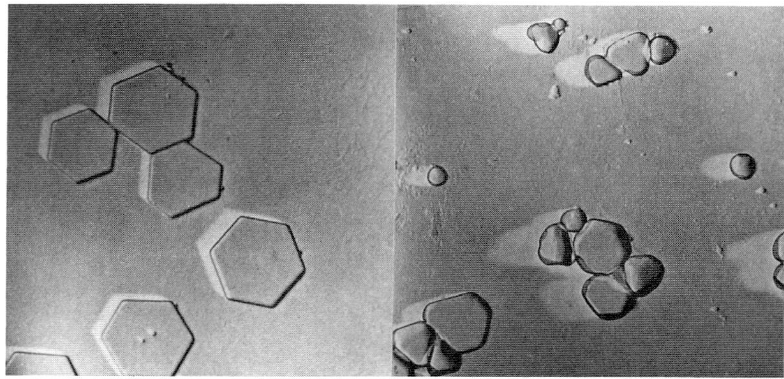

**Figure 9.** Photomicrographs of Tabular (left) and regular 3-dimensional (right) silver halide grains

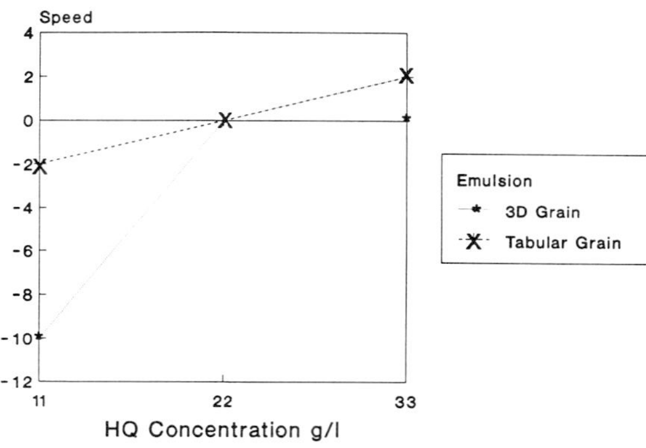


**Figure 10a**

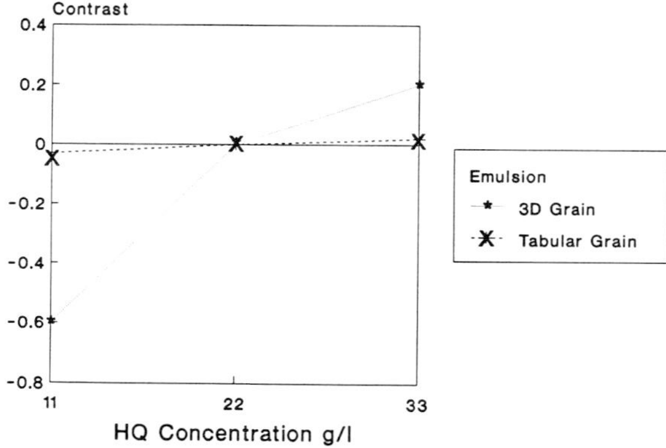


**Figure 10b**

## Effect of pH on Speed

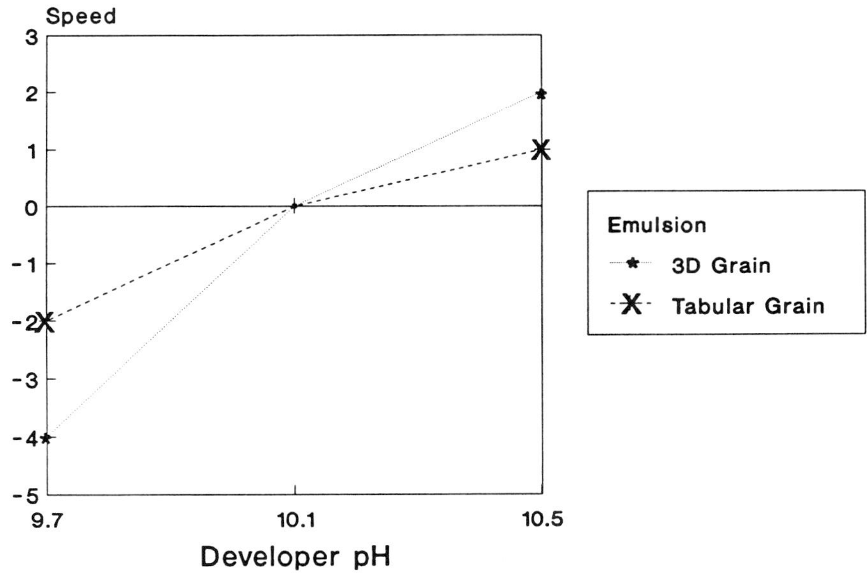


Figure 11a

## Effect of pH on Contrast

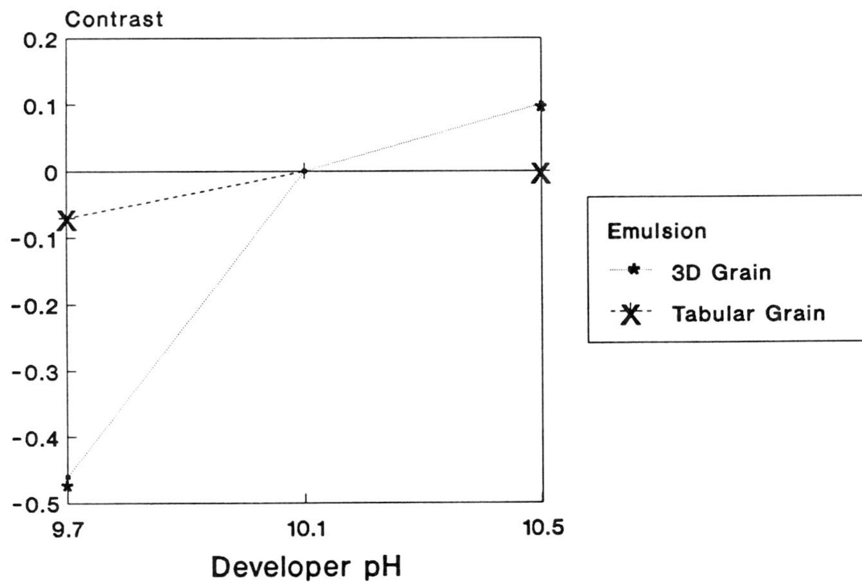


Figure 11b

## Effect of Bromide on Contrast

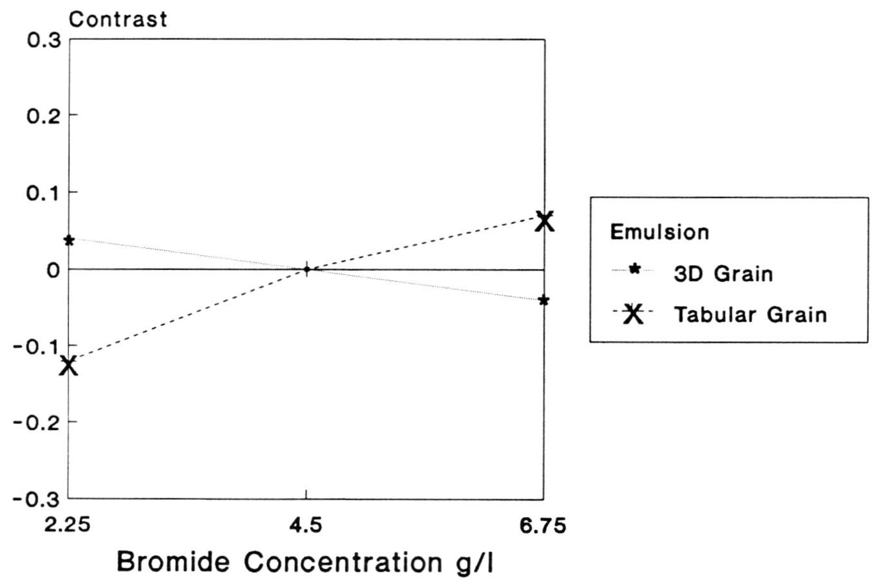


Figure 12a

## Effect of Bromide on Speed

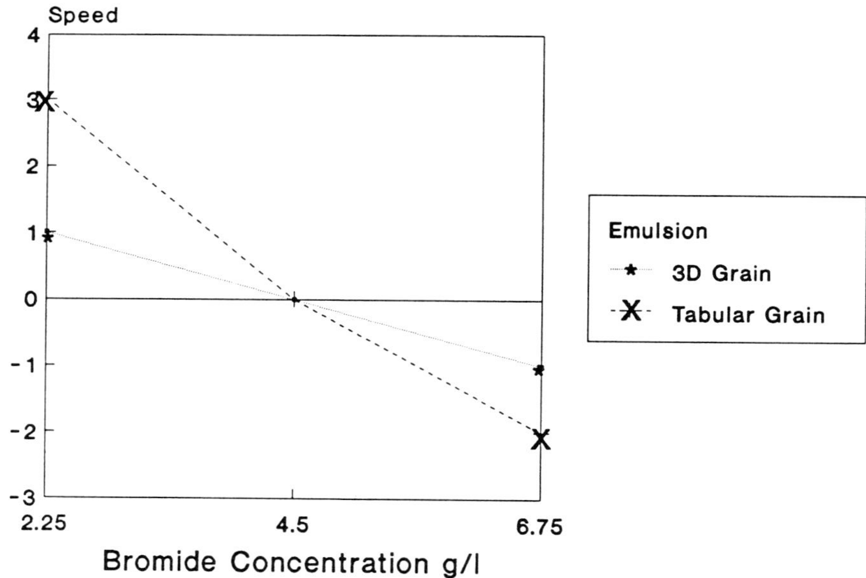


Figure 12b

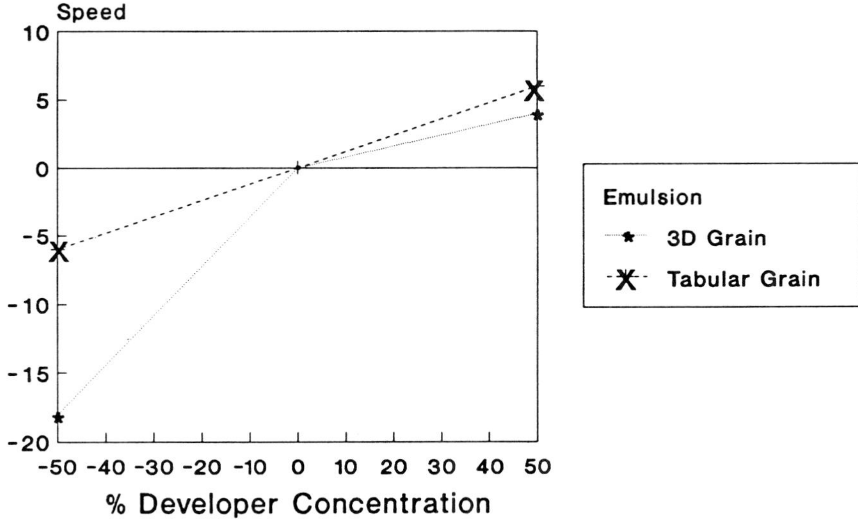



Figure 13a

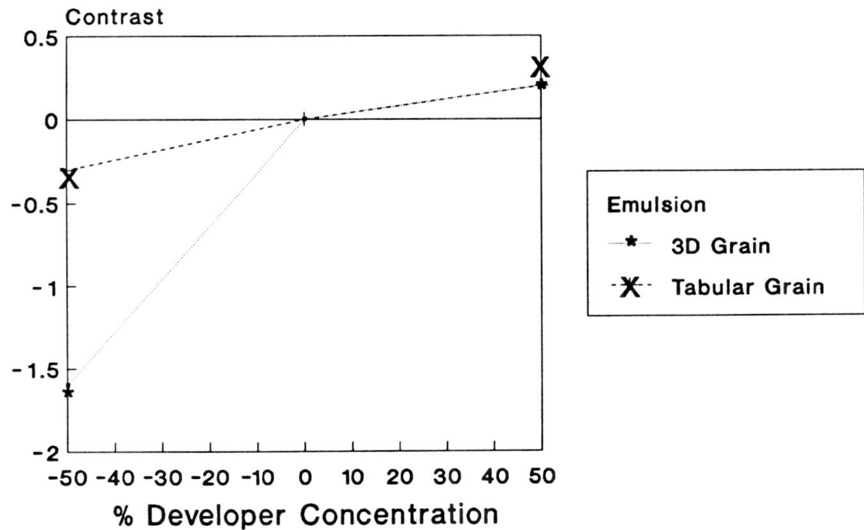



Figure 13b

## Analysis of Processing Chemistry

There are several approaches to monitoring developer composition and activity. These include the following:

1. Sensitometric quality control
2. Measurement of specific gravity
3. pH measurement
4. Component laboratory analysis

The first approach is to do control charting using daily process control sensitometric strips; if the process begins to fail, change chemistry. This approach may be the most cost effective and time effective as chemistry is relatively inexpensive compared to the total cost of the imaging system.

Measurement of specific gravity is a measure of the salt content of a solution, similar to what is used to measure the amount of sulfuric acid in your car battery. This is not a very accurate or specific test. For example, an important component that is normally added at low concentration could be missing and specific gravity measurement would never detect it.

pH measurements are also difficult and inaccurate because it is difficult to measure hydrogen ion activity in a solution with high salt content and special electrode and internal salts are needed to get accurate results.

The most accurate determination of developer composition is to submit a sample for laboratory analysis. This approach however is costly and not time effective.

## Co-optimization of Film And Chemistry

As has been previously described, silver halide films and photographic processing are intimately linked and require co-optimizing to achieve optimum results. A new film/chemistry/processor system was recently introduced to achieve very rapid processing with consistent quality and minimal process sensitivity. This system is the Kodak RA system and contains T-grain technology, redesigned chemistry and a new processor designed for very rapid processing.

The goal of this system was to reduce the total time required for the various stages of processing by of reducing the time in each stage. These stages include development, fixing, washing and drying. Improvement in rates of development were achieved by special features of the film. In addition there were changes to the chemistry and processor to further reduce cycle time in each stage.

## Features Enabling Processing
### Development

Microcrystal Shape: The Increased surface area of tabular grains in the film emulsion provide easier accessibility for developer components.

Silver Halide Composition: The silver halide emulsion was optimized for rapid development.

Film Chemistry: Use of DEA (Developing Enhancing Agent) reduces induction time of development.

Film Hardener: Forehardening of the film prior to development reduces film swell which in turn reduces diffusion path length.

## Fixing
Microcrystal Shape: Increased surface area provides faster fixing.

Silver Halide Composition: Halide content was optimized for high solubility.

Film Hardener: Low film swell reduces diffusion path length for faster fixing.

## Washing and Drying
Forehardened T-Grain Emulsion: Produces less film swell which results in lower chemical loading for better washing. Less chemical and water load results in faster drying.

**Table 3. Developer Comparisons**

**KODAK RP vs RA Developer**

| Component | RP | RA |
|---|---|---|
| Hydroquinone | Yes | Yes |
| Phenidone | Yes | No |
| HMMP | No | Yes |
| Bromide | No (Br in starter) | Yes |
| AF3 | Yes | No |
| AF5 | Yes | Yes |
| Glutaraldehyde | Yes | No |
| Sulfite | Yes | Yes |
| pH | 10.1(with starter) | 10.35 |
| # of parts | 3 | 1 |
| Starter | Yes | No |

Because of the changes in the film and process chemistry it was possible to design a new developer that is much simpler and easier to use. Table 3 shows a comparison of the older Kodak RP X-Omat chemistry and the new Kodak X-Omat RA/3D chemistry. Co-optimizing the film for response in process chemistry allowed for the possibility of significantly changing the process chemistry from a 3-part solution plus starter to a single-part developer. In addition, process time was reduced from 90 seconds to 38 seconds which provided increased productivity in busy medical centers. Only by co-optimizing film, chemistry and processor was this possible.

## Acknowledgments

This paper is the result of the work of many people. I would like to thank Alan Tsaur and Steven Hershey for their assistance in providing emulsion grain photomicrographs; Alan Fitterman for helpful discussions on process chemistry; and Peter Cumbo, who did the work on developer sensitivity studies and who was instrumental in the development of the RA process chemistry.

# Design Basics and Component Functions
# of Automatic Film Processors

**Kenneth W. Oemcke**
Health Sciences Division
Eastman Kodak Company
Rochester, New York

There are many variables that influence radiographic image quality. One of the prime contributors is the film processor. The elements of the film processor need to be carefully designed to provide the optimal processing parameters. This paper will describe each of the processing steps, define components in each step, and describe the basic principles of processor design.

The four prime steps in film processing are developing, fixing, washing, and drying. The most critical of these is the development step and must be given the most attention during the design phase. Development makes the latent image visible, therefore extreme caution must be taken to assure that no artifacts are induced on the film. The fixing section removes unexposed, undeveloped silver crystals thereby making the image permanent. The washing section removes all chemicals from the film emulsion to assure long term stability of the image. The drying section dries the film to allow immediate handling. In addition to these four sections there are many other factors to consider, such as, reliable transport, material selection, and safety regulations. Recent advancements in processor, film, and chemical technology, must also be considered during the design phase. Some of the latest processor advancements will be discussed at the end of this paper.

## Developer System

As stated before, the developer section is the most critical processing section for optimal image quality. The diagram below shows a typical processor developer system. There are four main sections of the developer system: replenishment, recirculation, temperature control and drain (Figure 1).

Each component, its function, typical values and design considerations is described below.

## Replenishment

**Replenisher** – This is the source of fresh chemicals and may come from tanks or a chemical mixer.

**Replenisher Pump** – This pumps the fresh chemicals from the replenisher supply to the developer processing tank. It should be adjustable to allow for different replenishment rates. Typical replenishment rates are 60 to 600 ml/min depending on the productivity of the processor or the processing time.

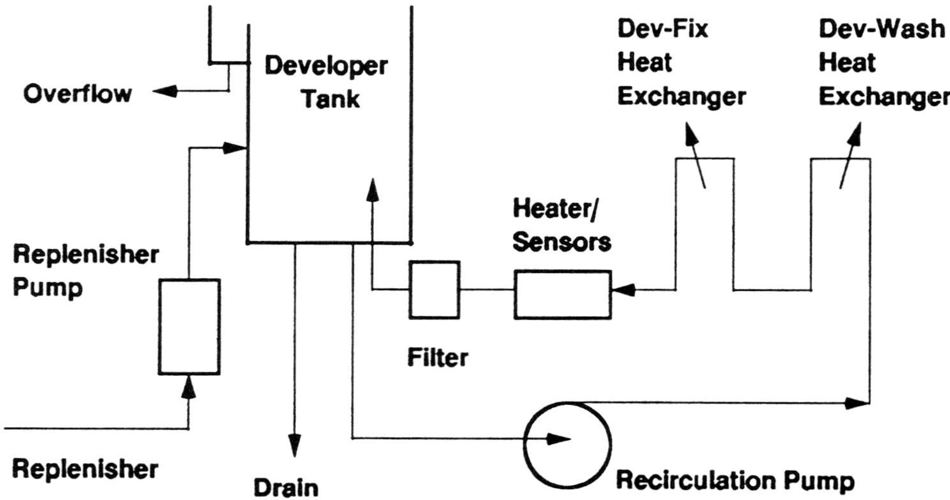


Figure 1. Developer System

## Recirculation

**Developer Tank** – This is the container for the developer solution and transport rack. It should be easy to clean and maintain. Typical volume ranges from 1 to 3 gallons.

**Recirculation Pump** – This is the component that continuously recirculates the developer for temperature control and mixing of fresh and seasoned chemicals. Typical range for the recirculation rate is 2 to 4 gallons/minute.

**Filter** – This keeps the developer clean so that optimal film quality is maintained. Typically the filter is 75 micron porosity with replacement recommended monthly or 5000 films.

## Temperature Control

**Developer-Wash Heat Exchanger** – This exchanger is used to help maintain the developer temperature. The air surrounding the developer tank can rise above the developer temperature due to heat from the dryer. This high air temperature causes a heat flow into the developer tank and raises the developer temperature. The developer-wash heat exchanger cools the developer solution and therefore helps maintain the developer temperature. Typically this is a thin-wall stainless steel tube in the bottom of the wash tank.

**Developer-Fixer Heat Exchanger** – This exchanger uses the developer to heat the fixer solution up to its minimum operating temperature. If the fixer has a heater, then the exchanger is not required. Typically this is a thin-wall stainless steel tube in the bottom of the fixer tank through which developer flows.

**Developer Heater/Sensors** – These are the critical elements for maintaining the developer temperature. Sensors are used to monitor the developer temperature and control the developer heater as needed. The sensor is either a thermostat or a thermistor. Typically, the heaters are rated between 500 and 1500 watts and are sized according to desired warmup times and replenisher amounts. Temperature of the developer is usually controlled in the 90 to 100°F range with a tolerance of ±0.5°F. Sensors are also added to the design for safety reasons, such as overtemperature and solution detection.

## Drain

**Drain/Overflow** – As replenisher solution is added, some developer must exit through the overflow to a floor drain or collection system. When cleaning the developer tank, the developer is drained by way of a drain valve. Sometimes the overflow and drain lines are combined and sometimes they are separate.

An important consideration that applies to all of the above components is service life. Considering that whenever the processor is on, the above components are in use, typical life is 10,000 hours for a 5 year life goal. This means that each component should be carefully selected and tested to achieve the reliability goals and service life set for the processor.

## Fixer System

The fixer system is similar to the developer system but somewhat simpler. The diagram below shows a typical fixer system of a processor. It contains the same four sections as the developer: replenishment, recirculation, temperature control, and drain (Figure 2).

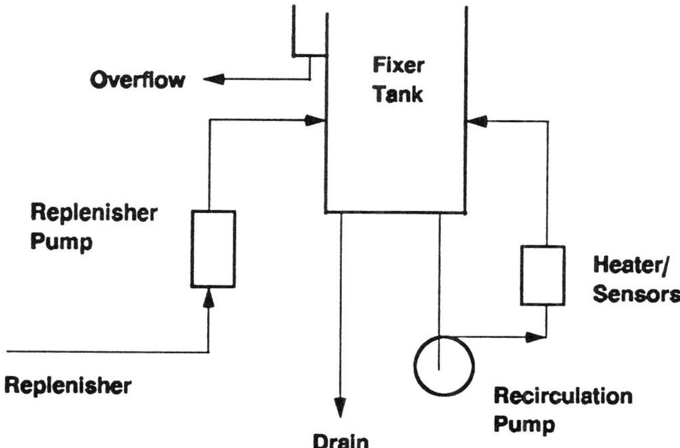


Figure 2. Fixer System

Each component, its function, typical values and design considerations is described below.

## Replenisher

**Replenishment Tank** - This is the source of fresh chemicals and may come from tanks or a chemical mixer.

**Replenisher Pump** - This pumps the fresh chemicals from the replenisher supply to the fixer processing tank. It must be adjustable to allow for different replenishment rates. Typical replenishment rates are 80 to 800 ml/min depending on the productivity of the processor.

## Recirculation

**Fixer Tank** - This is the container for the fixer solution and transport rack. It should be easy to clean and maintain. Typical volume ranges from 1 to 3 gallons.

**Recirculation Pump** - This is the component that continuously recirculates the fixer for temperature control and mixing of fresh and seasoned chemicals. Typical range for recirculation rate is 2 to 4 gallons/minute.

**Filter** - The fixer solution typically does not need a filter as does the developer.

## Temperature Control

**Developer-Fixer Heat Exchanger** - This exchanger uses the developer to heat the fixer solution up to its minimum operating temperature. If the fixer has a heater, then the exchanger is not required. Typically this is a thin-wall stainless steel tube in the bottom of the fixer tank through which developer flows.

**Fixer Heater/Sensors** - These maintain the fixer temperature. Sensors are used to monitor the fixer temperature and control the fixer heater as needed. The sensor is either a thermocouple or thermistor. Typically the heaters are rated between 500 and 1500 watts and are sized according to desired warmup times and replenisher amounts. Temperature of the fixer is usually controlled only up to a minimum temperature that may vary from 85-95°F. The fixer temperature may drift above the setpoint. A higher temperature only improves fixing and causes no problems. Sensors are also added to the design for safety reasons, such as overtemperature and solution detection.

## Drain

**Drain/Overflow** - As replenisher solution is added, the fixer must exit through the overflow to a floor drain or collection system. When cleaning the fixer tank, the fixer is drained by way of a drain valve. Sometimes the overflow and drain lines are combined and sometimes they are separated.

Again, an important consideration for the fixer components is service life and reliability. Typical life is 10,000 hours for a 5 year service life. Similar selection and testing as the developer components should take place.

## Wash System

The wash system is the last of the wet sections.  Below is a typical diagram of the wash system. It consists of the water input and drain sections (Figure 3).

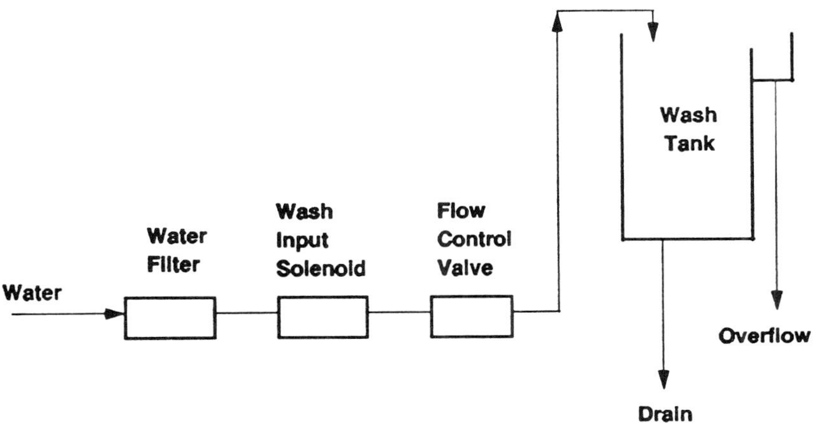


Figure 3. Wash System

Below is a short description of each component, its function, typical values and design considerations.

## Water Input

**Filter** - This is used to assure that particulate matter in the water does not adversely affect the water flow and cause dirt on the film.  Typically the filter is 50 micron porosity with replacement recommended every 1 to 3 months.

**Input Solenoid** - This is used to control water usage by allowing the water to be turned on and off, as needed.  The water is turned off during the standby mode with the exception of when cooling of the developer solution is needed. It is becoming important to use as little water as possible for environmental reasons.

**Flow Control Valve** - This is used to regulate and keep constant the flow of water into the processor as fluctuations occur in water line pressure.  Typical flow rate of the incoming water is 0.25 to 1.5 gallons/minute.

## Temperature Control

**Water Temperature** - Most processors do not require control of the water temperature within the processor as with the developer and fixer solutions.  There are however temperature limits on the incoming water.  Since the water is sometimes used for cooling the developer, an upper limit of 5 to 10°F below the developer temperature is desired. Typical low limit for the incoming water is 40°F.

## Drain

**Drain/Overflow** - As with the other solutions, when the water is replenished with fresh incoming water, the excess goes out the overflow.  When the tank needs cleaning, a drain valve is opened to drain the tank.  Most processors when turned off, now drain the wash tank in order to reduce algae growth.

Another critical concern in the wash water system is compliance with the many governmental regulations.  The primary regulatory concern is the siphoning of contaminated water back into the potable water supply.  For this reason, there are many regulations requiring such items as vacuum breakers or 20 mm air gaps. Los Angeles County, Cook County, and most of Europe are very stringent about meeting their regulations.

## Dryer System

The last step in processing an x-ray film is drying.  Figure 4 shows a typical dryer system.  It consists of air movement and temperature control sections.

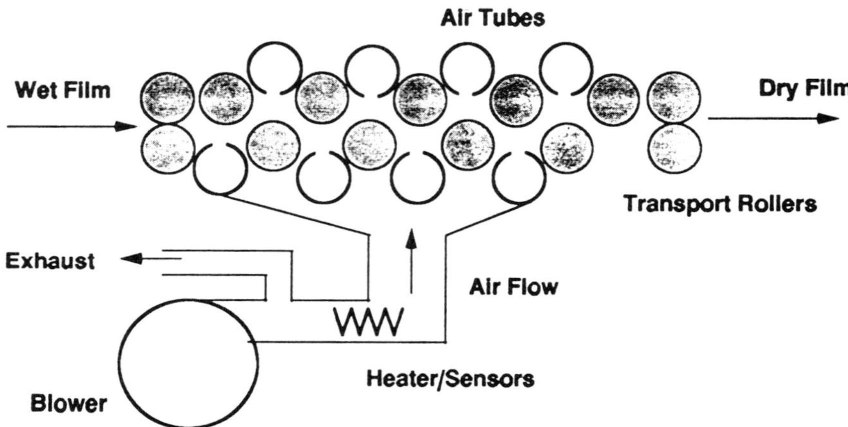


Figure 4. Dryer System

Below is a short description of each component, its function, values and design considerations.

## Air Movement

**Blower** - This is used to move the heated air to the film surface for drying to occur. Typical air flow capacity of the blower is 100 to 300 cubic feet per minute. Every effort should be made to reduce the noise of the blower in order to lessen any irritation to the operator.  Proper operation on 50 or 60 hertz power must be considered to make sure the unit dries on all worldwide power sources.

**Air Tubes** - The air tubes are the critical part of the air movement system. They are the component that uniformly distributes the air to the film surface.  They provide the air turbulence at the film surface thereby accelerating moisture evaporation from the film. Higher air flows typically give a greater heat transfer and therefore quicker drying.

**Air Exhaust** - As film is dried, the air in the dryer builds up with moisture. The air exhaust allows some of the humid air to be ducted away from the dryer and therefore stabilize the humidity in the dryer at an operable level. Typical values for the percentage of exhaust range from 25-100%.

## Temperature Control

**Heater/Sensors** - As with the developer and fixer, the dryer has a heater and the appropriate control and safety sensors. Typically the heater ranges from 1500 to 3000 watts and is sized to provide air temperatures from 100-160°F and rapid warmup times. The control sensor again is either a thermocouple or a thermistor. Safety sensors include an overtemperature sensor and sometimes an air flow switch. The air flow switch assures that air flows across the heater before turning it on.

## Transport System

The transport system moves the film through the developer, fixer, wash and drying sections. Various manufactures of processors use different methods of film transport but all generally have rollers and guide shoes. Rollers move the film and may be an opposed or staggered path. The guide shoes are used to turn the film in situations not easily accomplished by rollers. Figure 5 shows a typical transport system.

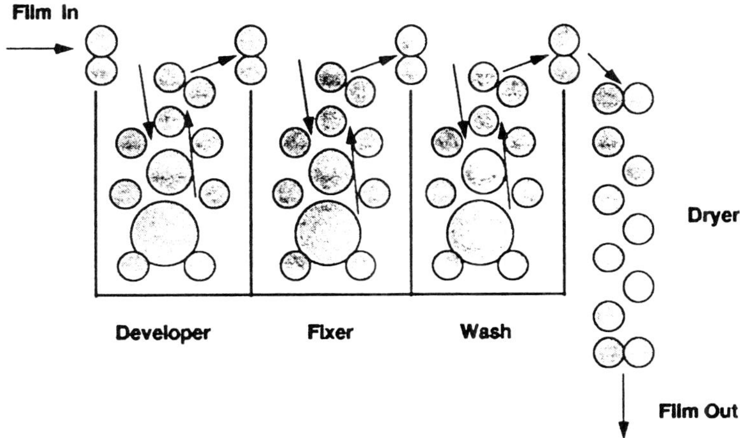


Figure 5. Transport System

The transport system has many design considerations that must be balanced. The transport must be very reliable. As many as 50,000 to 100,000 films of various sizes and types will be processed before a transport system is considered complete. This is naturally to make sure that patient re-exposure is not caused by a lost film due to a faulty transport system.

Extreme care must also be taken when designing the transport system to assure that film artifacts which may interfere with a diagnosis are minimized.

Maintenance of a processor is critical to its continued performance from a quality and reliability standpoint. Lack of proper maintenance can cause component failure and/or film artifacts. Processor manuals generally specify daily, weekly, and monthly maintenance procedures.

## Material Selection

Throughout the design of a processor, the selection of materials to be used is critical. Three primary materials are used throughout a processor: plastics, metals, and elastomers.

Plastics get used in applications such as: panels, rollers, and bearings. Processors that have the entire tank system made of plastic tend to be safer, more durable and lower cost than all metal tank systems. Plastic parts must be thoroughly checked for chemical compatibility so that the material does not degrade with contact with the chemicals. Also photographic activity must be checked to assure that it does not have an affect on the film development. Plastics frequently used in processors are ABS, polypropylene, and nylon.

Metals are used extensively throughout a processor in such applications as shafts, guide shoes, and electrical boxes. Any part that is in direct contact with the chemicals or fumes should be type 316 stainless steel. Components that are a safe distance from the chemical or fumes can be aluminum if properly protected with a coating.

The last primary material used in a processor is elastomers. They are used for rollers and gaskets. Elastomer materials such as silicon or ethylene-propylene-terpolymer (EPT) are used for rollers. Gaskets are used in areas that need sealing, like pump heads or dryer air flow paths. Again these should be checked for chemical compatibility and photographic activity to assure no problems occur.

## Safety/Regulations

There are numerous regulations that must be met and a variety of safety approvals that must be obtained. These allow the processor to be sold into various countries or counties around the world. Below are described the typical approvals that should be considered.

**Safety** - Approvals such as Underwriters Laboratory, Canadian Standard Association and German TUV are desirable. These regulations are primarily related to electrical safety. Processors designed and manufactured to meet these regulations, protect the operators against electrical hazards and reduce the chances of any electrical fires. Some regulatory items covered are high voltage to low voltage spacings, temperature rise of electrical components, clearances, safety interlocks,

**EMI** - EMI stands for ElectroMagnetic Interference.  These standards regulate emissions of radiated/conducted interference, and susceptibility of the processor to EMI interference.  Many worldwide standards exist for EMI.  Some are mandatory and some are voluntary.  Examples include: Federal Communication Commission (FCC) and German Post Vfg.  These standards assure that the processor will not emit EMI noise that might interfere with other neighboring pieces of equipment and that the processor is not susceptible to noise emitted by other equipment.

**Seismic** - The State of California has regulations concerning the stability of equipment when exposed to earthquake forces.  These assure that equipment is properly mounted and will not cause human hazards during an actual earthquake.  This approval requires a seismic mounting kit be designed and then approved by the State of California.  This kit must be installed on every processor installed in California.

**Water** - Various regulations control the manner in which the water enters the processor. As previously mentioned, European regulations require that water entering the wash tank have a 20 mm air gap to assure no mixing of the contaminated and potable water. Other regulations control what materials are used in the water inlet parts.

## Processor Advancements

Processors have gone through many advancements and improvements over the past few years. These have been primarily related to improving the productivity of the processor.  In the table below a comparison has been made between an old and a new processor, in this case a KODAK *RP* X-OMAT Processor, Model M6B and a KODAK X-OMAT 460 RA Processor.

### Processor Advancements

| Processor Type | M6B | 460 RA |
|---|---|---|
| Process Cycles | 1 (Standard) | 4 (Ext/Std/Rapid/kwik) |
| Capacity (films/hour) | 230 | 120/230/350/460 |
| Film Drop Time | 90 sec | 180/90/60/45 sec |
| Tank Fill Method | Manual | Auto |
| Replenishment Type | Length | Area |
| Operator Interface | Ready Light | Lights + LCD Display |
| Control | Discrete Logic | Microprocessor |
| Diagnostics | None | Included |
| Upgrades | Manual | Software |
| Languages | 1 | 12 |

Notice that the M6B has just one processing cycle whereas the newer one, the 460 RA, has four processing cycles. These faster cycles on the 460 RA give an increased processing capacity and shorter drop time. It also provides the newer extended cycle for mammography processing. The 460 RA also has a significant number of processing features such as automatic tank fill, area replenishment, and microprocessor control. The operator interface is also significantly improvde on the new processors, including a liquid crystal display which allows the operator to monitor and change all processing parameters via the display. The menus on this display are programmable in 12 different languages to allow the operators to see the display in their native language. With the microprocessor control, processor operation can be easily changed and updated by a software upgrade via a laptop computer. All in all, the newer processors have many new features, ranging from increased productivity to improved operator interface.

## Summary

Processor design is a critical component to providing optimal x-ray film quality. Every component has a specific function within the processor and must be properly selected for optimal operation. Component design should consider function, reliability, and life. Film quality is the ultimate goal of the processor design. Not only is the design phase critical, but also the testing and evaluation, in order to assure reliable operation and long life. The last and most important consideration for the owner of a processor is to maintain the processor at the manufacturer's recommended service intervals. The manufacturer typically includes in the processor manuals a complete list of daily, weekly and monthly maintenance. Following the recommended maintenance will insure a long life and continued optimal film quality.

# Mammography Processing Systems

## Thomas A. Batz and Arthur G. Haus

Health Sciences Division
Eastman Kodak Company
Rochester, New York

## Mammography Processing Systems

Following the manufacturer's recommendations for film processing in mammography is critical in terms of processor cycle time, proper chemicals, replenishment rate, temperature, and processor maintenance in order to achieve and maintain appropriate film speed, contrast and fog levels. The issues and concerns involved in mammography film processing are widely known but often misunderstood. Several of these key issues/concerns will be discussed with recommendations on how to improve film processing in mammography.

## Processing System Variable Overview

Topics on automatic film processing systems which will be discussed include: 1) the automatic film processor, 2) film, and 3) chemicals. These system components must be considered together as a system and therefore properly optimized in order to obtain appropriate image quality in terms of film contrast of the processed radiograph. The resulting film speed affects radiation dose to the patient.

## Film Processor

Automatic film processor variables include 1) processing cycle time, 2) temperature, 3) replenishment, 4) agitation and 5) drying.

### 1)Processor Cycle Time

Processing cycle time is usually defined as the time it takes for 1)the leading edge of the film to enter and exit from the processor, or 2) the leading edge of the film to enter and the trailing edge of the film to exit the processor. The latter definition will be used in this article. Processing cycles for mammography range from approximately 90 to 210 seconds. The so-called conventional or standard processing cycles for general-purpose processing in medical imaging are between 90 and 150 seconds (Table 1). Developer temperature and replenishment rates are determined by the processing cycle in order to achieve the desired sensitometric characteristics (contrast, speed, base plus fog) for the film being used.

## Table 1. Processing Conditions for Kodak Min-R Mammography Film[1]

| Kodak X-Omat processors | | M35<br>M35A<br>M35A-M<br>M20 | M6B<br>M6-N<br>M6A-N<br>M6AW | M7<br>M7A<br>M7B | M8 | 270RA[2] | 460RA[3] |
|---|---|---|---|---|---|---|---|
| **Kodak Film/Processing Cycle** | | | | | | | |
| Min-R E film, extended cycle processing | Proc. Time[4]<br>Dev. Time[5]<br>°F<br>°C | 207 sec<br>47 sec<br>95°F<br>35°C | 172 sec<br>47 sec<br>95°F<br>35°C | 192 sec<br>43 sec<br>96°F<br>35.6°C | N/A | 201 sec<br>53.2 sec<br>94°F<br>34.4°C | 170 sec<br>46.2 sec<br>95°C<br>35°C |
| Min-R H, Min-R M, or Min-R T films, standard processing | Proc. Time[4]<br>Dev. Time[5]<br>°F<br>°C | 140 sec<br>32 sec<br>92°F<br>33.5°C | 90 sec<br>24 sec<br>95°F<br>35°C | 122 sec<br>27 sec<br>94°F<br>34.4°C | 90 sec<br>21.5 sec<br>96°F<br>35.6°C | 100 sec<br>26.6 sec<br>94°F<br>34.4°C | 88 sec<br>23.8 sec<br>95°F<br>35°C |

[1] Kodak RP X-Omat chemicals recommended.

[2] The listed processing times are associated with a front film exit. Top film exit processing times are 214 seconds for extended-cycle processing and 107 seconds for standard-cycle processing.

[3] Some variation may occur in the listed times due to adjustable turnarounds.

[4] Processing time is based on 24 cm of film travel, leading edge entering the processor to trailing edge exiting the processor.

[5] Developer time is based on the leading edge of the film into the developer to the leading edge of the film into the fixer.

[6] Some M7 and M7A processors may have a longer standard processing time (140 seconds instead of 122 seconds). The temperature recommendation for all Kodak mammography films, standard processing, in this case is 92°F (33.5°C).

Recently there has been considerable interest in extended-cycle processing for some single-emulsion mammographic films. In extended-cycle processing, the processing cycle is longer than the standard cycle (Table 1) and, therefore, the film remains in the developer longer. Developer temperature is not altered significantly. For some single-emulsion films, the film contrast is higher and film speed is increased – resulting in an approximately 35% reduction in radiation dose (Figure 1). For double-emulsion films, the extended cycle process does not significantly affect film contrast and film speed and is, therefore, not recommended (Figure 2).

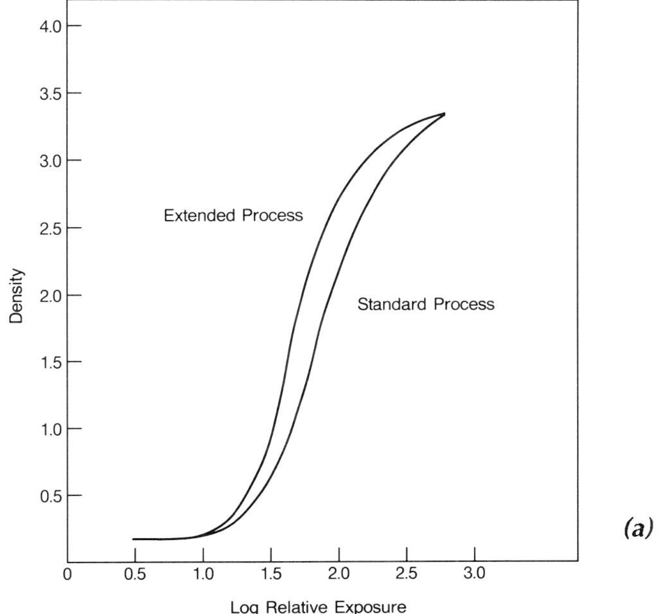


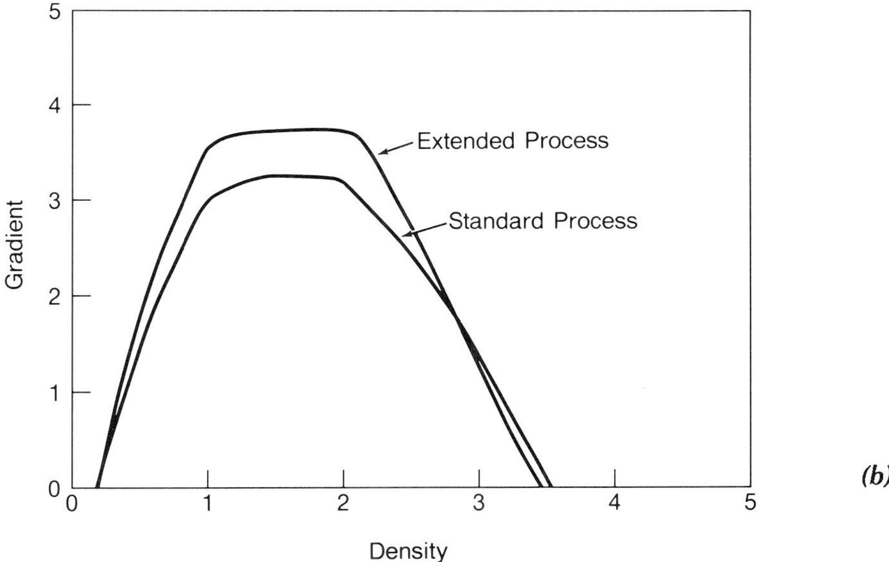


**Figure 1.** Graphs demonstrating relative film speed and film contrast differences for Kodak Min-R E film, in the standard-and extended-cycle processes. The characteristic H&D curves (Figure 1a) show that there is approximately a 35% exposure reduction for the extended-cycle process without an increase in film fog. The gradient versus optical density graph (Figure 1b) illustrates that film contrast is higher for optical densities from 0.30 to 2.70 for the extended-cycle process. The gradient is defined as the slope of the characteristic H&D curve at a specific optical density.

## 2) Developer Temperature

Developer temperatures in automatic film processors range from 33°C (91°F) to 39°C (103°F). The developer temperature depends on film type, transport speed and the manufacturer's recommendations. Developer temperature affects film speed (radiation dose), film contrast, and film base plus fog (Figure 2).

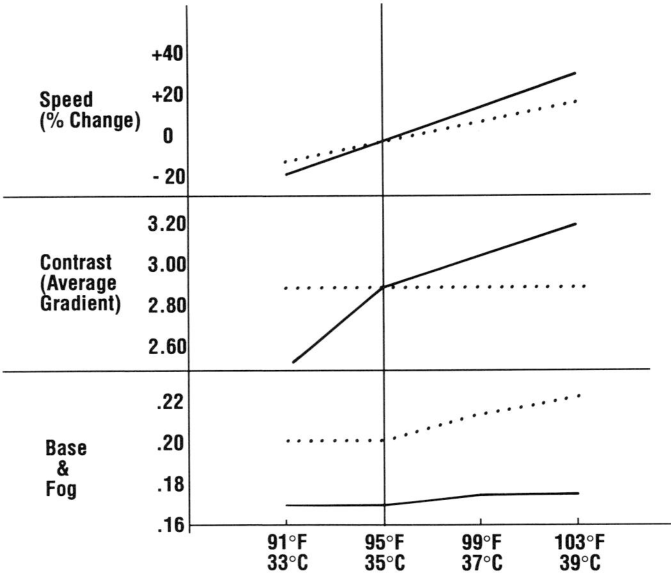


**Figure 2. Graph illustrating percentage of film speed change, film base plus fog plotted versus developer temperature for the single-emulsion Kodak Min-R E (solid line)and double-emulsion, tabular-grain Kodak Min-R T film (dotted line) with a Kodak processor using Kodak chemicals. The vertical line represents the recommendation for a standard processing cycle.**

The National Council on Radiation Protection and Measurement (NCRP) Report 99 on Quality Assurance and American College of Radiology (ACR) Mammography Quality Control Manual for Radiologic Technologists indicate that the developer temperature should be within ±0.5°F (±0.3°C) of that recommended by the manufacturer for the specific film-developer combination being used. The measurement accuracy, precision, and repeatability of the thermometer is most important. The thermometer used to measure developer temperature should have an accuracy at least equal to, or better than the variability recommended in the NCRP and ACR documents. In the radiology or medical imaging department, there are a variety of thermometers used to measure developer temperature. These thermometers vary in accuracy, precision, ease of reading, and cost. A recent study suggests inexpensive but accurate devices for measuring temperature of the developer solution. It is also recommended that the thermometers used to measure developer temperature be evaluated against a thermometer that has a calibration traceable to the National

Institute of Standards and Technology (NIST).

### 3) Replenishment

Replenishment is important for maintenance of stable developer and fixer activity. Proper replenishment 1) provides stable sensitometric results (film contrast, film speed, and base plus fog), 2) reduces/eliminates artifacts, and 3) provides long term (archival) keeping. Replenishment rates are sometimes divided into groups based on daily film volumes (Table 2). Low film use/day requires higher replenishment per sheet. Processors with very low film volume (such as surgery rooms) are very difficult to stabilize and to maintain consistency. Flooded replenishment is recommended under these conditions. A starter solution is added to the developer replenisher holding tank; the processor is replenished at specific time intervals independent of film volume in addition to replenishment per sheet of film processed. Flooded replenishment provides a stable fresh process. High film use/day requires lower replenishment per sheet.

**Table 2. Replenishment rates based on film volume for mammography films (standard or extended cycle) for Kodak M35, M6 and M7 X-Omat processors**

| Processed Film | Volume (use) | Sheet Film volume/8 hours | Developer replen. rate (mL/sheet) | Fixer replen. rate (mL/sheet) |
| --- | --- | --- | --- | --- |
| Intermixed film sizes | High | >150 | 20 | 30 |
| (18x24 cm and 24x30 cm) | Medium | 61-150 | 27 | 35 |
| | Low* | 30-60 | 35 | 40 |

* Flooded replenishment should be used when fewer than 30 sheets of film are processed.

For extended-cycle processing (mammography), film processor require even closer monitoring of replenishment. Film throughput (sheet films/day) is the basis for determining replenishment volumes; however, since the typical film sizes are 18x24 cm and 24x30 cm, the actual area of the film is less. Also note that if two 18x24 cm sheets of film are fed simultaneously, the replenishment rate per 18x24 cm of film should be doubled.

It is most important to consult with the manufacturer to correctly adjust and set up the film processor and replenishment rates in order to obtain results and consistency of those results. Film contrast, speed, and base plus fog values from processed sensitometric strips can be used to determine that replenishment rates are correct for a given film volume based on previously established values.

### 4) Agitation

Agitation maintains processing uniformity and temperature control. Agitation is provided by roller contact as well as chemical recirculation pumps. Film surface agitation is caused by roller contact. Tank solution agitation is caused by recirculation pumps.

### 5) Drying

The adjustable range of drying temperatures is from $38^{O}C$ ($100^{O}F$) to $71^{O}C$ ($160^{O}F$). Drying conditions depend on the environment. These may range from cool/dry to hot/humid. Many users tend to over-dry films. This may cause surface pattern artifacts on the film (water spotting, etc.) that may affect the radiologist's ability to read films. The dryer temperature should, therefore, be adjusted to as low as possible while still providing dry film as it exits the processor. This will also result in energy savings for the processor operation.

### Film Contrast

Film contrast characteristics determine how the x-ray intensity pattern will be related to optical density patterns in the image. Film contrast is affected by film type, processing conditions (solutions, temperature, time, agitation) fog level (storage, safelight, light leaks), and optical density level. Film contrast is defined in terms of the slope or steepness of the characteristic curve (Figure 3). The steeper the curve, the higher the contrast. High film contrast is obtained by using a high-contrast film and processing it optimally as recommended by the manufacturer.

Low film contrast can be the result of using a film designed to provide low contrast and processing the film as recommended (wide latitude, as used in chest radiography) or using a film with inherently high contrast capability and processing the film less than optimally (which should never happen).

The average gradient describes the average film contrast and is defined as the slope of a straight line between two points of specified densities. These densities are approximately the minimum and maximum useful densities in the clinical setting.

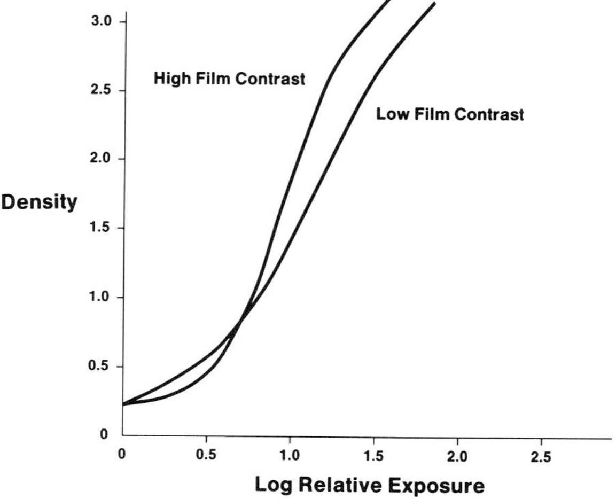


**Figure 3. Characteristic curves illustrating films with high and low contrast.**

**Film Speed**

The speed or sensitivity of a radiographic material is inversely related to produce a given effect. Speeds of radiographic films are often determined from the exposures required to produce a density of 1.0 above the base plus fog. Medical imaging films have different sensitivities or relative speeds. Factors which influence film speed (or the exposure required to produce a given density on the film) include: 1) film type, 2) type of screen, 3) film processing conditions, 4) ambient conditions, and 5) latent image fading.

### 1) Film Type

The composition of the film and the way it is manufactured affect film speed. The ingredients used in making the emulsion, the manner in which they are treated and combined, and the technique by which they are coated on the support all play a part in determining the sensitivity of the film.

### 2) Screen Type

Film emulsions are optically sensitized to cover a wide spectral range. Intensifying screens used in medical radiography have light emissions ranging from ultraviolet to green (approximately 300 to 650 nanometer). The manner in which the film responds to radiation of different energies or wavelengths is called its spectral sensitivity. It is most important that the spectral sensitivity of the film match the spectral emission of the screen in order to obtain appropriate film speed. The color of light transmitted by safelight filters is selected to provide only wavelengths for which the film has little sensitivity.

### 3) Processing Conditions

Among the most important factors affecting film speed are the conditions used in processing the film after exposure. The chemical formulation of the solution used, the way in which they are mixed and replenished, their temperatures, the manner in which they are agitated, the film's time of immersion, and washing and drying conditions all contribute to the film's speed and appearance.

### 4) Ambient Conditions

The film's sensitivity may also be affected by such factors as temperature, humidity, age, chemical fumes, and storage conditions. High temperatures, high humidity, and atmospheres containing chemical contaminants should be avoided insofar as possible. Protection from light leaks, excessive safelight exposure, and x- and gamma radiation must also be provided.

### 5) Latent Image Fading

If an exposure has been made on a film and processing is postponed for a relatively long time, the optical density obtained may be smaller than if processing had followed the exposure immediately. This effect is called latent image fading. It is caused by an instability of the latent image.

The size and stability of the latent image center is critical in achieving optimum sensitometric results. If the time between exposure and development is long, the potential exists for environment influences such as oxygen, moisture or other chemical agents to influence the latent image center. Oxidation can occur which causes the size of the latent image center to regress to a smaller size. The greater the period of time which elapses between exposure and development, the greater the potential for this regression process to occur.

Table 3 shows an example of percent film speed loss and film contrast changes for the time between exposure and film processing of 0, 4, 8, 24, and 48 hours. In screen-film imaging, film speed loss due to latent image fading can occur if the time between exposure and processing is delayed due to 1) transporting film from a van or satellite facility to a central location for film processing, or 2) if films are accumulated and batch processed at the end of the day. In order to minimize latent image fading in the clinical environment, it is important to be as consistent as possible day-to-day in the time interval between exposure and processing. Ideally, films should be consistently processed as soon as possible after exposure. To minimize time interval differences, process films in the order in which they are exposed. If films with slightly greater speed losses (due to latent image fading) are used and the time between exposure and processing is relatively long, the exposure technique can be adjusted on a one-time basis to obtain and maintain the appropriate density. For the film shown in the example in Table 3, if processing is delayed for more than 8 hours, it may be advisable to increase exposure time (AEC setting) in order to obtain proper optical density in the mammogram. Also note from Table 3, that there is very little change in film contrast due to latent image fading. For film processor quality control, it is recommended that film strips be processed immediately after exposure by the sensitometer to minimize the effects of latent image fading.

**Table 3. Example of latent image keeping data for a medical x-ray film***

| | 0 | 4 | 8 | 24 | 48 |
|---|---|---|---|---|---|
| Time delay between exposure and film processing (hours) | 0 | 4 | 8 | 24 | 48 |
| Percent film speed loss | 0 | 10 | 12 | 18 | 23 |
| Percent contrast change | 0 | 2 | 3 | 3 | 5 |

*Speed: determined at a density of 1.00 above base plus fog
  Average gradient: determined from the slope of the characteristic curve between densities of 0.25 and 2.00 above base plus fog

## 6)  Recommended Processing Chemicals

All film manufacturers have recommended chemicals (or equivalent) for their films. Many users consider chemicals from various manufacturers to be interchangeable. However, surveys have documented that film speed, film contrast and base plus fog respond differently to the various types of chemicals used (Figure 4). These effects also depend on the type of film being processed.

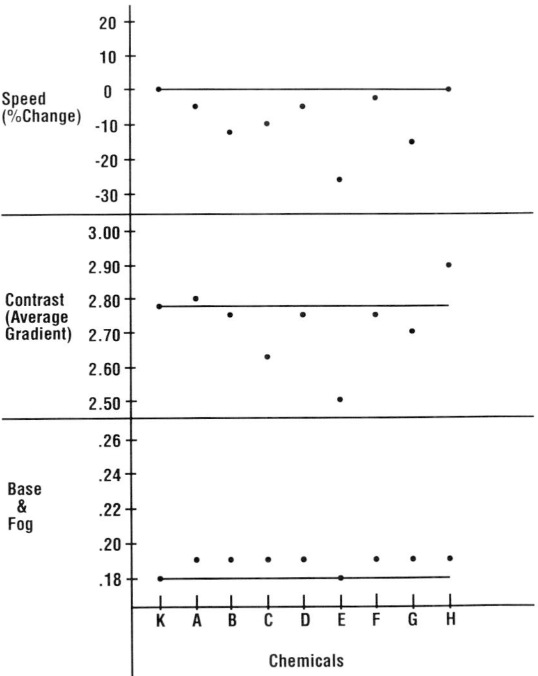


**Figure 4. Charts produced from film processing survey data which show film processing variations due to use of different chemicals; data shown are for a single emulsion film used for mammography. The letter K indicates processing data (and expected values) using Kodak processor and Kodak chemicals.  A horizontal line is drawn through the letter K. Letters A through H are data for different brands of chemicals.  Data were obtained  using film strips which were sensitometrically pre-exposed to light that simulates the light spectrum from Kodak Min R screens. Film speed differences, film contrast (average gradient) and base plus fog values were determined from the sensitometry data.**

## 7) Mixing Chemicals

In some cases, chemicals may not be mixed to the appropriate concentration in accordance with the manufacturer's recommendations. This variable is inherent since all chemical manufacturers distribute chemicals in concentrates. Solution service providers add water locally to complete the mixture.

Processing chemical variability can occur in the medical imaging market place due to a number of factors. Although most manufacturers use similar processing chemicals to achieve development and fixing, the concentration of these chemicals can vary, either initially or after being mixed by solution service dealers. This concentration variation can result in changes in film response of differing magnitude for certain film types. In addition, variability can also result from improper replenishment. Either overdevelopment or underdevelopment can occur, depending on the degree of replenishment or initial chemical concentration.

## 8) Chemical Storage

Concentrates of developer and fixer solutions are relatively stable when stored properly; however, they will deteriorate with time. Properly mixed developer and fixer solutions (concentrates plus water) will generally remain usable for approximately 4 to 6 weeks when stored properly at room temperature. It is most important that the developer/replenisher tank have a floating lid to minimize oxidation. In general, it is recommended that chemicals be used within two weeks from date they are mixed with water.

## Dedicated Processing for Mammography?

The American College of Radiology Mammography Quality Control Manual states:

"Due to the large number of combinations of film, chemistry, etc., it is extremely important to use the film, developer chemistry, the processor, the developer temperature, and immersion time <u>recommended by the film manufacturer.</u>"

The direction provided by the American College of Radiology (ACR) is obvious. More importantly, the ability of a mammography facility to meet the ACR guidelines for accreditation and maintain that accreditation will depend on the facility's adherence to the film manufacturer's recommendations.

The dedication for mammography can imply two separate approaches: 1) the most common of which is to process film in an extended processing cycle whereby film is immersed in the developer solution for 45 seconds in a film processor that is only used for mammography, and 2) dedication can be described again as a single film processor whose primary purpose is to process mammography film per ACR recommendations, typically in a 90-second total process time cycle (22-23 seconds developer immersion time).

The key considerations involved for proper decision-making on dedication for mammography include:

1) Number of exams per day – if exams/day are less than 15, the associated film volume will be less than 60 sheets of 18x24 cm film and would be considered low volume.

2) Film manufacturers generally require and recommend increased chemical

replenishment in low-film-volume-per-day processors to avoid chemical oxidation and evaporation due to the long periods of inactivity.

3) A film processor purchase price can range from approximately $5,000 to over $20,000 depending on need/preference.

4) The film processor service/maintenance costs can annually be 5-15% of purchase price.

5) Will the dedicated mammography processor be used for other film processing needs?

For example:

• Will it be used as a backup processor to another department in case of service/maintenance?

• Will it be used by other departments during their busy times?

• Will film from various film manufacturers be processed through the processor?

If your answer to any of these questions is yes, you WILL NOT have a truly dedicated processor and your mammography quality control will be severely challenged to maintain optimal results for speed, contrast and base plus fog. Additionally, your productivity and patient throughput/waiting time will be negatively affected.

Assuming cost/price justifications are resolved and you choose to dedicate your processor do it completely and maintain your process to assure consistent images.

Mammography film processing in mobile vans has recently generated many new issues. There are distinct advantages and disadvantages that need consideration:

### Advantages
• Convenience factor when films can be checked before patient leaves
• Phantom image verification on site
• No delay from exposure to processing (minimal film speed loss due to latent image keeping)

### Disadvantages
• Difficulty associated with maintaining quality processing
• Additional time to prepare/set up
• Waste management for effluents
• High potential for chemical oxidation/evaporation
• Time for processor and phantom QC
• Patient throughput influenced by associated film processing time
• High dependence on qualification, training and motivation of technologists in the van

## Recommendations

1. Purchase processing systems from a reputable manufacturer that offers a) full system product line, b) service support, c) technical support and d) educational support.

2. Follow the manufacturer's recommendations for film processing and chemicals based on how the films are used in the department.

3. Confirm that proper film contrast, film speed, along with base plus fog values are being obtained for each film in use in accordance with the manufacturer's specifications and tolerances. Request this information from the film manufacturer. Film contrast in terms of the average gradient and base plus fog can be determined directly using a properly calibrated sensitometer and densitometer.

4. Implement a processor quality control which uses a sensitometer, densitometer, and monitoring chart for routine monitoring of the film processor.

## Conclusion

In order to obtain optimum film contrast and maximum film sensitivity in radiographs and medical images, it is essential to consider the film processor, film type, and chemicals as a total system. It is important to follow the manufacturer's recommendations on film processing for each type of radiographic or medical film used. For film processor quality control, it is most important to confirm and maintain film contrast, film speed (sensitivity), and film base plus fog values as recommended and intended by film manufacturer.

## References


1. Haus AG, Cullinan JE. Screen-film processing systems for medical radiography: a historical review. *Radiographics* 1989: 1203-1224.

2. Schmidt RA, Doi K, Seiya M, Xu XW, Geiger ML, Lu CT, Mojtahedi MacMahon H. Evaluation of radiographs developed by a new ultra-rapid film processing system. *AJR* 1990; 154: 1107-1110.

3. Suleiman OH, Showalter CK, Koustenis G. Sensitometric evaluation of film chemical processing systems in the state of New Jersey. HHS publication FDA 82™ 8189, April 1982.

4. Galkin BM, Feig SA, Muir HD. The technical quality of mammography in centers participating in a regional breast cancer awareness program. *Radiographics*

1988;8:133-145.

5. Hendrick RE. Standardization of image quality and radiation dose in mammography. *Radiology* 1989;174: 648-654.

6. Rueter F, Conway BJ, Slayton RJ, Suleiman OH. NEXT 89: The abdomen/lumbo sacral spine projection. Proceedings of the 22nd Annual National Conference on Radiation Control Published by the Conference of Radiation Control Program Directors Inc. Frankfort, Kentucky, 1990.

7. Haus AG, Batz TA, Dickerson RE, Lillie RF, Oemcke KW and Lanphear JD: Automating film processing in medical imaging. In Siebert JA, Barnes GT, and Gould RG: Specification, Acceptance Testing and Quality Control of Diagnostic X-ray Imaging Equipment. American Institute of Physics, New York, NY, 1992.

8. Suleiman OH, Sensitometric techniques for the evaluation of processing, *Radiology* 1990, p.177, 132.

9. Suleiman OH, Shayton RJ, Conway BJ, Rueter FG. Effects of temperature, chemistry, and immersion time on x-ray film. *Radiology* 1990, 177P, 132.

10. Conway BJ, McCrohan JL, Rueter FG, Slayton RJ, Suleiman OH. Processing trends: Observation from 8 years national automatic film processing data (1982-1989) *Radiology* 1990, 177P, 173.

11. Kimme-Smith K, Rothchild PA, Bassett LW, Gold RH, Moler C. Mammographic film processor developer temperature, development time, and chemistry: effect on dose, contrast and noise. *AJR* 1989; 152: 35-40.

12. Tabar L, Haus AG. Processing mammographic films: technical and clinical considerations. *Radiology* 1989; 173: 65-69.

13. NCRP Report 99. Quality Assurance for Diagnostic Imaging Equipment. National Council on Radiation Protection and Measurements. Bethesda, MD 1988.

14. Hendrick RE, Dodd GD, Gray JE, Harvey M, Haus AG, Holland R, McCrohan J, McLelland R, Rossi R, Sulleiman DC, Sinninger M, and Wilcox P. American College of Radiology Program on Mammography Quality Control for Radiologists, Medical Physicists and Technologists. Published by the American College of Radiology.

15. Wilson WB, Haus AG, Nierman C, Lillie R, Batz TA. Evaluation of a clinical thermometer for measuring developer temperature in automatic film processor. Medical Physics (submitted).

16. Haus AG. Recent advances in screen-film mammography. Radiologic Clinics of North America 1987;25: 913-928.

17. Methods for the sensitometry of medical and dental x-ray films. ANSI PH2.9 - 1974. American National Standards Institute, Washington, DC.

18. Gray JE, Haus AG. Protocol for basic photographic processor quality control in Waggener RG and Wilson CR ed: Quality assurance in diagnostic radiology. American Institute of Physics, NY 1980; 39-48.

19. Gray JE, Winkler NT, Stears J, Frank ED. Quality control in diagnostic imaging. Aspen publishing, Rockville, MD 1982; 33-49 (1982).

20. Haus AG, Dickerson RE. Problems associated with simulated light sensitometry for low crossover medical x-ray films. *Medical Physics*, 1990 17(4):691-695.

21. Haus AG, Kimme-Smith C, Baker CW, Jones CD. A sensitometric method of on-site evaluation of film processing compared to manufacturers' expectations. *Medical Physics* (abstract), 1991 18(4):851.

# Performance Evaluation of Film Processors in the Clinical Environment

**Raymond P. Rossi**
Division of Radiological Sciences
Department of Radiology
University of Colorado Health Sciences Center
Denver, Colorado

## Introduction

Among the many items of equipment required for the production of radiographic images of high quality, the film processor is of critical importance. In order to obtain the optimum performance of film processors in the clinical environment, careful consideration must be given to a number of factors. These include: 1) selection of the appropriate film processor for the intended task; 2) identification and provision of necessary space and utilities; 3) initial installation of the processor; 4) optimization of processor performance for a given type or types of film; and 5) ongoing monitoring and maintenance of processor performance. In this presentation each of the above factors will be discussed from the perspective of the clinical radiology department and will be illustrated with actual examples. Particular emphasis will be placed on methods of ensuring the ongoing performance of the close film processor in the clinical environment.

Diagnostic radiology is beyond a doubt one of the most dynamic and exciting fields of clinical medicine. Continued efforts toward obtaining greater diagnostic information of clinical usefulness to the physician have lead to the development of technologically sophisticated imaging modalities such as digital radiography, computed tomography and magnetic resonance imaging.

Yet, with all the technological sophistication and in spite of continued efforts toward the implementation of picture archiving and communication systems and the filmless radiology department, the primary means of providing an interpretable image to the radiologist for all imaging modalities remains the recording of the radiological image on film.

The process by which the latent image recorded on film is rendered visible is, of course, photographic processing. During processing, the affected silver grains in the film emulsion are acted upon chemically to yield deposits of metallic silver which reflect the spatial intensity distribution of the x-rays exiting the patient or other signals which, in turn, reflect anatomical features of the patient.

In the modern radiology department, photographic processing is accomplished by automatic film processors; the performance of these devices is central to the production of consistent high-quality images. Regardless of how good the imaging equipment employed for the examination, or the degree of technical expertise of the staff, poor processing can only result in poor image quality. The quality and consistency of film processing is critical to the entire imaging process, cannot be overemphasized, and is not the place for false economy. Despite this fact, film processing is often overlooked and frequently ignored and may represent the weakest link in the imaging chain.

Any discussion of film processors must focus not solely on the processor as an isolated element; rather, it should view the film processor as part of a film processing system. This system consists of: 1) the imaging film; 2) the film processor; 3) the processing chemistry; and 4) the support utilities and facilities needed to obtain optimal performance of this system.

The ultimate goal of any film processing system is to consistently produce high-quality, artifact-free radiographic images. The film processing system must be properly selected, installed and optimized to obtain the design performance of the specific photographic product and should ideally function with minimum attention and intervention on the part of the user.

In order to achieve appropriate film processing in the clinical environment it is essential that: 1) the film processor selected be appropriate for the intended task; 2) the necessary space, utility and support system be identified and provided; 3) the processor be installed, evaluated and optimized for the film type(s) to be used clinically; and 4) an ongoing program to maintain and monitor the performance of the processor be established.

## Processor Selection

The selection of a film processor depends upon the specific application in which it will be used. In a busy department in which a single processor must serve multiple examination rooms, the volume of processed films will be large and the processor must have an appropriate film capacity. If both sheet and roll films are to be processed, it is essential to verify that the film transport system can provide reliable, jam-free transport for each type of film. Processor selection may also be influenced by the choice of a "daylight" processing environment versus a conventional darkroom processing environment because interface requirements may dictate that a specific processor or processors be used with the daylight film-handling equipment.

During the process of selecting a film processor, it is important to carefully review the manufacturer's specifications for space and utilities. Additionally, careful consideration should be given to the construction of the processor, its anticipated reliability and consistency of performance, and its serviceability. Overall processor serviceability can be enhanced by using a single model of processor throughout an entire imaging department.

## Space, Utility and Support System Requirements

Design of the film processing area necessitates that sufficient space be provided to accommodate the storage of upexposed film, work space, the film processor, the chemical replenishment system, the silver recovery system and the servicing and maintenance of the processor. The primary support utilities for a film processor include the electrical supply, the water supply, the chemical replenishment system, the silver recovery system, the waste water drain system and the ventilation system. Each of these items must be considered whether daylight or conventional darkroom processing will be used.

The electrical power supply for the processor must be of the proper voltage and current capacity and must provide the correct number of wires as specified by the processor manufacturer. The water supply must be within the appropriate temperature range and of adequate pressure and volume and should be filtered and pressure regulated prior to entry into the processor. Although the majority of film processors available today operate from a water supply at ambient temperature, appropriate temperature control for incoming water must be provided and will depend on local ambient water supply conditions. In northern climates, it is not uncommon for the temperature of incoming cold water in the winter to fall below the processor manufacturer's specifications (typically 4 to $6^O$ C); a mixing value must be installed to supply the processor with both cold and hot water lines. In southern climates, "cold" tap water can exceed the manufacturer's maximum allowed temperature (typically 30 to $32^O$ C); the installation of a water chiller will be required.

All processors require a chemical replenishment system to provide fresh developer and fixer chemistry to the working solutions in the processor tanks to compensate for the depletion of chemical activity as films are processed. This chemical replenishment system must be properly sized for the anticipated volume of processed films. When bulk holding tanks are used for chemical replenishment, their size should be chosen to provide an adequate amount of solution but should be as small as practical in order to minimize oxidization of the solution. Chemical automixers may also be used but they require continued attention and maintenance.

Recovery of silver from the spent fixer solution is essential. All discharge of fixer solution from the film processor must be passed through some form of silver recovery system prior to discharge to the drain. Common forms of silver recovery include: bulk collection of discharged fixer for subsequent central processing; chemical replacement canisters; and recirculating and non-recirculating electrolytic systems. Any of these systems can provide efficient silver recovery and provide environmentally acceptable discharge effluents, provided they are correctly sized to the specific processor installation.

The capacity of the floor drain for the processor must be sufficient to accommodate both the normal outflow of wash water and the outflow of water from the developer and fixer tanks during cleaning. The drain must also be resistant to chemical attack by the developer and fixer solutions.

Ventilation for the processor is important. Direct ventilation of the processors dryer exhaust is necessary to prevent chemical fumes from building up in the processor and causing contamination. When installed in a darkroom environment, the interior of the darkroom should be at positive pressure with respect to the processor so that chemical fumes are not pulled back from the dryer section through the processor. The darkroom itself should be properfly ventilated providing for at least six air changes per hour. In order to minimize the occurance of dirt and dust artifacts, particularity on mammographic film, all potential dust collecting surfaces, especially above the work counters in the darkroom, should be eliminated. Electrostatic air cleaners, painted drywall ceilings, and the location of vents for heating and air conditioning are all special considerations to minimize the collection of dirt inside cassettes.

## Initial Processor Installation and Evaluation

Prior to the actual installation of the processor it is important to verify that all the necessary utilities and support systems are installed in accordance with the processor manufacturer's specifications. The actual installation of the processor is usually performed by the vendor from whom the processor was purchased; however, final electric and plumbing connections may have to be performed by licensed trades people, depending on local building codes.

Initial evaluation of the processor and support facilities should be carried out by a representative of the facility and should begin with an evaluation of the darkroom. Verify the light tightness of the darkroom by turning all darkroom lighting off; check for white light leaks after allowing eyes to adapt to the dark for at least five minutes. Any white light leaks noted should be corrected before proceeding. Next, the adequacy of the darkroom safelighting should be verified by inspecting the safelight for proper bulb wattage and filter type and by performing a standard safelight fog test. Improper safelights, indicator lights on the processor and other equipment, and white light sources leaking into the darkroom can all combine to fog exposed film prior to processing and reduce the contrast in the image.

Assessment of darkroom fog can be made using a number of different methods. Regardless of the method used, exposed film must be used when performing a fog test. Evaluation of darkoom fog should be performed prior to completing any other tests involving processed film to avoid errors caused by film fogging. It is important to note that safelight filters fade with age and need to be replaced periodically. Some fluorescent lights exhibit an ultraviolet glow (invisible to the eye) after being turned off and can be a significant source of film fog; they are not recommended for use in darkrooms.

The final configuration of the work and storage space should be evaluated and an inspection performed to ensure that sufficient access has been provided for processor maintenance.

## Initial Processor Checks

Evaluation of the actual processor installation should begin by conducting an inspection to verify that: the processor is level, plumb, and stable; adequate access has been provided for required maintenance procedures; all specified and required utilities such as electrical power, water supply including flow restrictors, temperature control and filters and strainers are present and correct; air flow and ventilation is adequate; drain capacity and acid resistance are adequate; and silver recovery and water treatment systems are adequate.

Next, the internal tanks (developer, fixer and wash) should be filled with water to verify that there are no leaks in the internal processor lines. It is best to allow the processor to sit for several hours or preferably overnight so that small, slow leaks can be detected. The processor should next be turned on and, with the tanks still filled with water, the function of the recirculation system should be checked without the transport racks installed. Ripples on the surfaces in each tank verify the movement of fluid within the tank and the function of the recirculation pump. The developer, fixer and wash racks, but not the crossover racks, are then installed and, with the processor running, the function of the transport system is verified. Next, the crossover racks are installed and the function of the transport system is again verified. Finally, test film should be run through the processor to verify the adequacy of film transport.

Processor cycle time and developer immersion time should be measured using a stop watch. The processor cycle time is typically defined as the time the leading edge of the film enters the processor to when the trailing edge of the film exits the dryer section of the processor. The developer immersion time is typically defined as the time from when the leading edge of the film just enters the developer rack to when the leading edge of the film just exits the developer rack. It should be noted, however, that some manufactures refer to the development time and define this as the time from when the leading edge of the film just enters the developer rack to when the leading edge of the film just enters the fixer rack. These measured times should be compared to the specifications of the manufacturer.

Replenishment rates for developer and fixer should now be established, based on the recommendation of the film manufacturer for the anticipated volume of processed film. Use a graduated cylinder several times to ensure consistency of the delivered volume. For high-volume installations, replenishment rates are usually determined based on a specific volume of solution for a specified length of film travel. In low-volume installations, a flood replenishment system is frequently used where the replenishment system delivers a specific volume of solution on a periodic basis regardless of the volume of film processed.

The temperatures of the developer within the developer tank, fixer within the fixer tank, incoming water supply and dryer should be measured and adjusted to the values recommended by the film manufacturer for the specific processor and chemistry combination being used.

Temperatures must be measured and adjusted using a thermometer which is accurate to within $0.2^{\circ}$ F. Ideally, prior to measuring developer temperatures, compare the thermometer with another thermometer which has a calibration traceable to National Institute for Standards and Technology (typically available in clinical laboratories in hospitals). In practice, the typical digital readout clinical thermometer will fulfill this requirement nicely. After carefully measuring the developer temperature, adjust the reading of the external temperature display of the processor (if possible) to indicate the same temperature. The processor's temperature display can then be used for quality control purposes. If the processor does not have external temperature display, install temperature measuring probes in the processor for use in routine monitoring. The fixer temperature should also be measured and, in general, should be within $5^{\circ}$ F of the developer temperature.

Drain the water from the processor; fill the chemical tanks with the processing chemistry. Add developer starter in accordance with the instructions of the developer manufacturer. Initial seasoning of the chemistry is necessary to establish chemical equilibrium and should be carried out by processing approximately 50 sheets of 35 cm x 43 cm film which has been exposed to produce a gross optical density of approximately 1.5.

The temperature of the dryer should be adjusted so that the heat provided is sufficient to adequately dry a series of 8 sheets of 35 cm x 43 cm film which has been exposed to produce a gross optical density of approximately 1.5.

The processor should now be evaluated for freedom from artifacts. This may be accomplished by exposing and processing uniform, flat-field images such that the resulting optical density is in the range of 1.2 to 1.5. Each image should be carefully inspected for the presence of artifacts such as scratches, roller marks, streaks, spots, run back and pick off. In the event artifacts are noted, their cause should be identified and eliminated.

## Processor Optimization and Initial Sensitometry

Optimization of the film processing system begins with the appropriate selection of image receptor (e.g. screen and film) systems, processing equipment and processing chemistry. A systems approach in which the screens, films, processors and processor chemistry are all of the same manufacturer is useful. Although not essential, this approach has the advantage that in the event problems do arise there is only a single source to deal with, and this source should have maximum knowledge of the product.

Processing conditions should be optimized for the specific film type or types which are to be processed. Manufacturers' recommendations should be adhered to as the manufacturers have considerable expertise in obtaining optimal performance from their product.

Ongoing processor quality control and performance monitoring programs are designed to address sensitometric consistency of the base plus fog (B&F) level, mid-density (MD) level (speed), and density difference (DD) level of the development process. While it is important to establish that processing on a day to day basis is consistent, these typical quality control programs usually provide no indication of absolute sensitometry. That is, that the performance of the film-processor-chemistry combination is consistent with the design performance level intended by the film's manufacturer. Data collected annually since 1984 as part of the national survey "Nationwide Evaluation of X-Ray Trends" (NEXT) clearly indicates, especially in nonhospitals, that under-processing of films continues to be a significant problem.

Ideally, the installation and setup of a film processor should be such so as to obtain the performance intended by the film manufacture. Regrettably, no method is currently available which provides a convenient method by which the user can verify that the intended performance of the film has been achieved. Nonetheless, while absolute sensitometry in the field is not practical today, the odds that the film is being optimally processed are good if the film chemistry and processor are all the same manufacturer and the processor has been set up in accordance with the recommendations of the film manufacturer.

In order to provide a baseline for subsequent sensitometric monitoring of the processor, it is necessary to perform initial sensitometry of the processor. The equipment necessary for this includes a sensitometer, densitometer and a reserve supply of film of the type which will be used clinically. A number of sheets (e.g., 3 to 5) of film from the reserve supply should be exposed using the sensitometer and then processed. Each step of the resultant sensitometric image for each processed film is then read using the densitometer, is recorded, and the average value is determined.

Operating levels or normal values for the B&F, MD, and DD are then determined by selecting the appropriate steps of the sensitometric image. The B&F level is taken as the optical density of area of the film which has received no exposure. The MD level is taken as the optical density of the step of the sensitometric image which is between 1.00 and 1.30 OD. The DD level is taken as the difference in optical densities between two steps of the sensitometric image having optical densities of between 0.50 and 0.80 OD and between 2.10 and 2.30 OD for the low- and high-density steps, respectively. The results of this initial processor sensitometry provide the reference values for subsequent processor monitoring.

Currently, the ability to perform absolute sensitometry in the clinical environment is hampered by the lack of a calibrated sensitometer (e.g., a sensitometer with a known light intensity and exposure duration) and the lack of information from the film, processor, and chemistry manufacturers which explicitly defines the expected performance level of the product under a standard set of conditions in relationship to the output of a calibrated sensitometer. Efforts at overcoming these difficulties are currently be undertaken by at least one manufacturer and initial results are promising.

## Ongoing Monitoring and Maintenance of Processor Performance

A program of ongoing monitoring and maintenance of the film processor system is essential to ensure that the desired level of performance is maintained. Such a program includes sensitometric monitoring of the processor; periodic checks of the processing chemistry; and periodic preventive and, as needed, corrective maintenance.

Sensitometric monitoring of processor performance is performed using a sensitometer, densitometer and control film of a single emulsion number which has been set aside specifically for this purpose. Ideally the film used for sensitometric monitoring should be the same type as that which is most frequently used in the department. However, it is also essential that the film used be sensitive to changes in processing conditions. Many of the newer tabular-grain films are relatively insensitive to variations in processing conditions and should not be used. Single-emulsion, nontabular-grain films such as those commonly used in mammography are quite sensitive to processing variations and are recommended.

The exposing conditions of the sensitometer should match the type of film to be used. If a single-emulsion film is used, a sensitometer providing single sided exposure should be used. If double-emulsion film is used, a sensitometer providing double sided exposure should be used. The sensitometer should provide a sensitometric image with a sufficient number of steps that the density ranges discussed above for the MD and DD can be obtained. Experience indicates either an 11- or 21-step sensitometer is adequate.

The densitometer should be an internally referenced device capable of measuring diffuse density over the range of 0.0 OD to 4.00 OD with an accuracy of better than ±0.02 OD and a precision of better than ±0.01 OD. Our institution uses an X-Rite 303, an X-Rite 301 and a Kodak process control sensitomer; densitometers include an X-Rite 301 and a Kodak process control densitometer. The film used for processor monitoring is Kodak Min-R-E film which is a single-emulsion, non-tabular grain film; it was selected because it is quite sensitive to variations in processing conditions.

Routine sensitometric monitoring requires that the sensitomer be used to exposed a sheet of the control film which is then processed in the processor being monitored; the B&F, MD and DD are measured using the densitometer. The resultant values are compared to the normal values for these parameters established during initial processor sensitometry. The measured values of the B&F, MD and DD should be equal to the "Normal" value to within specified control limits, typically, $\pm 0.10$ to $\pm 0.15$ of the normal value for MD and DD and less than 0.03 of the normal value for B&F. In the event that a measured value falls outside of the control limit the test should be repeated; if the control limit is still exceeded, corrective action should be taken immediately. Usually if a control limit is exceeded and the processor temperature is corrected the problem lies with the chemistry. In this case, the most efficient approach is to change the processor chemistry.

In a facility with multiple processors, the sensitometric performance of the processors should be matched so that consistent radiographic results are achieved regardless of which processor is used to process the film. This is achieved by designating a specific processor as the "standard" or "master" processor and adjusting (usually through adjustment of developer temperature) all other processors to provide the same sensitometric results. In our facility, all processors are sensitometrically matched and use the same normal values and control limits.

Routine processor monitoring should normally be performed daily. Once sufficient history has been established regarding the sensitometric stability of the processor, the frequency may be decreased to three times per week. In our facility, routine monitoring of all processors is conducted three times a week – on Monday, Wednesday and Friday. Processors used for mammmography are monitored daily. Processor monitoring is carried out between 7:00 a.m. and 9:00 a.m. after it has been verified that all processors have been turned on and have reached operating temperature. Test films are exposed with the sensitometer, processed in the appropriate processor, measured to determine the B&F, MD level and DD level, compared to the normal values and examined to detect trends. Should sensitometric testing indicate that a control limit has been exceeded, the test is repeated. If the repeat test still indicates a control limit has been exceeded, the processor is removed from service until the cause of the poor performance is identified and corrective action has been initiated and completed.

Documentation of sensitometric monitoring results can be accomplished using control charts, log sheets or specialized computer programs; the method of choice depends on the specific facility. In our own facility, log sheets are used to record the daily data. Sensitometric results are summarized monthly by calculating the mean and standard deviation of MD and DD values for all processors. Standard procedures are used when changing control emulsion batches and checking the consistency between boxes within a given control emulsion. Processor chemistry is changed only when indicated by sensitometric monitoring and is rarely changed more frequently then every six months.

Evaluation of processor chemistry in the clinical environment is, in general, difficult to do and a comprehensive assessment can only be achieved by sending a sample to the manufacturer for analysis. Practical chemical checks which may be performed in the clinical environment include replenishment rate measurement, specific gravity measurement and pH measurement.

Once the appropriate replenishment rates have been established, based on manufacturer's recommendations, and stable sensitometric performance has been achieved, the replenishment rate should be periodically measured using a graduated cylinder to ensure consistency of delivered volume. Obtain from the chemistry manufacturer information on the proper specific gravity and pH. Specific gravity and pH of the chemical solutions can be measured using an hydrometer and pH meter, respectively, and may prove useful for detecting gross chemical mixing errors. Representative values of chemical characteristics for developer and fixer solutions are shown in Table 1.

**Table 1. Typical characteristics of processor chemistry**

|  | **Developer Levels** | **Fixer Levels** |
|---|---|---|
| -Specific gravity | 1.070 - 1.100 | 1.100 - 1.110 |
| -pH (fresh) | 10.4 - 10.8 | 4.0 - 4.3 |
| -pH (used) | 10.0 - 10.5 | 4.3 - 4.6 |
| -HQ | 20 - 30 g/l |  |
| -Bromide | 6 - 8 g/l |  |
| -Silver content |  | 0.4 - 0.8 troy oz. per gal. |
| -Clearing time |  | 7 s @ 85 F |

## Preventive and Corrective Maintenance

Preventive and corrective maintenance of the film processor is essential to ensure the reliability of performance. Specific startup and shutdown procedures should be available for each processor. If the processor is turned off overnight and over the weekend, the top of the processor should be opened to prevent the buildup of chemical deposits on the rollers. Following startup of the processor and prior to running clinical films, several sheets of cleanup film should be run to remove potential chemical buildup on the rollers. Crossover racks should be cleaned every day prior to the processing of clinical films. The main processor racks should be cleaned once a week. In a facility with a large number of processors of the same type, spare sets of racks can be purchased so that a rack swapping program can be implemented in order to minimize equipment downtime. During routine cleanings the processor should be inspected for potential  problem areas such as tubing leaks and gear wear; needed corrective action should be scheduled. Periodically the processor should be removed from service and a complete cleaning, mechanical and electrical inspection and adjustment carried out. Water and developer filters should be changed monthly and the entire replenishment system, including the bulk holding tanks, should be cleaned at least once a year. Silver recovery  yield and effluent discharge levels should also be monitored periodically.

## Summary

The production of consistently high-quality radiological images is critically dependent on the quality and consistency of the film processing system; the film processor is a central element of this system. Essential to achieving high-quality film processing are proper selection of the appropriate film processor based on its intended clinical application; identification and provision of space and utility requirements necessary to support the film processor; proper installation, setup and optimization of processor performance; and ongoing monitoring and maintenance of processor performance. Careful attention to each of these areas can greatly assist in achieving high-quality, artifact-free radiographic images on a consistent basis.

## Bibliography and Suggested Reading

1. Gray JE. Light fog on radiographic films: How to measure it properly. *Radiology* 1975; 115: 225-227.

2. Rossi RP, What a physicist wants from a processor with particular reference to small institutions. In: Proceedings of the Second Image Receptor Conference: Radiographic Film Processing, HEW Publication (FDA) 77-8036; 1977: 109 - 116.

3. Wagner LK. Acceptance testing and QC of film transport and processing systems. In: Specification, Acceptance Testing and Quality Control of Diagnostic X-ray Imaging Equipment. The American Association of Physicists in Medicine, New York, NY; 1991: 447 - 476.

4. Shanebrook RL, The design and function of automatic X-ray film processors. In : Acceptance Testing of Radiological Imaging Equipment. American Association of Physicists in Medicine, New York, NY; 1982: 92 - 103.

5. McKinney, WEJ. Initial start-up of automatic processors. In: Acceptance Testing of Radiological Imaging Equipment. American Association of Physicists in Medicine, New York, NY; 1982: 104 - 109.

6. Taylor D, Rossi RP, Hendee WR. A digital thermometer for use in sensitometric control of automatic film processors. *Applied Radiology* 1978: 95-96, and 99-100.

7. Suleiman OH. Sensitometric technique for the evaluation of processing. *Radiology* 1990; 177P: 132.

8. Conway BJ, McCrohann JL, Rueter FG, Slayton RJ, Suleiman OH. Processing trends: Observations from 8 years national automatic film processing data (1982 - 1989). *Radiology* 1990; 177P: 173.

9. Conway BJ, McCrohann JL, Rueter FG, Suleiman OH. Mammography in the eighties. *Radiology* 1990; 177: 335 - 339.

10. Suleiman OH, Slayton RH, Conway BJ, Rueter FG. Effects of temperature, chemistry, and immersion time on X-ray film. *Radiology* 1990; 177P: 132.

11. Tabar L, Haus AG. Processing of mammographic films: technicals and clinical considerations. *Radiology* 1989; 173: 65-69.12.

12. Kofler JM, Gray JE. Sensitometric responses of selected medical radiographic films. *Radiology* 1991; 181: 879 - 883.

13. Haus AG.Automatic film processing in medical imaging: System design considerations. In:Specification, Acceptance Testing and Quality Control of Diagnostic X-ray Imaging Equipment. The American Association of Physicists in Medicine, New York, NY; 1991: 420 - 446.

# Roller Transport Processing Artifact Diagnosis

**John H. Widmer and Ronald F. Lillie**
Health Sciences Division
Eastman Kodak Company
Rochester, New York

## Introduction

No one would want to return film processing to the pre-1956 era, that is, before the availability of roller transport processors. Today, no one could wait close to one hour to present a developed, fully fixed, washed, and dried film to a radiologist for interpretation. Patient care, throughput, and cost are just too important.

However, for all of its ability to deliver a quality film in a minimal amount of time, while removing human variations from processing, roller transport processors do have shortcomings. This is due in part to the basic, but sound, design philosophy of transporting film sinusoidally through each solution.

## Roller Transport System

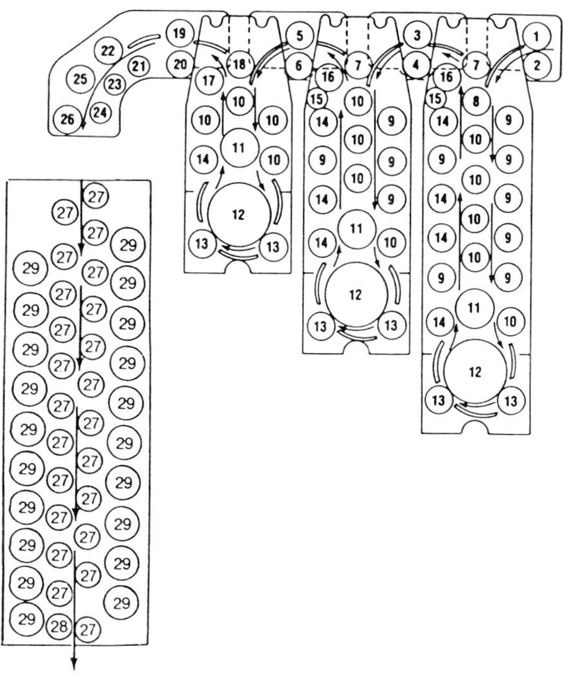

**Figure 1. Sinusoidal Roller Transport Path**

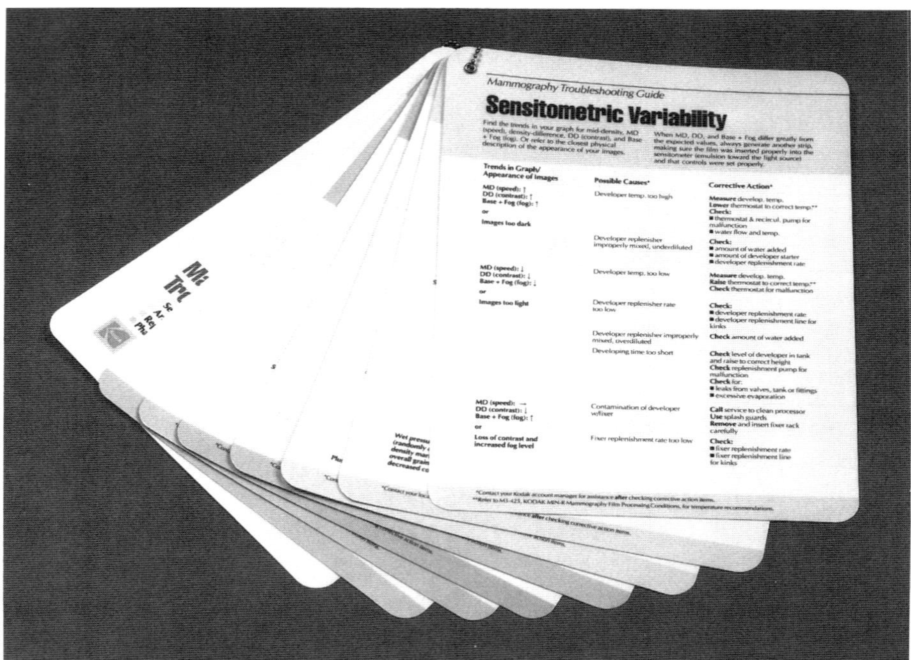


Figure 2. Typical Sensitometric Troubleshooting Publication

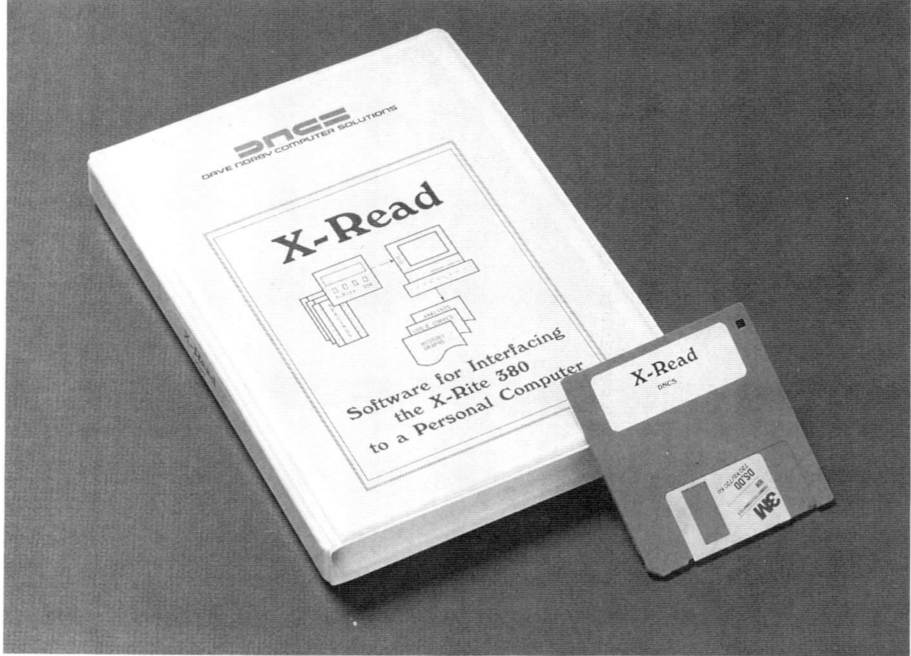


Figure 3. Typical Computer Software Troubleshooting Package

Additionally, there are numerous system variables that impact performance, such as: relatively complicated mechanisms for machine control, variations in film emulsion technologies, numerous varieties of photochemical formulations, extremes in operating environments, and the lack of proper care or maintenance.

Within the clinical environment, film processors are often thought of as "low tech", dirty, smelly, messy devices that should operate forever, unattended, and with no regular maintenance.

The curriculum for a radiologic technologist's training often ignores film processor care. Service personnel are often inadequately trained to service modern processors.

The purpose of this paper is to present information on how to recognize and reduce or eliminate unwanted artifacts on film processed in roller transport processors.

This paper will not discuss the more basic problem associated with processing sensitometric variability, since such publications are readily available from film manufacturing companies and others in the form of booklets, charts, and computer software packages (Figures 2 and 3).

## Discussion

What follows is a discussion with examples of 12 conditions describing degraded roller transport processing performance. The problems described have been observed in conjunction with processors made by a number of manufacturers. Note that, in most cases, the problem is best resolved by proper care, maintenance and the use of the appropriate high-quality photochemicals recommended by the film manufacturer.

(The authors have photographically enhanced some examples to improve their visualization.)

## 1. Drying Patterns and Water Spots  (Figure 4)

These are non-uniform areas on the processed and dried film that can readily be seen by reflected light. Severe drying patterns can be seen with transmitted light when the film is on the viewbox.

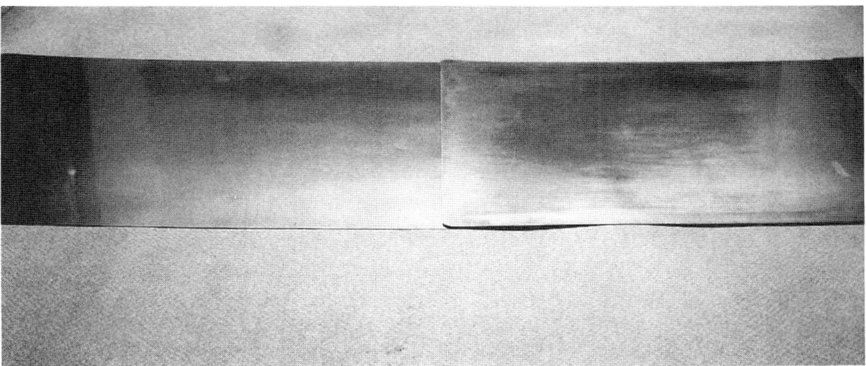

**Figure 4. Drying Patterns & Water Spots**

**Possible Causes Include:**
- Depleted photochemicals
- Poor squeegeeing at the exit of the wash rack
- Dirty rollers
- Missing dryer air tubes
- Plugged slots or orifices in the dryer air tubes
- Non-uniform airflow in the dryer
- Overdrying due to excessively high dryer temperature

**Possible Solutions Include:**
- Follow the manufacturer's instructions for preventive maintenance.
- Use high-quality photochemicals. All are not created equal!
- Use the film manufacturer's recommended replenishment rates.
- Reduce dryer temperature to the minimum required to dry the film.

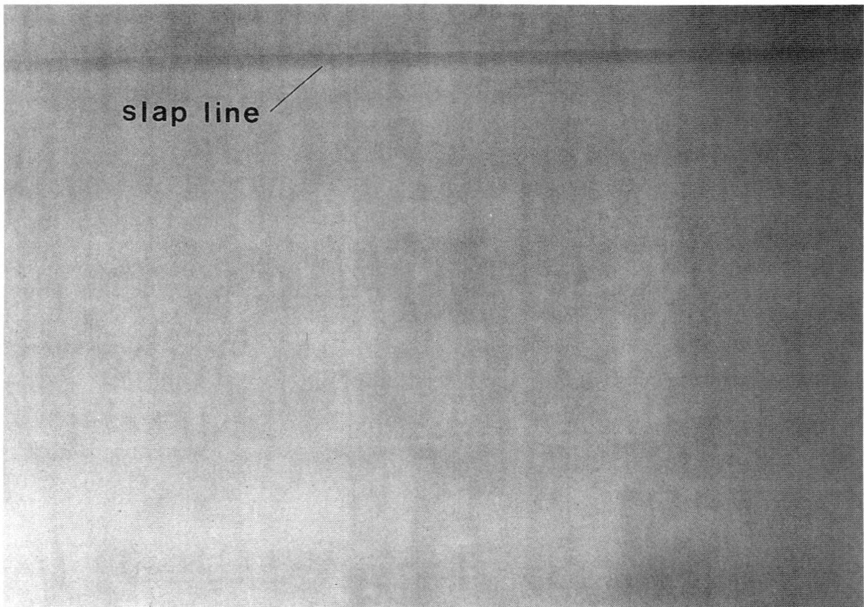


Figure 5. Slap Line

## 2. Slap Line  (Figure 5)

This is a plus-density, broad line, which is perpendicular to film travel direction; it is typically located 2 1/8 to 2 1/4 inches in from the trailing film edge.

### Cause:

- This artifact occurs at the top center roller of the fix rack when the trailing edge of the film abruptly releases from the developer-to-fixer crossover.

**Possible Solutions Include:**
- Check that the correct fixer is being used at the recommended replenishment rates.
- Confirm that the developer solution exit squeegees are operating uniformly.
- Use rollers recommended by the processor manufacturer.
  For Kodak X-Omat processors, note the use of a knurled roller in the fix rack.
- Verify that the film transport velocity is constant from developer to fixer solutions.

## 3. Shadow Images (Figure 6)

These are usually small, minus-density spots on the film. They are most visible on single-emulsion films.

**Possible Causes Include:**
- Dirt or dust on intensifying screens
- Dust or dirt in the air
- Dust or dirt on horizontal surfaces; such as counter tops

**Possible Solutions Include:**
- Clean intensifying screens.
- Clean darkroom area.
- Filter the darkroom air.

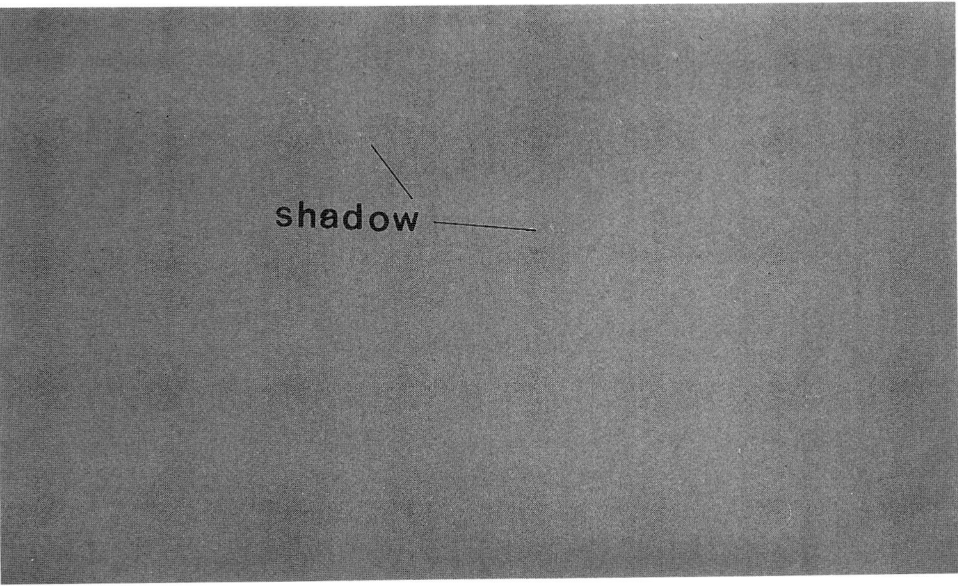


**Figure 6. Shadow Image**

## 4. Pick-off  (Figure 7)

These are small minus-density spots where the emulsion has been removed from the film base. This artifact is most readily detectable on single-emulsion films.

### Possible Causes Include:
- Rough rollers
- Non-uniform or inconsistent transport speed
- Photochemicals are not good

### Possible Solutions Include:
- Follow processor maintenance program
- Replace photochemicals and set replenishment rates to those recommended by the film manufacturer.

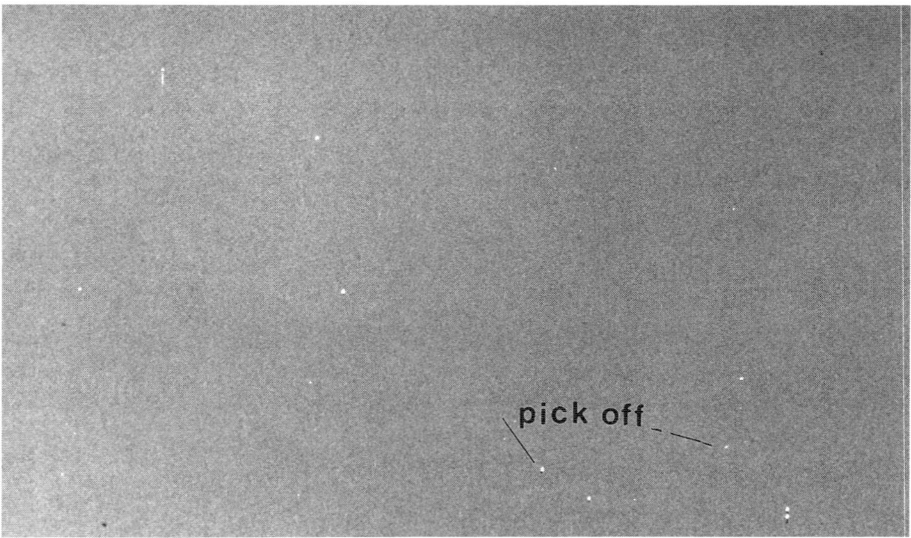


Figure 7. Pick-off

## 5. Skivings  (Figure 8)

This artifact occurs when emulsion is removed from the leading edge of a film sheet and is deposited – typically 3.14 inches (Pi) from that edge.

### Possible Causes Include:
- Inconsistent film transport velocity
- Inadequate developer or hardener-depleted developer solution

### Possible Solutions Include:
- Perform processor maintenance.
- Replace photochemicals and check replenishment rates.

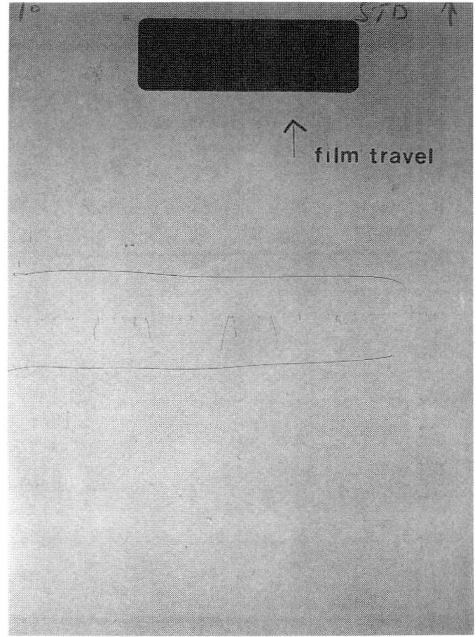


**Figure 8. Skivings**

## 6. Wet Pressure Marks (Figure 9)

This artifact appears as plus-density variations created from excessive pressure on the film emulsion while it is in the developer rack or the developer-to-fixer cross-over area.

**Figure 9. Wet Pressure Marks**

**Possible Causes Include:**
- Exhausted photochemicals
- Rough, blistered, or warped developer rack or developer-to-fixer cross-over rollers
- Overly sensitive film emulsion

**Possible Cures Include:**
- Change developer and verify proper replenishment rate.
- Repair or replace rollers.

## 7. Shoe Marks (Figures 10, 11, & 12)

Shoe marks are minus- or plus-density lines in the direction of film travel. When these marks are found on films processed through a Kodak X-Omat processor, they tend to be one (1) inch apart.

Figure 10. Shoe Marks (Plus Density)

- Plus density (Figure 10) : the problem is usually in the developer section and is associated with the guide shoes.

- Minus density, without emulsion surface damage (Figure 11): the problem usually occurs in the fix-to-wash cross-over area.

- If minus density, with emulsion surface damage (Figure 12): the interference may be anywhere in the film path.

**Possible Cures Include:**
- Adjust film guide shoes, cross-overs and turnaround assemblies.
- Be careful, not to drop or otherwise abuse racks, cross-over assemblies or other film transport components during maintenance or service activities.

Figure 11. Shoe Marks (Minus Density)

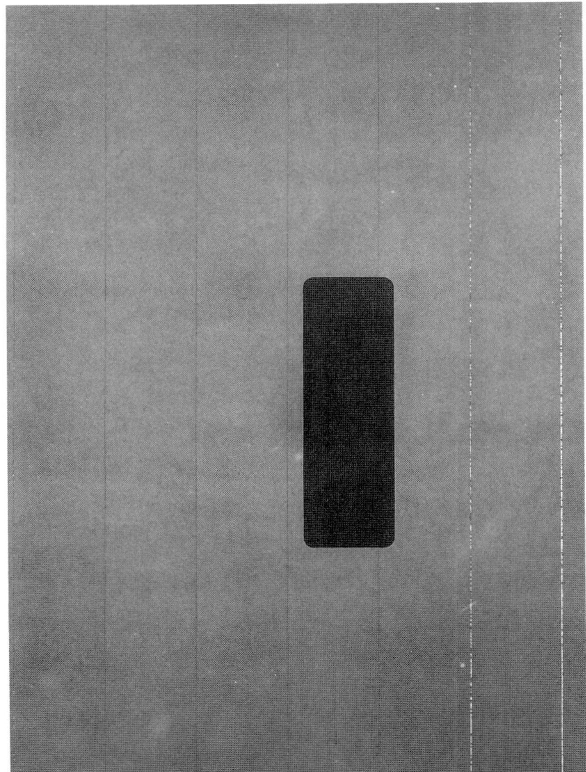

Figure 12. Shoe Marks (Minus Density With Emulsion Damage)

## 8. Seasoning Effects (Figure 13)

Seasoning effects are sensitometric changes that result as films are processed in roller transport processors that contain fresh, unused developer. These changes are normal as the chemicals approach equilibrium. Hydroquinone, pH, and antifoggant concentrations usually drop slightly, while bromide levels move either up or down. Starter solutions and optimized replenishment rates will reduce, but not completely eliminate seasoning effects.

You can expect increases in S (speed) index, C (contrast) index, Dmax, and average gradient as the developer processes the first 100 (plus) 35 x 43 cm films.

- Extreme changes may indicate that starter solution recommended by the manufacturer was not used.

- Lack of stability may be caused by under replenishment.

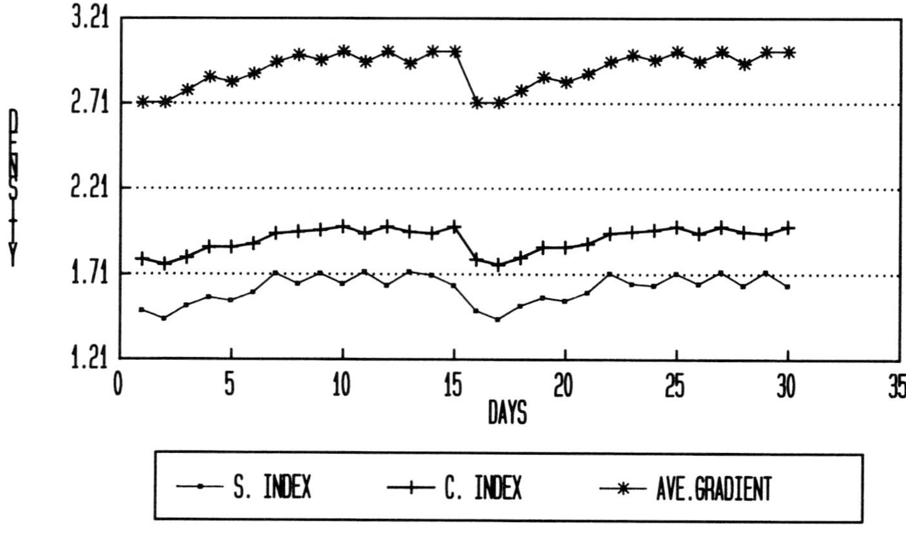


Figure 13. Seasoning Effects

## 9. Stub Lines / Hesitation Lines (Figure 14)

This artifact is exhibited as plus-density lines perpendicular to the direction of film travel.

**Possible Causes Include:**
- Non-uniform film velocity resulting from interference within the film path
- Warped or rough rollers

- Too loose or too tight rack drive chain
- Improper guide shoe positioning
- Inappropriate photochemicals

**Possible Solutions Include:**
- Repair or replace rollers.
- Adjust rack chains.
- Change photochemicals.
- Check replenishment rates.

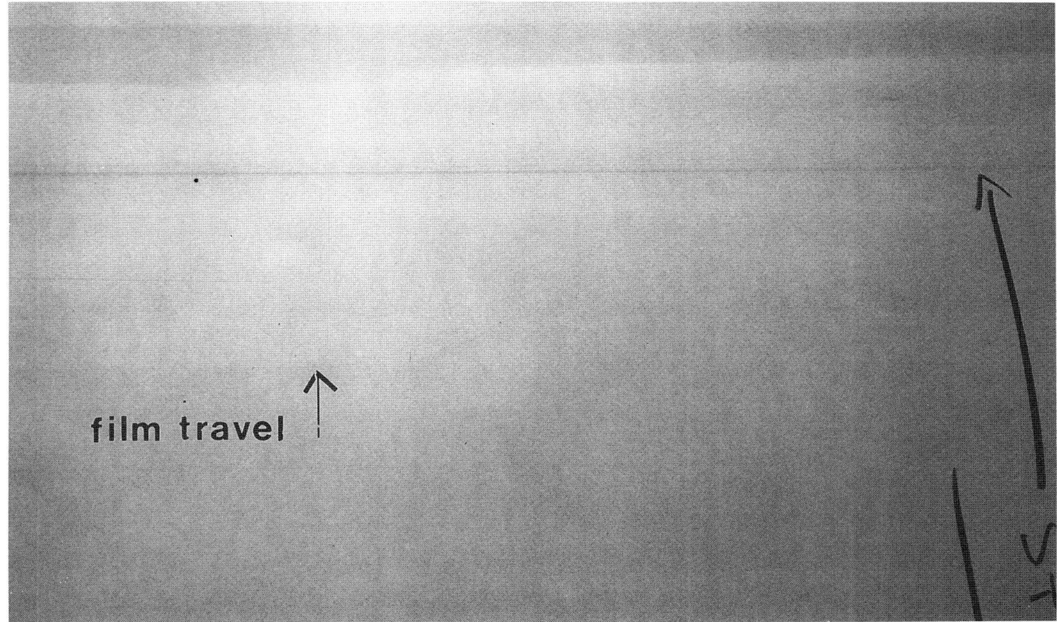


**Figure 14. Stub Lines/ Hesitation Line**

## 10. Runback (Figure 15)

This artifact is a plus-density dribble or scallop on the trailing edge of the film. This defect is typically created between the exit of the developer-to-fix crossover and the entrance to the fix rack. Developer solution on the trailing edge of the film runs down the emulsion as the film enters the fixer and causes increased and uncontrolled development in that area.

**Possible solution:**
- Check squeegeeing at the exit of the developer rack or in the developer-to-fix crossover rack; replace worn or damaged parts.

**Figure 15. Runback**

## 11. Delay Streaks  (Figure 16)

Delay streaks appear as non-uniform areas on the leading edge of the first film fed into the processor after the processor has been unused (or in standby) for an extended period of time. They are caused by oxidized developer on the developer-to-fixer crossover assembly which reacts with fixer fumes. The resulting deposition on the crossover rollers prevents uniform development on the film's leading edge.

**Possible Solutions Include:**

- Process a sheet of cleanup film whenever the processor has not been used for long periods.
- Never switch developer and fixer crossover assemblies.
- Make sure the processor's exhaust is operating properly. There should be airflow into the processor across the feed tray.

**Figure 16. Delay Streaks**

## 12. Chatter (Figure 17)

This artifact appears as a variation in film density which is perpendicular to the direction of film travel through the processor. The spacing between each density transition is generally constant or uniform.

### Possible Causes Include:
- Too loose or too tight developer rack drive chain or gears
- Too loose or too tight developer-to-fixer crossover assemble drive mechanism

### Possible Solutions Include:
- Adjust developer rack or developer-to-fixer crossover assembly drive system (follow the manufacturer's recommendations).

- Perform periodic maintenance as recommended by the processor manufacturer.

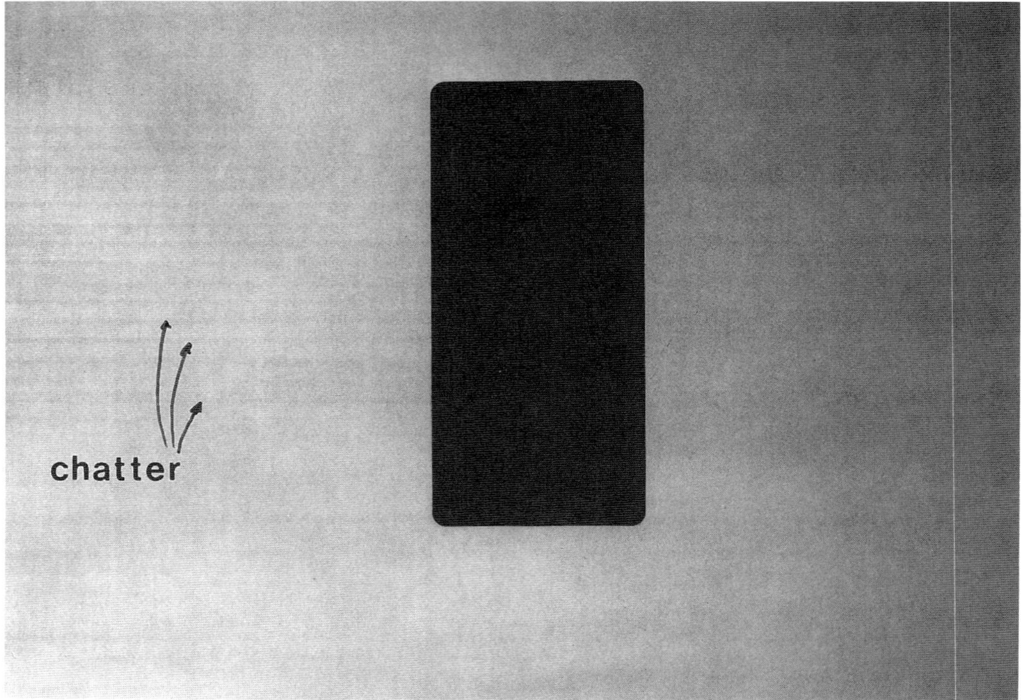



**Figure 17. Chatter**

Film processing systems have the ability to provide the health care supplier with images which meet the total range and the resolution of the most advanced imaging system.

This is accomplished with system components that on the surface may seem very unsophisticated in today's electronic world.

Film, processor and photochemical designers and manufacturers have been most diligent in their resolve to improve performance and productivity with minimum price escalation.

Eastman Kodak Company's most expensive X-Omat processor today sells for less than $30,000, which is approximately the same price of the first Kodak X-Omat processor, model M of 1956. After 36 years of inflation, that same processor would sell for $180,000 today.

Despite such efforts, diagnostic imaging film processing systems sometimes produce processing artifacts. When recognized, these artifacts can be eliminated or reduced to an acceptable level.

## The keys to quality film processing include

1.  Purchase quality systems including the recommended high-quality expendables.

2.  Install and maintain those items as recommended by the manufacturer.

3.  Provide personnel with appropriate training.

4.  Have your processor regularly serviced by qualified service technicians.

5.  Be vigilant in checking losses in performance and make appropriate corrections.

## Acknowledgment

1.  Messrs. Davenport, Dyer, Jerimich and others of the Visual Communications Services Staff (VISCOM), Building 82, Eastman Kodak Co. Research Laboratory, for their generation of enhanced 35 mm slides and photographs.
2.  Mr. Dave Norby, of Dave Norby Computer Solutions, for the permission to show his software package as an example available for monitoring and diagnosing processing systems.
3.  The technicians, past and present of the Health Sciences Systems Performance Laboratory for their generation and donation of illustrated artifacts.

# Film Processing: A Team Approach

**Robert J. Pizzutiello**
Upstate Medical Physics, Inc.
Victor, New York

When asked to consider the effect of film processing on diagnostic imaging, it would be easy to conjure mental images of H&D Curves, daily sensitometric process control plots, and other mathematical models – all of which we use. It is important to remember, however, that the day-to-day manifestation of these models is simply: clinical images.

The clinical images which appear on illuminators in radiology department around the nation are routinely considered "acceptable". They are evaluated as such because they meet our goal in diagnostic radiology: to produce the highest quality images at an appropriately low radiation dose. From time to time, however, an image appears which is deemed "unacceptable". Someone has determined that the image is not as good as it should be. The challenge is to discover what is wrong with this image, and how it can be made better. This is the practical context into which the elements of film processing are interwoven.

Within the limited perspective of a discussion of film processing, it might be easy blame any given imaging problem on sub-optimal film processing. In the big picture, however, this is only one of many factors which affect image quality. In order to review the elements which contribute to image quality or degradation, consider the following anthropomorphic journey.

Imagine yourself as one of a cohort of photons, just produced in the target of an x-ray tube. As you exit the x-ray tube, you may be described by your "quality", quantity, and spectral characteristics. Upon entering the patient, the effect of this mass of tissue upon you becomes overwhelming. The simple location of absorbing structures within the patient – their composition, whether closer or farther from the film surface – has much to do with your ultimate fate. Some of your number are absorbed by tissue structures and are lost forever. Others are scattered and, like fawns separated from the herd, may never find their way back to the fold. Those who do emerge from this gauntlet of tissue interaction are aware that they have been inexorably changed, and they carry the lessons learned from this encounter. But escape is only an illusion. The Crystalline Reaper meets you, demanding that you relinquish your life's breath so that thousands of lesser energy progeny may carry your message. You comply with the inevitable, hoping that your experiences will be passed onto film and, through optimal processing, produce an image worthy of interpretation by a competent creature of flesh and blood.

Clearly, there are many factors which contribute to image quality or degradation. The radiology community has invested substantial resources into optimizing many of these factors which relate to the x-ray photon distribution, patient factors and the creation of the latent image. Even if all these factors are optimized, poor processing will <u>always</u> produce poor images.

From an historical perspective, recall the original method of manual film processing using the "hand tank" method. It is useful to remember that a great many x-ray films are processed even today using this manual technique in dental offices. A small portion of my practice involves inspecting dental offices for the State of New York. I continue to encounter an occasional office in which a dentist elected to shorten the "turnaround time" by decreasing developer time and increasing the x-ray exposure. This clearly unacceptable practice demonstrates the need to maintain control over time, temperature and developing chemistry, even in a process so simple as manual developing.

The modern era has seen the domination of automatic film processors in all higher-volume imaging environments. Maintaining optimal image quality involves controlling multiple factors, including the film processor. Hence, a multi-disciplinary approach is required to detect, investigate, diagnose and correct problems which manifest themselves as poor images. To demonstrate the need for this multi-disciplinary approach, I will share two examples from my own clinical experience with mammography systems.

Five or six years ago, I was testing a dedicated mammography unit. In the process, a phantom image was produced with an artifact – a wavy line – across the field of view. The consensus in the office was that this was the result of a "processor problem" and that the processor service representative would be called to correct it. Motivated by my own suspicious nature and curiosity, I investigated further.

Using a uniform phantom, images were made and processed with alternately the wide, then the narrow edge of the film parallel to the film path. The absolutely consistent appearance of the artifact suggested a cause other than the processor. We asked the x-ray company service engineers to investigate the problem. They discovered an accumulation of oxidation on the surface of the molybdenum beam filter, which was the cause of the artifact. In this case, the film processor was simply a red herring, leading away from the true cause of the problem.

Most recently, my partner and I responded to a problem identified by an astute radiologist who was reading mammograms from two clinics using brand new, identical x-ray machines and film-screen systems. Site A had recently switched to an extended processing system and a dedicated processor. The radiologist described the clinical images from Site A as being inferior to those from Site B. Comparison of ACR accreditation phantom images revealed a noticeable loss of perceptibility of speck groups in the Site A images when compared with Site B images. The radiologist promptly demanded measurement and replacement of the x-ray tube, as he suspected an enlarged focal spot to be the cause of the problem.

We suspected the origin of the problem to be processor-related, since we had only just recently measured both focal spot sizes upon installation, within the past three months. We re-measured both focal spots and found, to our embarrassment, that the focal spot size at Site A was indeed well beyond specifications. The tube was scheduled for replacement.

Doubtful that this was the real cause of the problem, however, we compared phantom images from Site A with those from another client using extended cycle processing. Careful evaluation revealed a noticeably higher noise level in the images from Site A. Perceptibility of spec groups was similar, however, due to an apparent increase in the contrast from the Site A images. We again reviewed the daily processor sensitometry control charts for Site A's extended cycle system. We could find no unusual values. During this review the technologist remarked that the temperature display on the processor seemed to vary by a few degrees during the course of the day.

We verified this temperature fluctuation. Although the temperature was consistently within 0.2 degrees Celsius early in the morning (when processor QC was performed), it varied during the day. Further investigation revealed that the processor was a lower-end, three-minute, tabletop model which had never been designed for the close thermal tolerances required for mammographic processing. The processor was promptly replaced with an extended cycle processor specially designed for mammography. As a result, the image noise and detail perceptibility returned to the high level required to meet everyone's standards.

The moral of both these stories is the same. Most imaging problems present themselves as sub-optimal images with unknown cause. Although a key element in the imaging process, the film processor is not always the cause of the problem. A team approach, utilizing the radiologist, radiologic technologist, medical physicist, x-ray machine service representative, film processor service representative, film and film processor manufacturer is needed in order to investigate the cause(s) of imaging problems. Only in this way will the goal of producing the highest quality images at an appropriately low radiation dose be achieved.

# The Role of the Processor Manufacturer in Film Processing

**Susan E. Hartman**
Health Science Division
Eastman Kodak Company
Rochester, New York

The automatic film processor is not a stand-alone device. It is an integral part of a highly complex film processing system that also includes film, chemistry, accessories and service support. The ability to optimize and integrate all components to provide a system that meets or exceeds customer expectations is the ultimate goal of the film processor/system manufacturer.

There are three major factors that contribute to the success or failure of the film processor manufacturer: product availability, quality and cost.

**1.** Product availability refers to the manufacturer's ability to deliver new products to the customer when needed. It also applies to current product. When an order is placed, the customer expects to receive that product within a relatively short period of time.

Availability begins with new product development. A key factor in developing a new product is timing. In most cases it is important to anticipate what the customer is going to need two or three years before the customer really needs it. This is extremely difficult due to both the dynamics of the marketplace and those of the regulatory agencies.

Most processor manufacturers supply products on a worldwide basis. Thus, it is also important to understand differences and commonalties of customers' needs on a regional basis. The European region often has different needs than those of the United States. The needs of developing regions such as Latin America, Africa and Asia Pacific also need to be considered.

Technological opportunities are also important (see Figure 1). There may be current technologies that can be applied to new product development including applied, core, or even external technologies. These technology opportunities should be combined with new business opportunities and marketing opportunities through a very structured process. Through this process, programs are identified and prioritized. After prioritization, the programs are selected and the next phase will begin — the marketing and manufacturing timeline. All this is based on the needs of the marketplace.

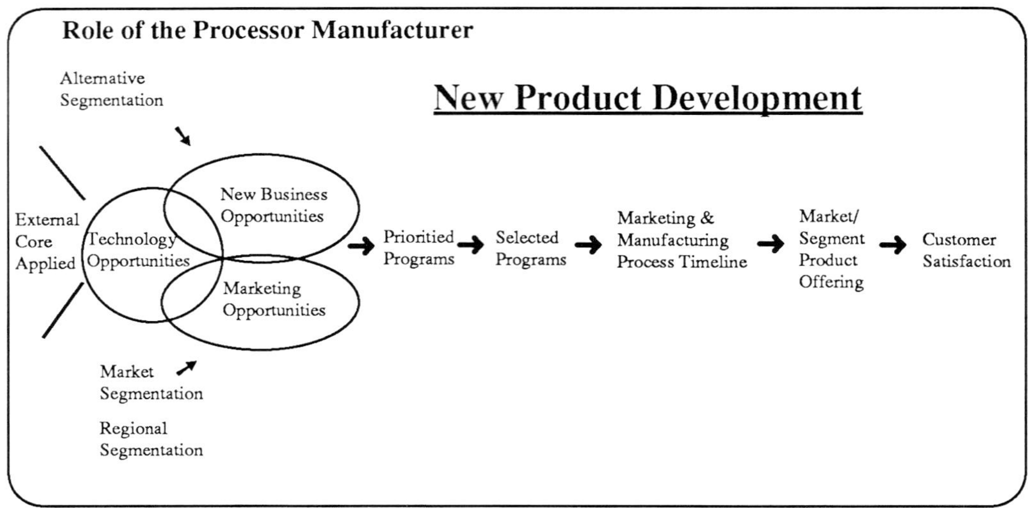


**Figure 1**

The timeline reflects a structured process consisting of a number of phases in a development program (see Figure 2).

The marketing and manufacturing timeline developed for processors begins with phase 0. Before progressing from one phase to the next, it is important to pass through a "gate" which ensures that the product team has delivered on specific product or program deliverables such as performance specifications for a particular product. The project team includes design, marketing, product planning and customer equipment service personnel. This team works together on specific program deliverables so that the final phase will be customer availability of that product. Depending on the complexity and specifications of the product, this process can take from six months to three years.

The second part of product availability is assuring that the product gets to the customer when the customer wants it. The logistics of supplying a worldwide market are complex and challenging (see Figures 3 and 4).

Product inventory goals are addressed along with marketing demand and customer service goals to generate product demand plans which are then translated into a production master schedule. Once the schedule is in place, material requirements planning begins which encompasses every component of the product. The schedule then goes to the suppliers so they can integrate the demand into their schedule. For many processor parts, long lead times of up to 20 weeks are common. Once the parts are ordered and received, inspection is required to ensure that parts meet specifications. Parts then go into the inventory control system to supply the customer parts service needs or go directly to the assembly area. Assembled products are then sent to packing/shipping, to the warehouse or directly to distribution where a customer order has already been received. The product is then shipped to the customer.

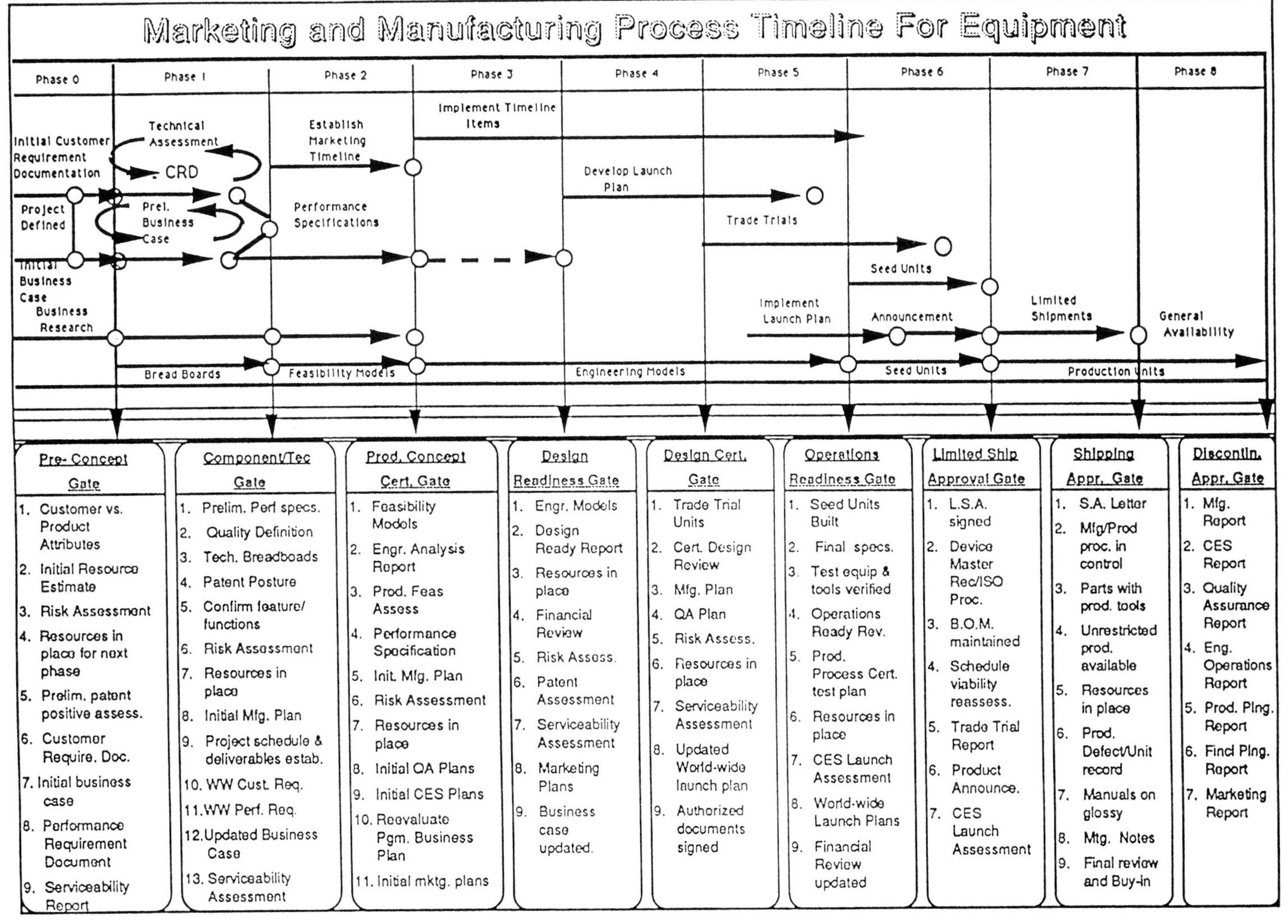


Marketing and Manufacturing Process Timeline For Equipment
Phase 0
Phase 1
Phase 2
Phase 3
Phase 4
Phase 5
Phase 6
Phase 7
Phase 8
Initial Customer Requirement Documentation
Project Defined
Initial Business Case
Business Research
Technical Assessment
CRD
Prel. Business Case
Establish Marketing Timeline
Performance Specifications
Implement Timeline Items
Develop Launch Plan
Trade Trials
Seed Units
Implement Launch Plan
Announcement
Seed Units
Limited Shipments
General Availability
Bread Boards
Feasibility Models
Engineering Models
Production Units
Pre- Concept Gate
1. Customer vs. Product Attributes
2. Initial Resource Estimate
3. Risk Assessment
4. Resources in place for next phase
5. Prelim. patent positive assess.
6. Customer Require. Doc.
7. Initial business case
8. Performance Requirement Document
9. Serviceability Report
Component/Tec Gate
1. Prelim. Perf specs.
2. Quality Definition
3. Tech. Breadboads
4. Patent Posture
5. Confirm feature/ functions
6. Risk Assessment
7. Resources in place
8. Initial Mfg. Plan
9. Project schedule & deliverables estab.
10. WW Cust. Req.
11. WW Perf. Req.
12. Updated Business Case
13. Serviceability Assessment
Prod. Concept Cert. Gate
1. Feasibility Models
2. Engr. Analysis Report
3. Prod. Feas Assess
4. Performance Specification
5. Init. Mfg. Plan
6. Risk Assessment
7. Resources in place
8. Initial QA Plans
9. Initial CES Plans
10. Reevaluate Pgm. Business Plan
11. Initial mktg. plans
Design Readiness Gate
1. Engr. Models
2. Design Ready Report
3. Resources in place
4. Financial Review
5. Risk Assess.
6. Patent Assessment
7. Serviceability Assessment
8. Marketing Plans
9. Business case updated.
Design Cert. Gate
1. Trade Trial Units
2. Cert. Design Review
3. Mfg. Plan
4. QA Plan
5. Risk Assess.
6. Resources in place
7. Serviceability Assessment
8. Updated World-wide launch plan
9. Authorized documents signed
Operations Readiness Gate
1. Seed Units Built
2. Final specs.
3. Test equip & tools verified
4. Operations Ready Rev.
5. Prod. Process Cert. test plan
6. Resources in place
7. CES Launch Assessment
8. World-wide Launch Plans
9. Financial Review updated
Limited Ship Approval Gate
1. L.S.A. signed
2. Device Master Rec/ISO Proc.
3. B.O.M. maintained
4. Schedule viability reassess.
5. Trade Trial Report
6. Product Announce.
7. CES Launch Assessment
Shipping Appr. Gate
1. S.A. Letter
2. Mfg/Prod proc. in control
3. Parts with prod. tools
4. Unrestricted prod. available
5. Resources in place
6. Prod. Defect/Unit record
7. Manuals on glossy
8. Mtg. Notes
9. Final review and Buy-in
Discontin. Appr. Gate
1. Mfg. Report
2. CES Report
3. Quality Assurance Report
4. Eng. Operations Report
5. Prod. Plng. Report
6. Finel Plng. Report
7. Marketing Report

Figure 2

A highly structured process, Manufacturing Resource Planning (MRP2), is used to make sure all resources of an organization are in place. It is made up of a variety of closely integrated functions, including business planning, sales and operations planning, master production scheduling, materials requirement planning and capacity requirement planning. Outputs of these functions are linked closely with financial reports such as business plans, inventory projections, and purchase commitments with suppliers.

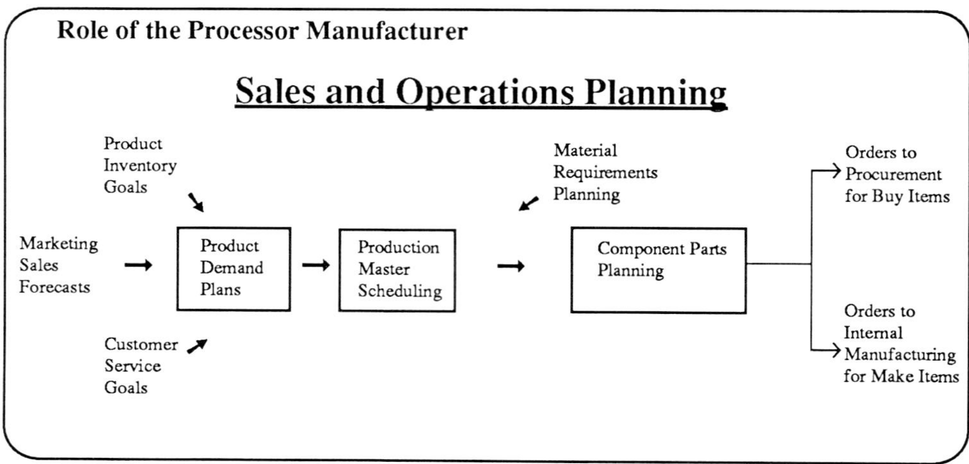


Figure 3

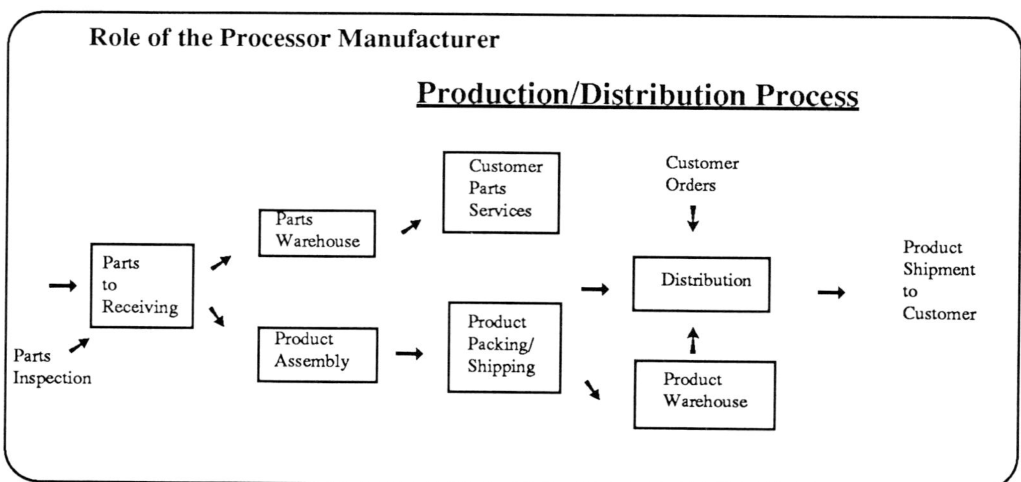


Figure 4

**2.** The second success factor, quality, is very critical to all manufacturers. Quality is a degree of excellence that applies to both the product and level of support/service that the manufacturer provides. The quality of a manufacturer is demonstrated at several different levels.

Quality management assures that the technical, administrative and human factors affecting the quality of an organization's products and services are under control. The system's effectiveness is routinely demonstrated and monitored. All manufacturers agree that this is important but, even more critical, the Food and Drug Administration (FDA) believes it is extremely important. FDA good manufacturing practices (GMP) define a quality assurance program for medical device manufacturers. Since radiographic medical  processors are classified as Class II medical devices, they are governed by FDA regulations.

The International Standards Organization (ISO) has authorized a new series of standards called the ISO 9000 series which is becoming a practical commercial necessity in the European marketplace. ISO 9000 Standards require that quality management is demonstrated internally at the manufacturer's site, externally to the customers, and to the British Standards Industry which audits manufacturers' quality management systems to make sure ISO 9000 standards are met.

ISO 9000 standards are implemented on several levels. ISO 9002 standard applies to manufacturing process certification and includes a number of criteria which monitor the quality management system. ISO 9001 standards apply not only to manufacturing but also to design and customer service. ISO 9001 requires extensive design control documentation. (The marketing and manufacturing timeline illustrated in Figure 2 is an example of design control documentation).

ISO 9000 standards thoroughly cover management responsibility, contract review, document control, purchaser-supplied product, product identification and traceability, process control, inspection and testing, and test equipment calibration. Corrective action and quality records are also addressed. Finally, internal quality audits, training and statistical techniques are required by ISO standards.

Aside from ISO or FDA requirements, quality assurance and quality control functions are ongoing throughout the manufacturing and support organizations to ensure that product meets documented quality standards. Training certification, documented work instructions, and dispositioning discrepant material are all part of quality standards. Engineering change control is used to get input from different parties before costly changes occur. Every product is tested to a predetermined set of specifications and the information is stored as part of the medical device history record. Every new manufacturing process is stringently tested to make sure that it produces a quality product that meets the customer's needs.

Corrective action is a detailed process (see Figure 5) used to identify, solve and prevent the recurrence of problems associated with equipment manufacturing service or use. Problems are communicated by warranty feedback cards which are returned by the customer or dealer, by failed components which are returned by service providers, by internal assemblers and auditors, and by the manufacturer's sales personnel. The result of corrective action is improved product, improved processes, cost savings and, most importantly, customer satisfaction.

As an electrical product, the x-ray film processor must adhere to a number of product safety standards. Among these are electromagnetic interference requirements, UL certification in the U.S., CSA certification in Canada, TUV VDE certification for the European Community and a number of ANSI standards. These certifications help to ensure that a quality product is being shipped to the customer.

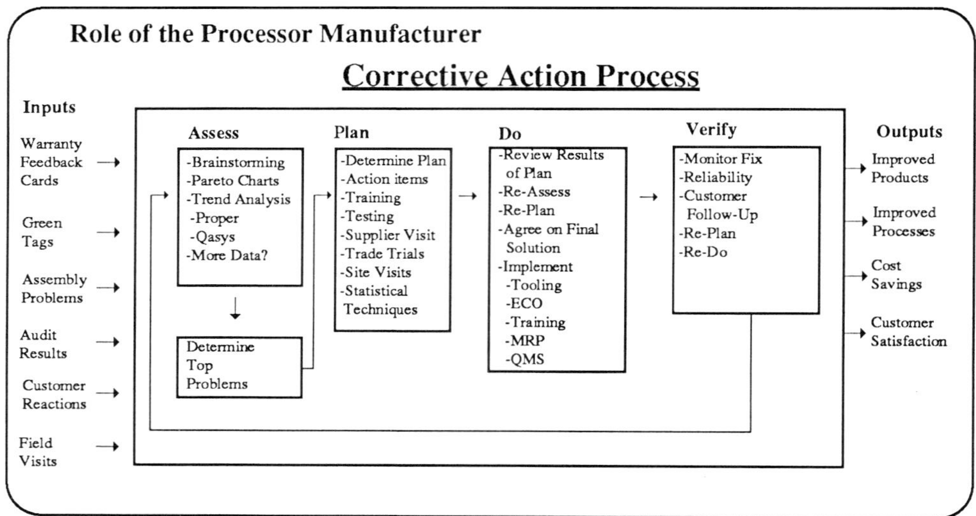


Figure 5

**3.** The third factor contributing to the success of a processor manufacturer is the ability of the manufacturer to provide quality products that meet the customers' expectations and, simultaneously, generate positive earnings for the manufacturer. Positive earnings for the manufacturer are obviously important but, more importantly, the customer must perceive a positive cost/benefit ratio associated with the purchase of the product.

There are a number of factors that contribute to overall processor cost. These include component parts costs, assembly and engineering labor costs and costs associated with repair and scrap. In addition, research and development costs are critical to ensure a continuous stream of new products that meet the customers' changing needs. Finally, costs associated with regulatory agency approvals, product warranty, customer support and inventory management are added to the overall product cost. The processor manufacturer is continually challenged to manage the total cost structure.

This presentation has focused on three success drivers for the processor manufacturer – product availablity, quality and cost. Each of these impacts either positively or negatively the role that the film processor manufacturer plays in the medical imaging marketplace.

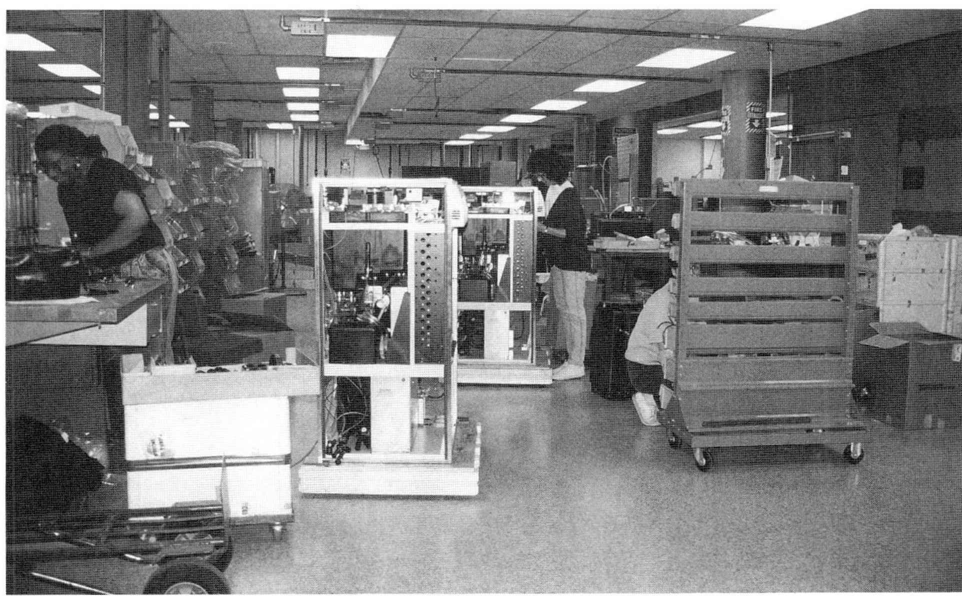

Figure 6. Shows part of the X-Ray Film Handling and Processing Systems Department, Health Sciences, Eastman Kodak Company. All Kodak X-Omat processors are manufactured at this facility.

# The Role Of The Dealer / Service Organization
# In Film Processing

**A. L. Snyder and David C. Forsee**
F&S Medical Systems
Sellersburg, Indiana

August 1974, brought the medical imaging industry its first major regulatory "nudge" with the implementation of federal regulations regarding performance standards for ionizing-radiation-producing equipment.

These new regulations, administered by the Bureau of Radiological Health (BRH) and enforced by the Food and Drug Administration, were the subject of a great deal of controversy of review by the industry. It is certainly an understatement to say these new regulations created concerns, misconceptions, and some over-reaction as to the intent.

Prior to 1974 the industry was essentially unregulated. Father time, the ultimate judge, has proven the 1974 regulations to be very beneficial and the catalyst to some major technological advances in the medical imaging industry. The greatest impact on medical imaging dealers was the development of a new awareness of their responsibilies to their customers and especially to the patient.

Little did the medical imaging dealer realize what lay ahead for the industry. All the indicators were there, but like the ostrich, many dealers chose the "mind set" of ignore it and it will go away and it's "business as usual".

It certainly is not "business as usual." Today's imaging dealer is being forced to conduct business in an every growing quagmire of new regulations, increasing emphasis on quality control, cost containment programs, and even an underlying and growing resentment from the general public toward the medical industry in general.

It is no longer a "nudge"; the medical imaging dealer is being literally shoved into a new era of regulation, evaluation, and forced attrition.

Medical imaging in the 1990's!....confronting new technology, ever changing regulations, cost controls, greater public scrutiny, and all the while expected to produce the highest quality images possible. No less should be expected and this is where the Dealer/Service Organization plays its major role.

## Who is the Imaging Dealer of the 1990's?

Dealers, as a rule, are independent business people. With this independence comes the latitude to make immediate decisions regarding business activity, vendors, new products, staff training, and, foremost, the needs of the customer.

The imaging dealer of the 1990's will be the dealer who uses this decision-making process to meet the inherent responsibilities of a medical imaging dealer/service organization.

A list of the characteristics of the imaging dealer of the 1990's would perhaps read as follows:

- Places top priority on the technical training of the service staff.
- Insists the service personnel be good communicators.
- Environmentally conscious and knowledgeable.
- Quality control program in place within the dealer's facility to insure delivery of the highest quality product.
- Good working relationship with the vendors.
- Quickly responds to a customer's problem with either a solution or a source for a solution.
- Flexible....can respond to changes in environmental regulations, quality control requirements, and be supportive to the customer.
- Financially stable.

The list, which no doubt could be longer, has to be prioritized in a very subjective manner. However, the fact remains that during the 1990's, only those dealers acknowledging, and responding, to the items listed will survive.

Changes affecting the medical imaging industry are occuring rapidly, are very dynamic, and much too complex to embrace the attitude of "business as usual." The imaging dealer of the 1990's will be responsive to the consumer's needs, be a highly skilled professional, have extensive knowledge of environmental regulations, be prepared to service the consumer's environmental needs, and, foremost, be dedicated to helping the customer produce the highest quality images possible.

## The New Attitude Toward "Film Processing"

Witness the following scenerio:

"Rock A. Billy travels to his favorite stereo store and, after much consternation, purchases the best stereo receiver/amplifier in the store. Billy spends just over $2000 for his music machine.

On his way home, he stops at ACME ELECTRONICS and forks over $40 for a pair of speakers that are smaller than the average wristwatch.

Finally, at home, he proceeds to connect all this newly acquired equipment. Power on.......disappointment!!!

He cannot believe the poor quality of the sound system's final product."

Film processing, all related activities, and products, can no longer be the "$40 pair of speakers" in a radiology department where hundreds of thousands of dollars are expended on equipment and personnel.

In the past, many dealers have been guilty of treating film processing as a "necessary evil." As a result, service response, training, and the general attitude toward film processing was analogous to the attitude of Cinderella's stepmother toward Cinderella.

Suffice to say, "the glass slipper has been found." Film processing has come of age and the realization that "poor film processing capabilities yield poor image quality" has become the anthem of all radiology departments.

Imaging dealers have indeed acquired a new attitude regarding film processing, image quality, and the role they must play in obtaining optimum image quality. The attitude change may be attributed to many things....accreditation....environmental regulations....changing technology....etc. Regardless, film processing has finally achieved the level of importance in the medical imaging industry it was always due.

Imaging dealers choosing to maintain the old attitudes regarding film processing will not survive the 1990's.

Any imaging dealer may be judged on the level of importance they place on film processing and image quality by asking a few basic questions:

- Is there a training program in place?
- What is the background of the service technicians?
- Do you participate in available certification programs?
- If you offer pre-mixed chemistry, what are the qualifications of the personnel doing the mixing?
- Parts inventory....is it adequate?

A person takes their new GO-MOBILE (cost $23,000) to the local GO-MOBILE mechanic. The odds are very likely they would be intensely interested in his qualifications and dedication to performing quality service.

In general, imaging dealers now are investing more in training and other efforts to meet their obligations to quality service in film processing/image quality.

## The Imaging Dealer's View of Film Processing in the 1990's

Rest assured that today's imaging dealer no longer views film processor service merely as changing the chemistry, rinsing the tanks, scrubbing the racks, sending an invoice for services rendered. The dealer's view of film processing, processor service, and other related services has undergone a major metamorphosis. All for the better.

The "new view" of film processing is directly related to the change in attitude discussed previously. Film processing can no longer be treated as the "stepchild" of a radiology department or a dealer's service organization.

Viewing the industry indicators, one can semi-accurately develop a view of what is ahead for film processing in the 1990's:

- Performance standards for film processors
- Certification requirements for service personnel
- Certification of dealer/service organizations
- Accreditation standards for other procedures
- Intensified emphasis on environmental compliance
- Changes in film processor technology, chemistry, and film
- Increased financial commitment to processor service

**Performance standards** - common sense dictates that if standards are enforced for x-ray apparatus, then the very piece of equipment (the film processor) which controls the final step in achieving good image quality must also meet minimal performance standards. This is not matter of "if," just when.

**Certification of Service Personnel** - to establish performance standards for equipment not required service personnel to meet certain training standards is somewhat analogous to allowing the local auto mechanic to service a Boeing 727. This certification concept applies equally to film processor services personnel as well as to those servicing x-ray apparatus.

An interesting question....why should a physician, technologist, or other health care professional be required to meet certain professional standards while the equipment used to provide services to the patient is serviced by personnel who have no enforced standards of qualification?

**Certification of Dealers** - logic dictates that if service personnel are required to meet certain standards, their employer should be subject to the same scrutiny. Parts inventory, training schedules, financial stability, customer satisfaction, number of qualified (certified) service personnel would all be elements used to evaluate the dealer.

**Accreditation of Other Procedures** - mammography is the first radiology procedure for which specific standards have been established for final image quality. This is due primarily to increased public awareness and the large amount of publicity this procedure has received.

A spot on the lung is a health concern.

The ability to detect the smallest bone fracture is a health concern.

As public awareness grows, and health care professionals strive to maintain the integrity of their profession, the certification of all radiology procedures is predictable.

Welcome to medical imaging of the 1990's.

**Environmental Compliance** - this is no longer optional. The medical imaging industry has been identified as a user – and producer – of hazardous materials and waste.

More than any other factor, film processing of the 1990's will be impacted by the requirement to comply with local, state, and federal environmental laws and regulations.

**Technology Changes** - equipment is becoming more technically sophisticated; film and screen technology is changing. Alternate image processing modalities are becoming available - laser imagers. 3-D imaging, a variety of digital systems for both acquisition and post processing of images. Advances in processing cycle times – 90 seconds to 45 seconds.

Film processing of the 1990's will involve all the new modalities. For the dealer, this translates to training....training....and more training.

**Financial Support** - the dealer of the 1990's will be required to make a major financial commitment to training of service personnel, the customer's cost containment programs, associated test equipment, and in-service programs.

## What the Consumer Should Expect from the Dealer

Every consumer should establish certain guidelines to evaluate an imaging dealer:

- Does the dealer respond with service in a timely manner?
- Are the service personnel adequately trained?
- Does my dealer have an ongoing training program for service personnel?
- Is the service on the film processor adequately documented and left on-site?
- Are the charges incurred for these services respresentatives of the charges levied by other dealers in a given geographical area?
- Does the dealer maintain a service history of the film processor?
- Is the dealer trained and knowledgeable relative to environmental regulations?
- Does the dealer answer questions, or at least place the consumer in contact with someone who can?

## Consumer Education

One of the major roles a 1990's imaging dealer will play is that of an educator. This role will take the form of a homogeneous variety of activities. The first is to utilize service personnel who can communicate with the consumer. The most repetitive contact any dealer organization has with any customer is through the activities of the delivery and service personnel.

The consumer expects any representative of the dealer to at least be able to have a minimal command of the English language. The day of the muted service person has passed.

The customer contact person (i.e., delivery, service) must be able to communicate with the customer. Consumer education begins with having highly trained and communicative personnel assisting the account.

As a dealer, we are privy to information and data which may, or may not filter to the level of the end user. Therefore, it becomes incumbent on the dealer to maintain good communication with each customer and to apprise the customer of changes which impact their planning,  job functions, accreditation, and methodology of patient care.

Dealers have an inherent responsibility to keep their customers informed. The information may be commuicated in serveral formats – knowledgable service personnel, newsletters, in-service programs. The basic theme for the dealer is "trained personnel" and developing a form of communication with the dealer's customer base to adequately meet the responsibility of consumer education.


## Problem solving

The day of any form of an adversarial role between the vendor, consumer, and dealer will cease. The problems confronting the consumer, relative to image quality, requires the mutual cooperation between the dealer, vendor, and customer.

As an end user of the product and confronted with the need to produce radiographic images of certifiable quality, it would behoove every customer to involve, insist, and demand that both the dealer and the manufacturer be involved simultaneously in arriving at a solution to any image quality or film processing problem.

- The role of the imaging dealer in the 1990's is multifaceted:
- Increased emphasis on technical training.
- Total familiarization with environmental compliance.
- Acceptance of quality control as a standard practice.
- Image quality becomes the prime concern, not number of images pro duced.
- Prepare for the new technology in film processing.


Business in the medical imaging industry must now be conducted on the basis of quality and added value.

The imaging dealer who has, in the past, conducted business on "I am a nice guy" concept will fall from grace unless a commitment to the new dealer role is made.

# The Role of the X-ray Equipment Manufacturer in Film Processing

**Rita W. Heinlein***

Mammography Consultant
Clarksville, Maryland
*Formerly with GE Medical Systems, Hanover, Maryland

With the increased focus on quality control, especially in mammography, it is imperative that those involved have a thorough understanding of all aspects of the imaging chain. The x-ray equipment and the processing conditions are the two links in the chain that most affect image quality. Unfortunately, too many people see a clear division of responsibility between the dealer and associated film manufacturer and the manufacturer of the exposure equipment. This division has resulted in finger pointing, each side saying, "If there is a problem, it is their fault, not ours!" The fact of the matter is that the roles of all these organizations cannot be neatly separated: radiography requires equipment and film to produce a latent image and processing to convert that latent image to a visible image. If any one is missing or inadequate, radiography is not possible. This interdependency must be carried through to the relationship among the exposure equipment manufacturer, the film/processing manufacturer, and the dealer organization and the role they each play in producing quality mammography. The goal of any radiographic procedure and especially of mammography is to produce images with excellent resolution and high contrast, at the lowest possible exposure to the patient. Producing such images requires a complex interaction of many factors as discussed by A. Haus (Table 1). If any one of these factors is changed, others are usually affected. It is necessary to understand how each of these factors will impact the resolution and contrast which must be achieved in order to optimize the image as well as the impact on the dose level.

The impact of processing conditions on mammographic image quality cannot be underestimated. Image contrast can be affected by developer temperature that is too low, extended versus standard processing time, insufficient replenishment of the developer, light leaks in the darkroom, type of chemistry used, improper safelight, etc.

For these reasons, daily sensitometric monitoring of the processor is mandatory. It is also for these reasons that the service engineer (for the mammography equipment) needs to review the sensitometry prior to calibrating the phototimer during installa tion of the unit and prior to any servicing to correct an image quality problem. Whenever the quality of mammography is substandard, the first possible source of trouble to be checked is film processing. This is based upon the fact that processor chemicals undergo change more frequently than does the mammography unit, due to mechanical or electronic failure. Therefore, a review of the sensitometric chart by the technologist prior to calling for service or by the service engineer may resolve the problem more efficiently. For example, a service engineer was called in to evaluate a mammography unit because of "light images." After three hours, the engineer reported he could find nothing wrong with the unit. When he and the technologist looked into the processor, they found the new developer had oxidized. Replacing the developer solved the "light image" problem.

## Team Approach

Image quality can be degraded by problems originating with the mammography equipment as well as in the darkroom and with the processing.The first step in resolving the problem is an investigation to determine the cause (Table 1). If films were overexposed or underexposed, a determination must be made concerning: AEC or kVp calibration, variation in mR/mAs, correct filtration, replenishment of chemistry, or time and temperature of development. If there is a loss of image contrast, it could be an equipment problem: kVp out of calibration, aged tube, incorrect filter, problems with the compression device, or faulty grid. It could be a processing problem: improper replenishment, variation in the time or temperature, developer added without starter, or changes in film manufacturing.

Artifacts on the film could be caused by the mammography unit or by the processing equipment; for example, grid lines, mottled filter, variations in the compression paddle, roller marks, pick-off, chemical stains, guide shoe marks, or dirt on the feed tray.

Although the investigation to determine the cause of the image problem starts with the technologist, it must involve the coordinated efforts of the equipment manufacturer, the dealer representative and the film/processor manufacturer. It is only through a collaborative approach initiated and controlled by an informed user that all appropriate imaging factors will be optimized to produce high-quality mammograms.

**Table 1. Factors affecting radiographic image quality***

| Radiographic Sharpness | | Radiographic Noise | |
| --- | --- | --- | --- |
| **Radiographic Contrast** | **Radiographic Blurring (Unsharpness)** | **Radiographic Mottle** | **Radiographic Artifacts** |
| Subject Contrast<br>Absorption differences<br>   Thickness<br>   Density<br>   Atomic number<br>Radiation quality<br>   Target material<br>   Kilovoltage(kVp)<br>   Filtration<br><br>Scattered Radiation<br>Beam collimation<br>Compression<br>Air gap<br>Grid<br><br>Film Contrast<br>Film type<br>Processing<br>   Chemistry<br>   Temperature<br>   Time<br>   Agitation<br>Photographic density<br>Fog<br>   Storage<br>   Safelight<br>   Light leaks | Motion Blurring<br>Patient<br>immobilization<br>Exposure time<br><br>Geometric Blurring<br>Focal spot size<br>Focal spot object<br>distance<br>Object-image receptor<br>distance<br><br>Screen-Film Blurring<br>Phosphor thickness<br>Light absorbing dyes<br>and pigments<br>Phosphor particle size<br>Screen-film contact | Film Granularity<br><br>Quantum Mottle<br>Film speed<br>Film contrast<br>Screen absorption<br>Screen conversion<br>efficiency<br>Light diffusion<br>Radiation quality<br><br>Structure Mottle | Processing<br>Streaks<br>Spots<br>Scratches<br>Dirt<br>Stains<br><br>Handling<br>Finger marks<br>Scratches<br>Static<br>Crimp marks |

* Reproduced with permission from: Haus AG: Screen-Film Processing Systems and Quality Control in Mammography: Symposium on the Physics of Clinical Mammography. (Eastman Kodak publication N314).

## References


1. Kimme-Smith C, Bassett L, Gold R: Workbook for Quality Mammography. Williams & Wilkins, 1992.

2. Kopans D: Mammographic Equipment – What Do You Need?: Breast Imaging, The Team Approach II. Boston, MA, October 23-25, 1992.

3. Haus AG: Screen-Film Processing Systems and Quality Control in Mammography: Symposium on the Physics of Clinical Mammography sponsored by the American College of Radiology, July 25-27, 1990, St. Louis, MO (Eastman Kodak publication N314).

4. Haus AG, Cowart RW, Dodd GD, et al: "A Method of Evaluating and Minimizing Geometric Unsharpness for Mammographic X-ray Units." *Radiology* 128:775, 1978.

5. Sickles EA, Weber WN: High Contrast Mammography With a Moving Grid: Assessment of Clinical Unit. *AJR* 146:1137, 1986.

6. Swann CA, Kopans DB, McCarthy KA, et al: Mammographic Density and Physical Assessment of the Breast. *AJR* 148:525, 1987.

7. Feig SA: Screen-Film Mammography: Equipment, Technique, Quality Control in Breast Imaging: Categorical Course Syllabus for the 88th Annual Meeting American Roentgen Ray Society. San Francisco, CA, May 8-12, 1988.

8. Haus AG: Technologic Improvements in Screen-Film Mammography. *Radiology* 174:628-627, 1990.

9. Haus AG: Recent Advances in Screen-Film Mammography. *Radiologic Clinics of North America* 25:913-928, Sept. 1987.

10. Haus AG: Evaluation of Image Blur (Unsharpness) in Medical Imaging. *Medical Radiography and Photography* 61:42-53, 1985.

11. Tabar L. Haus AG: Processing Mammographic Films: Technical and Clinical Considerations. *Radiology* 173:65-69, October, 1989.

12. Mammography Quality Control Manual. American College of Radiology, Committee on Quality Assurance in Mammography. 1992 Edition

# The Role Of The Radiologist In Film Processing

**Stephen A. Feig and Benjamin M. Galkin**
Breast Imaging Center
Department of Radiology
Thomas Jefferson University Hospital
Philadelphia, Pennsylvania

The radiologist should not be a passive film reader but must be involved in every phase of image production to render proper interpretation. Radiologist involvement is especially important in mammography film processing due to the need for high contrast to perceive the relatively narrow inherent range of breast tissue densities without excessive loss of skin and subcutaneous structures; high resolution to demonstrate microcalcifications and spiculations which may be less than 1 mm in size; adequate speed to permit reduced doses for mass population screening; short exposure times to prevent motion unsharpness on routine and magnified studies; adequate exposure levels for penetration of dense fibroglandular tissues and low noise levels which do not significantly interfere with image information. Although this paper will reflect the viewpoint of a radiologist and a medical physicist who specialize in mammography, much of its content will be applicable to film processing in other areas of radiology as well.

## Rationale For Radiologist Involvement In Film Processing

Why should the radiologist be involved in film processing? First, because proper processing is absolutely necessary for accurate interpretation. Secondly, because evaluation of film processing is an important part of the American College of Radiology (ACR) Mammography Accreditation Program. Moreover, processor performance will reflect the radiologist's professional reputation. Finally, because the radiologist is medicolegally responsible for the technical quality of radiographs.

## Effect of Image Quality on Interpretation

An example of the need for proper processing in mammography is shown in Figure 1. The initial mammogram (1a) from another facility was sent to one of us for consultation after the patient came for a routine visit to a gynecologist at our hospital. There had been no reported mammographic abnormality. The clinical findings were also normal. Although the image had poor contrast and consequently low resolution, one could appreciate a density in the mid breast which needed better imaging. The mammogram was repeated at our breast imaging center and disclosed a spiculated mass in that same area (1B). Subsequent biopsy confirmed a 0.8 cm infiltrating carcinoma. Ironically, the initial study had been performed on the same type, state-of-the-art mammographic unit which we had at our own facility. In fact, their unit was newer than ours and was working properly.

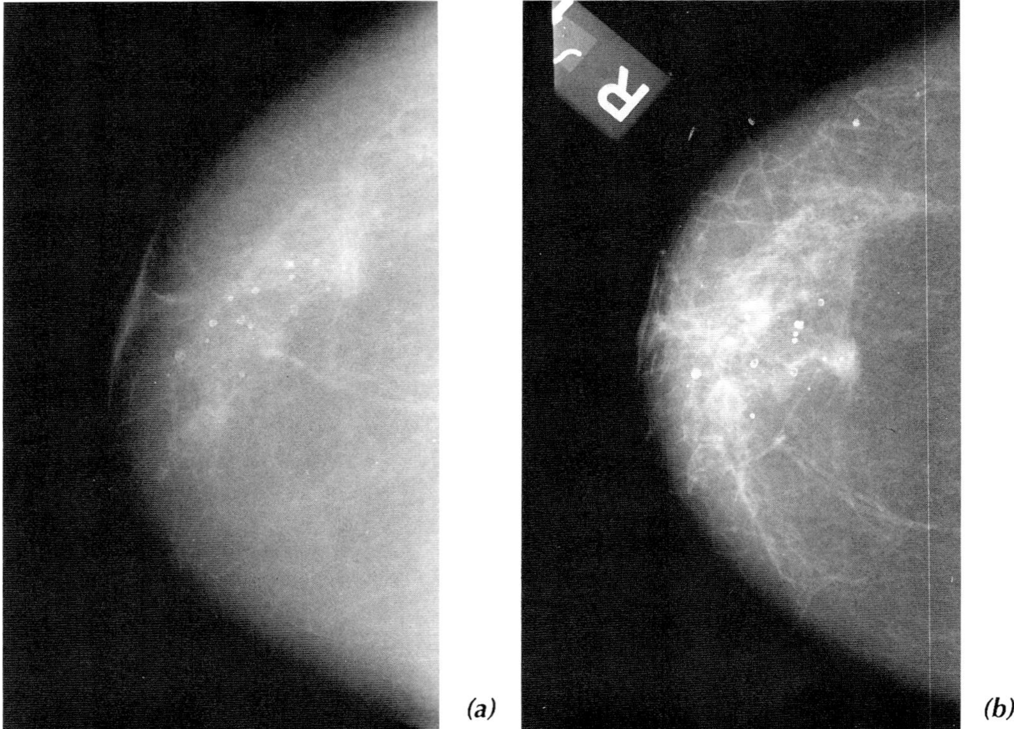


**Figure 1. Spiculated mass is hardly suggested on poorly processed film (a) but easily visualized on properly processed image (b).**

Such an episode has significance beyond the immediate case. A widely circulated poster from the American Cancer Society makes "a positive point about breast cancer" – that it can be detected by screening mammography when it is no larger than the point depicted therein (Figure 2). However, even under ideal circumstances, mammography cannot always find such early cancers. The likelihood will depend very strongly on image quality components, especially processing. Mammography is not a brand name product which is the same regardless of where it is obtained. Detection sensitivity will vary considerably according to technical quality.

Practically every mammographic screening project conducted around the world over the past 20 years has shown increased survival or decreased mortality. However, the amount of benefit and even its presence will depend on a number of factors (Table 1). Any of these factors can influence screening results, but certainly if there is inadequate technique – especially processing – the study may not show good results even if every other factor is appropriate. The conclusion may be appreciated when results from major screening trials are reviewed.

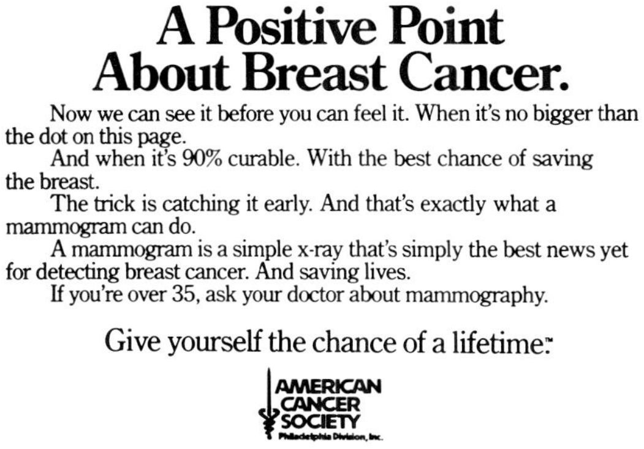

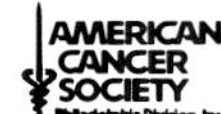


**Figure 2. American Cancer Society public service poster**

**Table 1.   Factors Affecting Mammography Screening Trial Outcome**
- Film Processing
- Mammographic unit
- Positioning and compression

- Screening interval
- Number of views

- Size of study and control populations
- Proper randomization of study and control groups
- High compliance of study group
- Negligible screening rate among control group
- Proper mammographic interpretation

One example would be a comparison of the results of the Health Insurance Plan of Greater New York (HIP) Study which used the mammographic techniques of the 1960's with those of the American Cancer Society (ACS), National Cancer Institute (NCI) supported, Breast Cancer Detection Demonstration Project (BCDDP) conducted with the improved mammographic techniques of the mid-1970's (Table 2).[1,2] In both studies, physical examination and mammography were performed on every woman. In both studies, approximately 40% of the cancers among women age 50 and older were detected by mammography alone. In the HIP study, only about 20% of cancers detected among women aged 40 to 49 were detected by mammography alone, a great drop off from the percent detection for older women. In the BCDDP Project, the percent of cancers detected by mammography alone in this younger age group increased to 35%. This change has been attributed mainly to improvement in mammographic technique. Thus, the greatest improvement in cancer detection from better technique was seen among women aged 40 to 49 who tend to have more glandular breasts than older women.

**Table 2.   Comparison of HIP (1963-1968) and BCDDP (1974-1981):**

Improvement in Mammographic Detection

Cancers detected by mammography alone

|  | Total | 40-49 yrs. | 50-59 yrs. |
|---|---|---|---|
| HIP | 34.4% | 19.4% | 41.5% |
| BCDDP | 40.0% | 35.4% | 42.1% |

Cancers detected by physical examination alone

|  | Total | 40-49 yrs. | 50-59 yrs. |
|---|---|---|---|
| HIP | 47.0% | 61.0% | 40.0% |
| BCDDP | 9.0% | 13.0% | 6.7% |

Minimal cancers

| HIP | 8.0% |
|---|---|
| BCDDP | 25.0% |

Source Refs,[1,2]

Another difference between these two studies relates to the sensitivity of mammography in detecting very early cancers. Minimal carcinomas (defined here as any cancer less than 1 cm even if it is invasive) and every *in situ* carcinoma constituted about 8% of the cancers detected in the HIP study vs 25% in the BCDDP Project. The lower detection threshold is best explained by better mammographic technique.

The effect of improvement in technique during the course of a single study may be seen in results from the Edinburgh Screening Trial. Concomitant with a significant improvement in technique from the initial screenings to the later ones, there was a markedly increased detection sensitivity rate on the later screenings and a pronounced drop in the proportion of interval cancers that occured between screenings (Table 3). These key observations were commented on by the investigators themselves in their first 7-year report.[3]

**Table 3. Screening Sensitivity and Interval Cancer Rates in the Edinburgh Trial**

| | Screening Round | | | | | | |
|---|---|---|---|---|---|---|---|
| | 1 | 2 | 3 | 4 | 5 | 6 | 7 |
| Sensitivity(%) | 92% | 72% | 91% | 62.5% | 97% | 69% | 97% |
| Proportional Incidence of interval cancers | 28.1% | 36.0% | 16.6% | 26.7% | 4.6% | 24.7% | 5.2% |

Protocol:      Mammography and clinical examination years 1,3,5,7
Clinical examination alone, years 2,4,6

Source: Ref. [3]

The Swedish Two-County Trial run by Dr. Laszlo Tabar had excellent technique. This study attained the same mortality reduction with single-view mammography alone at 2-3 year intervals in the 1980's as had been achieved in the HIP Project in the 1960's with annual two-view mammography and physical examination.[4]

The Canadian National Breast Cancer Screening Study, especially in the early years of the project, had numerous technical problems: old equipment, non-dedicated processing, no grids. [5-7] There was improvement in technical quality later on, but for the first five screenings there were serious technical problems which are reflected in their early results. So far, no benefit has been shown to the women in any age group who were screened. [8]

In summary, results from the U.S.A., Great Britain, Sweden and Canada all indicate that technical quality is necessary for proper interpretation and the ultimate goal of breast cancer mortality reduction.

## Variation in Processor Performance

A number of recent studies have shown substantial differences in film speed and contrast among processors at different facilities [9-11] as well as variability in the day-to-day performance at a given facility.[9] One survey involved 32 facilities which had been enrolled in a regional breast cancer awareness program in the Delaware Valley[9] without any real prior test of the technical quality of their films. Participating facilities were required to have dedicated mammographic units but there were no requirements for compliance with film processing standards.

As part of the study, pre-exposed test strips of film were distributed to each facility. They were asked to process one strip every day for 15 consecutive work days. Densitometric measurements were then made of the base plus fog, medium density and high density areas. It was found that there was considerable variation in average mid-density values from one center to another. This was not solely or even mainly attributed to the differences in film-screen systems since the density of the test strip varied even among facilities using the same screen-film system (Figure 3).

When the day-to-day performance of an individual center was evaluated, some of the processors had very good stability; others had significant variation (Figure 4). Overall, about 37% of the centers showed variation which was greater than the recommended limit for processor stability of 0.1 density unit. As a consequence of this study, documentation of processor sensitometry was added as a requirement in the ACR Mammography Accreditation Program.[12]

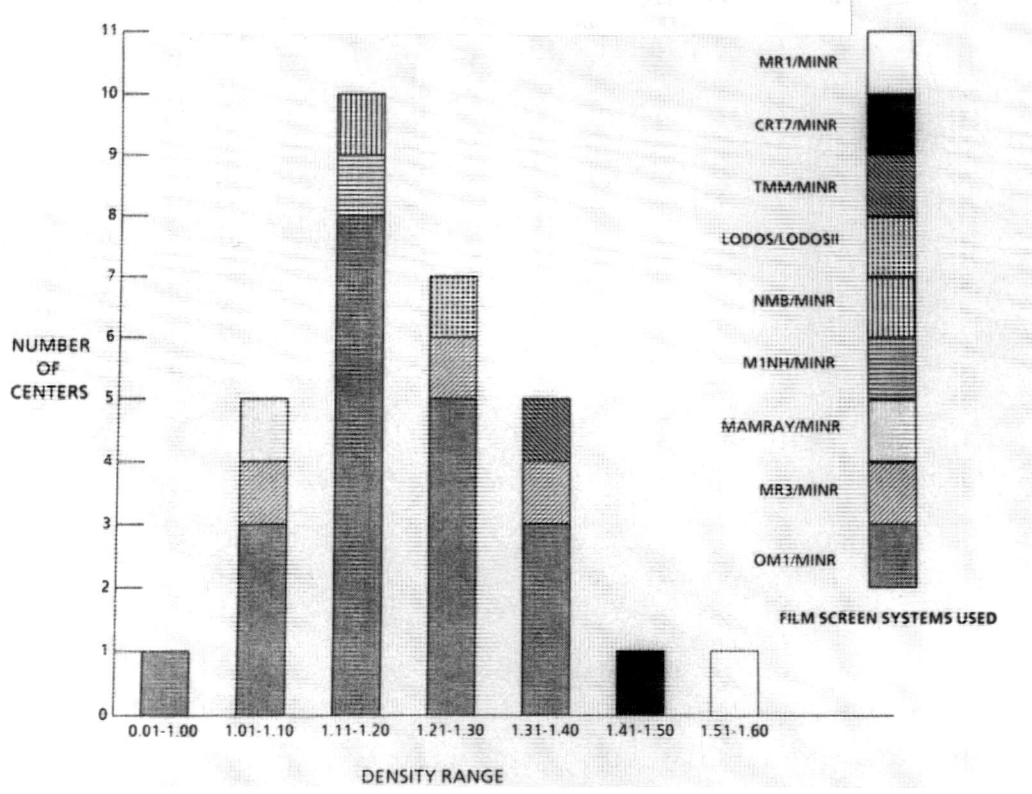


Figure 3. Average optical density of medium density test area of pre-exposed films developed at different mammography centers (From Ref. 9, with permission).

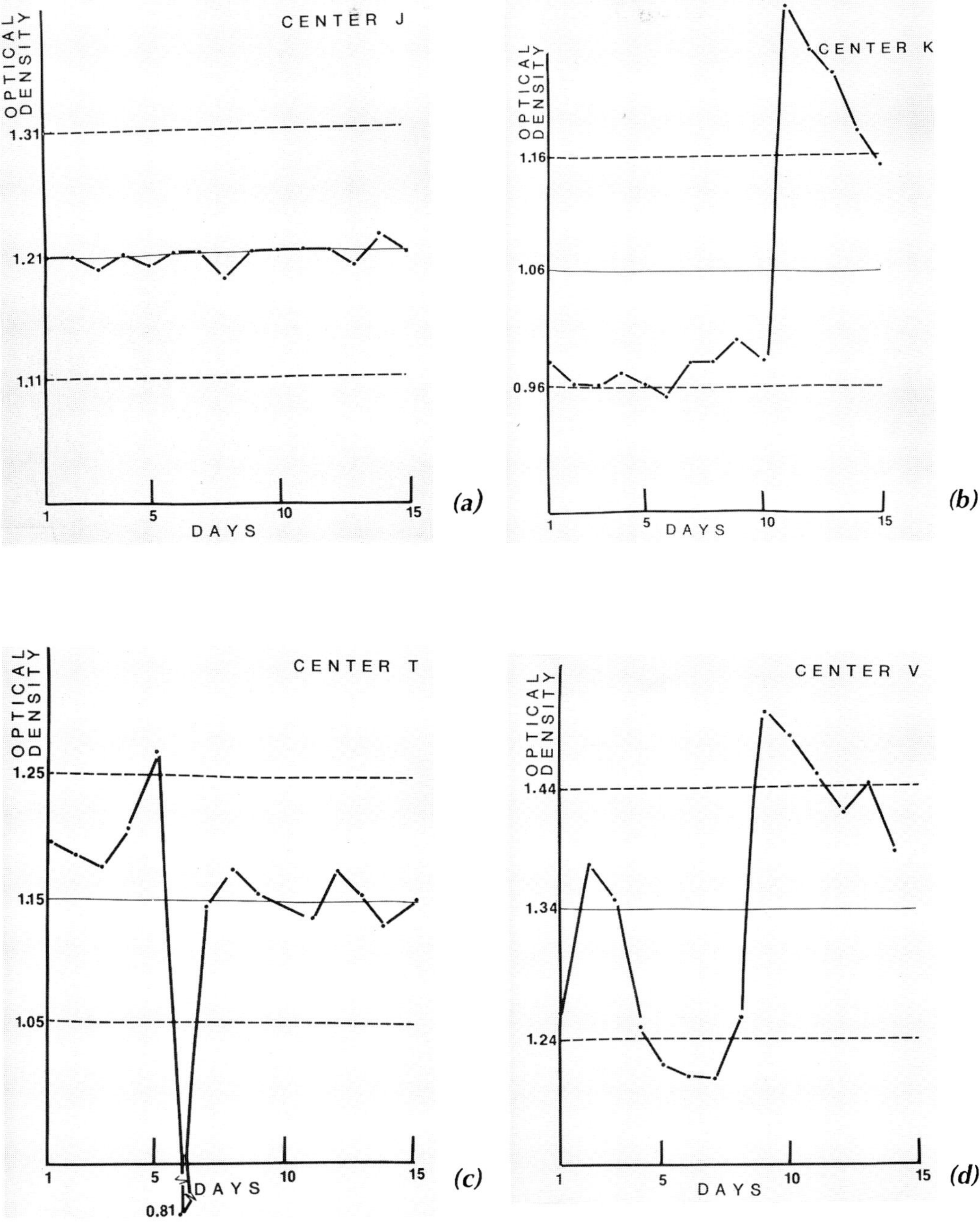



**Figure 4. Processor control charts from four facilities, all of which used Kodak Ortho M film and Min-R screens. (A) Shows good processor stability, (B-D) show poor processor stability (From Ref. 9, with permission).**

## Table 4.  Criteria for ACR Mammography Accreditation Program

Clinical image evaluation

- Positioning
- Compression
- Exposure level
- Resolution
- Contrast
- Noise
- Exam identification
- Artifacts

Phantom image evaluation

- Reading scores for fibers, specks and masses
- Density
- Artifacts

Dosimeter assessment of average glandular dose
Processor sensitometry records
Site survey questionnaire

- Practice setting and demographics
- Training, certification, experience of radiologists, radiologic technologists and medical physicists
- Mammographic x-ray unit, image receptor system, processor and processing conditions
- Routine number of views, technique factors
- Responsibility and frequency of quality assurance tests
- Patient reporting and follow-up mechanism
- Policy for retention of mammograms

## ACR Accreditation

The radiologist should also be interested in processing because it is important for ACR accreditation. The criteria for accreditation are outlined in Table 4. Most of them are directly or indirectly related to processing. Among the clinical image criteria, the exposure level, contrast, noise, presence or absence of artifacts, and even to some degree the resolution are dependent on processing. Only positioning and compression are unrelated. Results of phantom image evaluation reflect the performance of the x-ray unit, screen-film system and processor. Dose for a given patient is largely a result of screen-film system, processing, compression and grid. Dose is only slightly affected by other features of the x-ray unit. Processor sensitometry records became a requirement for the 3-year ACR accreditation in January 1992 and are now required in the annual renewal process as well. Dedicated mammographic processing *per se* is not a present requirement. However, performance standards requirements for contrast, dose, etc., are more easily fulfilled if processing conditions are those recommended by the manufacturer of the screen-film system being used.

## Professional Reputation

Today, as more and more films are sent from one institution to another either for a second opinion or for referral for surgery or radiation therapy, the quality ot these radiographs will affect the reputation of each radiologist's practice. At our own breast imaging center, we routinely see films from many other local facilities. We have a good idea of the technical quality of their studies, not based on solitary cases, but through seeing many examples of their cases over and over again. These referral patterns will influence our opinion of other facilities and, in turn, will affect our own reputation as well. We should want our film quality to be something we can take pride in.

## Medicolegal Responsibilities

Delay in diagnosing breast cancer has become one of the leading causes of malpractice claims in the entire country.[13] It is now the fastest growing cause of malpractice suits for the radiologist. There are a number of reasons for this disturbing trend. For one thing, breast cancer is very common. Secondly, if a clinician misses a breast lump which is cancerous, it may be difficult to prove in retrospect that the lump could have been palpable and that it was suspicious enough at the time to biopsy. If a radiologist misses a breast cancer, there is mammographic documentation which can then be evaluated retrospectively by an "expert." Not all missed cases are as obvious as the one recently publicized by television reporter Diane Sawyer on the American Broadcasting System's "Prime Time" television show. There are subtle findings which even the best radiologists may miss. Even when the mammographic findings are not truly suspicious, the plaintiff's attorney can try to hire someone to say, " Yes, I can see it there and it should have been biopsied." The radiologist's attorney will then try to produce another "expert" to defend his/her client's interpretation. The case then becomes a contest between "expert" witnesses, each striving to establish credibility with the jury.

When a radiologist is accused of malpractice, the plaintiff's lawyer will try to establish a number of elements that are related to the law of negligence.[14-16] First, the attorney will state that the radiologist had a duty not only for proper interpretation, but also in providing a technically adequate study. After establishing that the radiologist interpreted a study which was not technically adequate, the plaintiff's lawyer will try to show that the cancer could probably have been detected earlier if the technical quality of the mammogram were up to standards. Then he/she will attempt to establish that either survival, treatment options, or quality of life was affected because of the delayed diagnosis.

Even at a facility having ACR accreditation, the radiologist may still be medicolegally liable for a study in which breast cancer is not shown due to substandard technical quality. In legal terms, ACR accreditation may not be dispositive in such a case.[14-16] Certainly ACR accreditation is helpful, but it may not necessarily save the radiologist if the study is technically poor.

## The Radiologist's Responsibilities In Film Processing

### Setting Image Quality Objectives

Each radiologist should have a set of image quality objectives. Although he/she should appreciate the acceptable range for image parameters such as contrast and density, there is room for individual preference within this range. Certainly, no radiologist should passively accept his/her current image quality without being aware of the other options. Since improvement in contrast, density, resolution, mottle, skin and subcutaneous tissue visualization, and dose may be mutually exclusive objectives, each radiologist should individually rank these parameters in terms of personal preference.

### Selection of Processing Options

Having set image quality objectives, the radiologist can then proceed to select the appropriate processing factors. Does he/she prefer dedicated or nondedicated, standard or extended, on-site or off-site processing? Is the current processor chemistry satisfactory or should it be changed to a different brand?[17] Is the lower contrast, higher dose and lower density from a nondedicated vs dedicated processor[18] or 90-second vs 2-minute vs 3-minute processing acceptable?[17,19-20] Is the convenience of an off-site processor and/or batch processing an acceptable trade-off for the higher dose and/or lower density?[21] All of these considerations have to be carefully weighed by the radiologist.

If the radiologist selects extended processing, the dose will be lower and the contrast will be higher than with 90-second processing. However, film mottle will be doubled. Visualization of skin and subcutaneous tissues will be diminished. Examination time will be longer. Unless the processor can switch back and forth easily from one cycle to another, extended processing may not be suitable for the workflow in a busy radiographic section. The relative weight given to each of these advantages and disadvantages will depend on the individual radiologist's preferences as well as the circumstances at the imaging facility. There is no single best type of processing cycle for everyone.

Selection will also depend on the type of mammographic film being used. The effect of extended processing on relative speed (an indicator of dose) and average gradient (an indicator of contrast) for three different single-emulsion films is shown in Table 5. It can be seen that the dose reduction and contrast improvement from extended processing are greatest with Kodak Min-R-E film. There is less incentive to switch to extended processing for other films including double-emulsion Kodak T-Mat M film. [19] Therefore, selection of processing cycle should be influenced by the type of film being used.

**Table 5. Effect of Processing Time/Temperature on Sensitometric Indicators of Dose and Contrast for 3 Mammography Films**

|  | Relative Speed[1] | | Average Gradient | |
| --- | --- | --- | --- | --- |
| Processing time/temperature | 90 sec/94 F | 180 sec/95 F | 90 sec/94 F | 180 sec/95 F |
| **Film** | | | | |
| Kodak Min-R E | 100 | 128 | 3.0 | 3.6 |
| Kodak Min-R M | 117 | 141 | 2.8 | 3.0 |
| Dupont Microvision[2] | 85 | 96 | 3.1 | 3.4 |

1. All speeds compared with Kodak Min-R E film, 90 sec, 94 F processing
2. Version released in 1990
Data from Ref.[22]

Differences in response to extended processing can be explained by differences among the film emulsions. A double-emulsion film such as Kodak T-Mat film contains the same amount of silver as single-emulsion film, but it is divided between the two sides of the film. Since the emulsion can now be half as thick, the film is more fully developable in a shorter period of time. Accordingly, the benefit of extended processing is less with double-emulsion film. Similarly, the benefit of extended processing will be less on a film such as Dupont Microvision film where the grain size is relatively smaller and the silver is closer to the grain surface.

Radiologists should also be involved in the selection of a film processor. This responsibility should be accomplished more easily and objectively in the future when a set of criteria for processor performance is issued by the ACR.

Some processors can automatically switch back and forth from 90-second to extended cycles. Others can be modified to do so by means of an adaptor kit. Still other processors can be permanently changed to extended processing following installation of a gear change kit.

Selection of type of processor chemistry is also important since it will affect both film speed and contrast.[17]

## Selection and Supervision of the Q-A Technologist and Medical Physicist

The radiologist should also be responsible for the selection of a Q-A technologist and medical physicist who are motivated, reliable and fastidious and have the specialized knowledge to perform their tasks as described in the ACR Mammography Quality Control: Technologist Manual[23] and the Medical Physicist Manual,[24] respectively. Selection of appropriate individuals to fill these positions is really key to the success of the program. The Q-A technologist and medical physicist should have enough time and proper test equipment to perform these duties in a careful, thoughtful and unhurried manner.

Then, of course, the radiologist should lead or at least oversee the team effort in performing routine Q-A functions and in solving any technical problems by investigating their causes and taking corrective actions.[25] He/she should show interest and enthusiasm in processor Q-A, making it apparent that processing Q-A is a high-priority function. The radiologist should oversee such tasks as daily sensitometry, processor cleaning, preventive maintenance and chemical replenishment. He/she does not have to be there every time these occur, but must ensure that they are being performed as often as necessary and ought to know exactly how they are performed. He/she should review processor sensitometry results with the Q-A technologist at least weekly and should personally read the phantom radiographs every month. The radiologist certainly has to know the principles and practice of film processing and quality control. Besides the ACR Q-A Manuals, a number of other textbooks and practice manuals should be helpful in this regard.[23-29] Above all, the radiologist has to provide encouragement, supervision and support to everyone who is involved in the Q-A process.

## Selection of a Processor Service Company

Processor service companies differ in their reputation and in the quality of service they offer in terms of their willingness and ability to provide replenishment, cleaning and preventive maintenance as often as needed; reliability in adhering to their schedule; carefulness in adding chemicals; thoroughness in cleaning processors; skill in observing, reporting and solving mechanical problems. Most service companies are reputable, but some have been known to dilute chemistry or to substitute cheaper chemistry for brand name chemistry in order to cut costs. The radiologist should also determine if his/her processor service company is providing adequate service to produce the desired standard results from the chemistry being used. The means of determining this will be discussed later in this paper.

If the radiologist is not satisfied with the service which he/she is getting from the present company, he/she should first speak to the serviceperson and then to the manager, rather than switching to another company as the first step. The radiologist might think that another company can be expected to provide better service because another radiology practice group has been satisfied by them. However, the other group's impression might be based on their individual serviceperson who might not be representative of the general level of service offered by the company. Showing interest and letting the company know that the radiologist is aware of what they do, when they are supposed to do it, and how well they do it, are very important in getting them to perform their functions properly. The radiologist should get to know the companies, their personnel and the quality of their service and then select the one that performs its job best.

## Monitoring Clinical Image Quality

The radiologist has a unique role in this regard. Especially if he/she reads films from several mammographic rooms on line, the radiologist will probably appreciate artifacts and other technical problems before the technologist does. The radiologist also is in an ideal position to monitor clinical image quality because he/she should always compare the mammographic image to prior images for purposes of interpretation. In doing so, the radiologist should also observe how the technical quality of the current study compares to that of a previous one. If the contrast or density has changed for the worse, the radiologist should initiate an investigation to determine the cause.

## Future Responsibilities

Several developments could result in even better processor performance in the future and would entail only slightly additional responsibilities for the radiologist. One would be a comparison of an H&D curve for film processed at each clinical facility  to one of the same type film processed under optimized conditions at the manufacturer's laboratory. This is discussed further in the chapter titled "A Method of Verifying that Film is Providing Appropriate Speed and Contrast in the Clinical Environment" by Moore, et. al.  Another proposed Q-A measure would be a comparison of a stepped wedge density pattern on the clinical image to one on a control film.[30,31] After the mammogram is performed, a stepped-wedge pattern along with the patient's identification is flashed near the edge of the film (Figure 5) in the darkroom. The film is then processed. A record of processor performance is thus incorporated in each individual mammographic film. The stepped wedge image on the clinical mammographic film is then visually compared to a standard stepped wedge image. The system can be used to visually monitor processing throughout the day.

To evaluate this system further, an experiment was carried out to determine if radiologists could correctly assess processing changes by visual means rather than from densitometric readings.[32,33] Could a radiologist look at a pair of stepped wedge images and perceive very subtle differences in density?

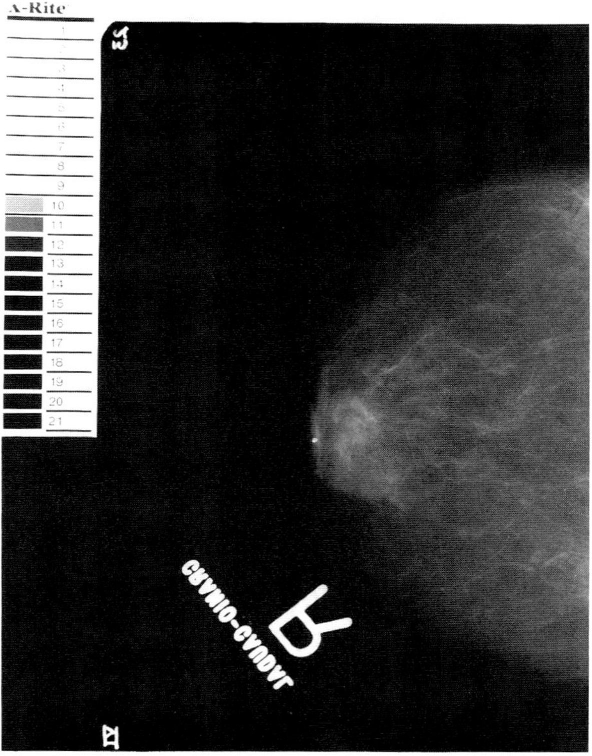

**Figure 5. Film containing clinical mammography image and stepped wedge pattern.**

In order to perform this experiment, it was necessary to use several different processing conditions. Films were exposed with a sensitometer and then developed using processors whose performances could be expected to differ from one another and from the one used for mammography. For this purpose, films exposed with a stepped wedge were developed in processors in our breast imaging center, nuclear medicine, radiation therapy, general radiology, angiography sections, etc. Each image was then compared visually by six different radiologists to an arbitrarily chosen standard stepped wedge image. It was found that each radiologist could ascertain a difference as low as 0.1 density unit. This indicated that a continuous visual monitoring system such as this is feasible in conjunction with daily sensitometry/densitometry.

If such a system were put into practice and the radiologist observed that density and/or contrast on a clinical mammogram was too low, he/she could then rule out or rule in processing as a potential cause. If the stepped wedge density comparison indicated proper processing, then the image deficiency would have to be due to some other cause such as suboptimal compression, x-ray exposure or to the film itself.

This system might also be used in an accreditation program in conjunction with phantom scores. If a stepped wedge image of this type was exposed along the side of the phantom image, it could be used to determine whether phantom image deficiencies might be due to processing.

## Conclusion

Processing is critically important in mammography because it may well be the weakest link in the imaging chain which can prevent early detection of breast cancer. Our goal should be to optimize processing to make sure that we are missing less and less in order to maximize the sensitivity of mammography and reduce breast cancer mortality. To this purpose, the  radiologist as well as the medical physicist, the technologist, industry, and radiologic organizations must all assume added responsibilities.

## References

1. Beahrs OH, Shapiro S, Smart CR: Report of the working group to review the National Cancer Institute - American Cancer Society Breast Cancer Detection Demonstration Projects. *J Natl Cancer Inst* 62:640-709, 1979

2. Baker LH: Breast Cancer Detection Demonstration Project - 5 year summary report. *CA-A Cancer Journal for Clinicians* 32:194-225, 1982

3. Roberts MM, Alexander FE, Anderson TJ, *et al*: Edinburgh trial of screening for breast cancer: Mortality at seven years. *Lancet* 335:241-246, 1990

4. Tabar L, Fagerberg G, Duffy SW, *et al*: Update of the Swedish Two-County Program of mammographic screening for breast cancer. *Radiol Clin of North Am* 30:187-210, 1992

5. Baines CJ, Miller AB, Kopans DB, *et al*: Canadian National Breast Screening Study. Assessment of technical quality by external review - *AJR* 155:743-747, 1990

6. Kopans DB:  The Canadian Screening Program: A different perspective. *AJR* 155:748-749, 1990

7. Merz B: Author of Canadian breast cancer study retracts warnings. *J. Natl Cancer Inst* 84:832-834, 1992

8. Miller AB, Baines CJ, To T, Wall C: The Canadian National Breast Screening Study [In] Cancer Screening [Ed by] Miller AB, Chamberlain J, Day NE, Hakama M, Prorok PC. New York: Cambridge University Press 1991, pp45-55

9. Galkin BM, Feig SA, Muir HD: The technical quality of mammography in centers participating in a regional breast cancer awareness program. *RadioGraphics* 8:133-145, 1988

10. Hendrick RE: Standardization of image quality and radiation dose in mammography. *Radiology* 174:648-654, 1990

11. Conway BJ, McCrohan JL, Rueter FG, *et al*: Mammography in the eighties. *Radiology* 177:335-339, 1990

12. Hendrick RE: Quality Assurance in mammography: Accreditation, legislation, and compliance with quality assurance standards. *Radiol Clin of North Am* 30:243-255, 1992

13. Physician Insurers Association of America: Breast Cancer Study, Lawrenceville NJ, 1990

14. Potchen EJ, Bisesi MA, Sierra A, Potchen JE: Mammography and malpractice. *AJR* 156:475-480, 1991

15. Brenner RJ: Medical legal aspects of screening mammography: A primer [In] Syllabus, Categorical Course in Breast Imaging [Ed by] Feig SA. Reston, VA: American Roentgen Ray Society 1988 pp 121-128

16. Brenner RJ: Medicolegal aspects of breast imaging. *Radiol Clin of North Am* 30:277-286, 1992

17. Kimme-Smith C, Rothschild PA, Bassett LW, *et al*: Mammographic film processor temperature, development time, and chemistry: Effect on dose, contrast, and noise. *AJR* 152:35-40, 1989

18. Haus AG: Technologic improvements in screen-film mammography. *Radiology* 174:629-637, 1990

19. Tabar L, Haus AG: Processing mammographic film: Technical and clinical considerations

20. Skubic SE, Yagan R, Oravec D, *et al*: Value of increasing film processing time to reduce radiation dose during mammography. *AJR* 155:1189-1193, 1990

21. Kimme-Smith C, Bassett LW, Gold RH, *et al*: Increased radiation dose at mammography due to prolonged exposure, delayed processing and increased film darkening. *Radiology* 178:387-391, 1991

22. Kimme-Smith C: Mammography screen-film selection, film exposure, and processing [In] Screen-Film Mammography: Imaging Considerations and Medical Physics Responsibilities [Ed by] Barnes GT, Frey GD. Madison WI, Medical Physics Publishing, 1991, pp 135-158

23. American College of Radiology Committee on Quality Assurance in Mammography: Mammography Quality Control: Radiologic Technologist's Manual. Reston VA: American College of Radiology, 1992

24. American College of Radiology Committee on Quality Assurance in Mammography: Mammography Quality Control: Medical Physicist's Manual. Reston VA: American College of Radiology, 1992

25. American College of Radiology Committee on Quality Assurance in Mammography: Mammography Quality Control: Radiologist's Manual. Reston VA: American College of Radiology, 1992

26. McKinney WEJ: Radiographic processing and quality control. Philadelphia: JB Lippincott, 1988

27. Wentz G: Mammography for Radiologic Technologists. New York: McGraw Hill, 1992

28. Andolina VF, Lille SL, Willison KM: Mammographic imaging: A Practical Guide. Philadelphia: JB Lippincott, 1992

29. Eastman Kodak Company: Mammography Quality Control Manual. Rochester NY: Eastman Kodak, 1990

30. Galkin BM, Feig SA, *et al*: Processor Control in Mammography. *Radiology* 173 (P):353, 1989.

31. Galkin Benjamin M., Method and apparatus for testing radiographic film

processors, United States Patent #5,063,583., 1991.

32. Feig SA, Galkin BM, Mendelson EB, *et al*: Evaluation of visual and quantitative methods for mammographic processor control. Program of the Ninetieth Annual Meeting. The American Roentgen Ray Society. Washington DC, 13-18 May 1990, paper number 113, p.162

33. Feig SA, Galkin BM, Mendelson EB, *et al*: A new method for processor control in mammography. Scientific exhibit no. 500. Program of the Ninetieth Annual Meeting, The American Roentgen Ray Society, Washington DC, 13-18 May 1990, paper number 113, p.312

# The Role of the Medical Physicist in Film Processing

**Joel E.Gray**
Department of Diagnostic Radiology
Mayo Clinic and Foundation
Rochester, Minnesota

## Introduction

The medical physicist serves multiple roles in the quality assurance and control programs in a modern diagnostic imaging department. First, and foremost, the medical physicist is responsible for the quality control program and the technical quality of the diagnostic images. Many of the tasks associated with such a program may be delegated to other physicists or radiologic technologists. The medical physicist also serves as a consultant to the radiologists, technologists, service engineers, and administration regarding the technical operation of the department. It is in this role which the responsibilities of the medical physicist in film processing will be discussed.

The medical physicist is responsible for many facets of the film processing programs in addition to conventional quality control. These responsibilities include, but are not limited to, the following:

- Monitoring of the processor quality control program including periodic review of QC charts and logs
- Selection of appropriate screen-film combinations, photographic chemistry, developer temperature, and immersion time
- Selection and quality control of sensitometers, densitometers, thermometers, etc.
- Storage of photosensitive materials
- Mixing and storage of chemicals
- Acceptance testing of photographic processors
- Silver recovery and pollution control

## Monitoring Processor Quality Control

It is essential that the medical physicist understand how to carry out processor quality control – and experience is the best teacher. Every physicist should carry out processor quality control on several processors for at least a month. This will provide insight into the problems associated with processor QC as well as the time and effort required of the QC technologist. Basic information regarding processor QC can be found in the literature.

Processor control charts are one of the primary tools in a processor QC program. A control chart (Figures 1, 2, and 3) is a plot of a measured variable (on the y axis) as a function of time (on the x axis). The measured variable, for example the mid-density (MD), has an operating level (the level at which the process should be operating), an upper control limit (UCL), and a lower control limit (LCL). The control limits indicate the point at which immediate action must be taken when the measured variable reaches, or exceeds, the respective limits. In other words, if the measured variable reaches or exceeds the limits, then the process is no longer considered to be "in control".

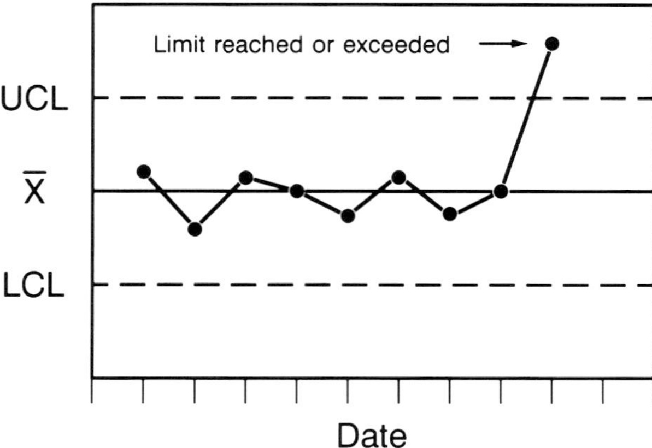


Figure 1. Control chart showing the lower limit (LTC), the operating level (or average value), and the upper control limit (UCL). Whenever the LCL or UCL is exceeded, immediate corrective action required.

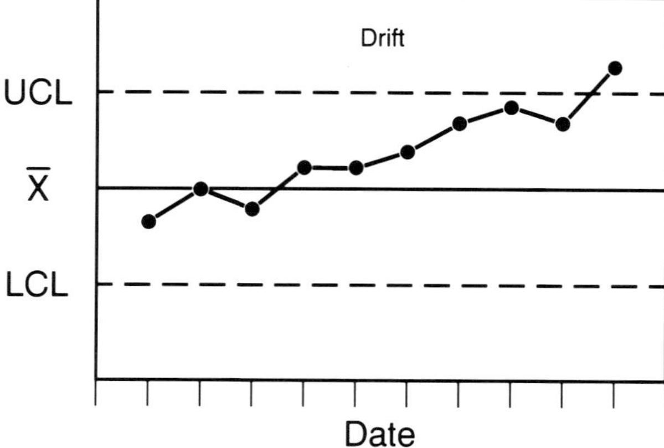


Figure 2. Control chart demonstrating drift and process which is out of control. Whenever drift is noted, i.e., whenever there are three or more consecutive data points moving in the same direction, the process is considered to be out of control and immediate corrective action is required.

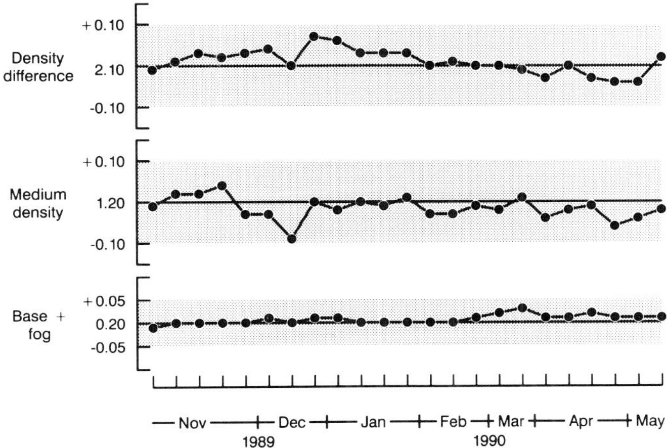


**Figure 3. Typical photographic processor control chart showing the stability of the process which can be achieved.**

For film processing, the selection of the operating level is critical since there are no specifications available from the film manufacturer which indicate what density levels should be obtained for a specific film, exposed with a sensitometer, and processed according to recommendations. Consequently, a specific procedure must be followed, using fresh chemistry, in order to establish the operating level.

The UCL and LCL are normally established statistically or based on experience with a process. In the case of photographic processor quality control, we know that the UCL and LCL should be set at 0.10 in density for the mid-density and density difference. For the base-plus-fog level (B+F) no LCL is needed. The UCL should be 0.03 for mammographic film and 0.05 for all other medical imaging films.

In addition to determining if a data point has reached or exceeded the control limits, one must look for trends in the data. Typically a trend is defined as a series of three or more points which are moving in the same direction (Figure 2). This usually indicates that the process is out of control even though the data points are still within the UCL and LCL. Since this process is "out of control," immediate corrective action is required.

It is essential that sensitometric control strips be exposed and processed, and that the densities be read and plotted *daily, immediately before clinical films are processed.* To be effective, quality control requires immediate feedback. If the strips are processed and the densities are read or plotted later, then the program is merely providing *quality monitoring, not quality control.*

Most important, it is essential to use the appropriate film for monitoring the photographic processor. The type of film processed in the processor for clinical applications should also be used for monitoring the processor. If more than one type of film is processed in a single processor, then it is necessary to monitor the processor with each type of film. Each film type may respond differently to changes in the processor because of the processing by-products from different films. In addition, some films are inherently less sensitive to changes in the developer chemistry and temperature than others. Consequently, sensitometric strips of one film type may indicate that the processor is in control while the processor may be out of control for another film type.

There are many problems and pitfalls associated with film processor QC of which the medical physicist should be aware. First of all, it is necessary to reduce the variability associated with the processing of sensitometric strips as much as possible. The lightest, or least exposed, end of the strip should be fed into the processor first. This minimizes the effect of "bromide drag" which results from the development by-products, reducing the developer activity on trailing steps of the sensitometric strip. The development by-products, primarily bromide ions, retard development and may not be efficiently removed from the film surface by some film processors.

The strip should be placed on the same side of the processor feed tray each time since there may be a slight temperature differential from one side of the processor to the other, or there may be differences in developer agitation. For single-emulsion films, the emulsion side should be oriented the same each time, i.e. emulsion up or down, to avoid slight agitation differences. Sensitometric strips should be exposed and processed immediately each day to avoid any changes in the latent image characteristics with time. If a delay between exposure and processing is necessary, then it should be the same each day.

Film is produced in batches and it is impossible to duplicate the film characteristics from batch-to-batch. Consequently, one or more boxes of the same emulsion number should be set aside for quality control purposes. Whenever it is necessary to change emulsion batches, it is essential to do a "crossover" comparison. Several sheets of the old emulsion number film should be processed at the same time as a similar number of sheets of the new emulsion number film. The mid-density value, density difference, and base-plus-fog levels of the two should be compared. If necessary the operating levels should be adjusted to reflect the differences in the emulsion batches (specific steps are provided in reference 1).

If the photographic process is "out of control," i.e., one of the control limits has been reached or exceeded, or a trend is apparent, then corrective action is required immediately. The developer temperature should be checked first. If it is correct, then the developer solution should be changed, replacing it with fresh solution and the specified amount of starter solution if recommended by the chemistry manufacturer. Developer is relatively inexpensive – a few dollars per gallon – so it is not cost effective to attempt to bring the processor back into control any other way. In other words:

**Don't mess around, change the chemistry!!**

## Selecting the Correct Screen-Film and Processor Combinations

For any application, it is essential to select the screen-film combination which is optimal for the clinical examination. This includes the correct matching of the screen and film in terms of spectral match, i.e., green-emitting screen with green-sensitive film, and film type, i.e., single screen with single-emulsion film.

Another important selection is the processing chemistry, photographic processor, solution temperature, and processing or immersion time.

### Use the chemicals, processor, solution temperature, and immersion time recommended by the film manufacturer!

This is essential in order to assure that the film-processing system is optimized. The film manufacturers cannot be expected to test their film with every possible combination of processing chemistry, processor, temperature, and immersion time available, especially if the chemistry is mixed locally by an x-ray equipment dealer. In addition, slight changes in film emulsion and developer chemistry will be made from time to time by the manufacturer. Such changes may affect some products adversely while improving other products.

In addition to proper selection of processing chemistry and conditions, it is essential to assure that a sufficient number of films are being processed in the processor each day. The recommended replenishment rates established by the manufacturer assume that a certain amount of film, of a specific type (dual- or single-emulsion), exposed to a typical average density, is being processed each day. Normally the replenisher rates are established assuming that 25 to 50, 14 x 17-inch, dual-emulsion films, or the equivalent, exposed to an average density of about 1.25, are processed each day. If this is not the case, then the films should be processed in a processor where such volume is achievable or processor stability cannot be assured.

There are two options which may help stabilize processing conditions. First of all, a "standby system" should be installed on the processor. This system automatically turns off all processor functions, except the developer temperature control, when the processor has not been used for a predetermined period of time. This reduces developer oxidation, power and water consumption, and processor wear. In fact, all processors should be equipped with such systems. Second, one may use flood replenishment. This technique adds a set amount of developer and fixer replenisher to the processor at specified time intervals. The intent is to completely replace the developer solution every 8 to 16 working hours. This, obviously, increases chemistry consumption but also provides a stable processing environment which may be impossible otherwise. (The developer replenisher in this case is a combination of the conventional replenisher and the amount of developer starter solution specified by the chemistry manufacturer, e.g., fresh developer solution.)

## Selection and Quality Control of Sensitometers, Densitometers and Thermometers

The equipment used for film processor quality control must be selected carefully. Most importantly, the quality control equipment must also be monitored by a quality control program.

The sensitometer should be selected so that its exposure matches the characteristics of the film being exposed. If green-sensitive film is being exposed, then the sensitometer should emit primarily green light. If red- or infrared-sensitive films are being used, then the sensitometer match presently available is one which utilizes a tungsten light source. Some newer films are designed to work with ultra-violet emitting screens. Unfortunately, there is no sensitometer available which can produce a spectrum which matches the emission from these screens. In this case the closest match would be with a sensitometer with a blue emission spectrum.

If dual-emulsion film is being exposed, then a sensitometer which exposes both sides of the film simultaneously is required. This is particularly important with films which have low, or no, crossover exposure. If a single-sided sensitometer is used with such dual-emulsion films the characteristic curve will have a unique shape and, due to this shape, the film may be less sensitive to changes in the developer solution than if it were exposed with a dual-sided sensitometer.

The densitometer should use a "white" light source and geometry as specified in the appropriate standard. There have been some changes in the standard for illumination and collection geometry over the past few years. Densitometers designed under the old and new standards may exhibit some differences in measured density, especially at lower densities. This should not pose a problem for quality control purposes but one should be aware that comparing density measurements with different densitometers may give somewhat different results.

Temperature measurements should be made with an accurate thermometer. i.e., one with a specified accuracy of $\pm 0.2°F$ or better. These thermometers can be relatively expensive. However, oral medical thermometers, which cost about $10.00, are available with this accuracy. Care must be taken when using oral thermometers to assure that the "peak hold" feature does not give an erroneous reading. In addition, the user must be aware that these thermometers will not register temperatures below the specified minimum.

The temperature indicated by thermometers built into processors should not be trusted unless the thermometer has been compared to, and calibrated with, a thermometer of known accuracy. However, the built-in thermometer can be used as a quick means to check the stability of the processor.

Quality control of sensitometers is difficult. Many do not provide easy access to the light sources so it is difficult or impossible to measure the light output. In addition, most photometers do not provide an "integrate" mode, and those that do may not be sensitive enough to measure the small amount of light emitted by the sensitometer during a typical exposure. The easiest means of providing processor quality control for sensitometers is by a direct comparison between two sensitometers using film. This method will at least indicate if there is a significant change in the relative output of the sensitometers since the last evaluation. Most importantly, if the output of one sensitometer is suspect, then a quick comparison with a second sensitometer will at least indicate if major problems exist. Sensitometers should be cross compared at least annually.

Densitometer quality control is quite simple and should be carried out on a monthly basis and the results recorded on a control chart. Calibrated step wedges are normally provided when the densitometer is purchased. These should be stored in a safe place and used sparingly, i.e., annually, to verify the condition of the densitometer. Uncalibrated step wedges can be purchased and calibrated to the "standard" wedge. These "secondary standards" can be used on a monthly basis to monitor the densitometer accuracy. In addition, one may wish to have a "tertiary standard" available for daily checks of the densitometer. In this case it is not necessary to use a step wedge. The tertiary standard may consist of only a few densities, one of which should be in the range of 1.20 to 1.50. For monthly QC checks it is suggested that at least four steps covering the normal density range be monitored, e.g., densities of 0.25, 1.00, 2.00, and 2.75.

## Storage of Photosensitive Materials

Photographic materials are photosensitive. This means that they are sensitive to light, heat, humidity, chemical contamination, mechanical stress, and radiation. Film should be stored at temperatures below $75^O$ F and preferably between $60^O$ and $70^O$ F. Open packages of film should be stored in an area where the humidity is between 40 and 60%.

Photographic materials should be stored away from chemical fumes or radiation. Radiation includes radionuclides, radioactive wastes, and direct or scattered x rays. Since films are pressure sensitive, boxes of film should always be stored standing on end. Two or three boxes of films stacked horizontally can result in pressure artifacts.

## Mixing and Storage of Chemicals

There are four key words in working with photographic chemicals:

### Follow the manufacturer's instructions!

If specific temperatures are given for the water used to dilute concentrated chemicals, then the water temperature should be at the specified temperature. The exact amount of water specified for dilution should be used.

Sensitometric testing is the only way to determine if the chemistry has been mixed properly. Although specific gravity and pH have been suggested, neither of these measures provides a complete analysis of the chemistry, especially the sensitometric activity. The specific gravity only indicates the amount of material in solution. A solution of sugar water can have the same specific gravity as a properly mixed developer solution. The pH is not a good measure of developer activity since developer is a highly buffered solution. In addition, not all of the components are equally sensitive to changes in pH. In one study, contamination of the developer with fixer solution (about 30ml of fixer in 10,000 ml of developer solution) showed virtually no change in pH while changes, i.e., increases, in the mid-density of about 0.50 were evident. Sensitometric testing is the only method available to determine if the photographic developer activity is correct. It is prudent to sensitometrically test batches of freshly mixed chemicals, especially if the chemicals are mixed in bulk and distributed to many processors in the radiology department.

Chemicals, either concentrated or diluted working solutions, should not be allowed to freeze. All chemicals should be stored at temperatures between $60^{\circ}$ and $70^{\circ}$ F. Chemicals should not be stored in direct sunlight. Discoloration or sedimentation of photographic chemicals indicates that some components have oxidized or have precipitated out of solution. In either case, the chemicals should not be used and should be returned to the dealer. Working solutions should be used within one to two weeks in order to avoid any oxidation or deterioration in the quality of the chemicals.

Unfortunately, most institutions pay very little attention the photographic chemistry they purchase. How does the institution know exactly what they are purchasing? How does the dealer determine if the sensitometric activity of the developer is correct? Photographic chemistry is relatively inexpensive, usually less than 5% of the total film and chemistry budget. Consequently, it is not prudent to purchase such a critical component, one which is the final element in the diagnostic imaging chain and the one which is most likely to cause problems, on a low bid basis. Any institution which is quality minded should purchase the concentrated photographic chemistry *recommended by the film manufacturer* and carefully mix the working chemistry solutions according to the manufacturer's instructions.

## Acceptance Testing of Photographic Processors

Acceptance testing of photographic processors is the most overlooked step in most quality control programs. An excellent discussion of processor acceptance testing is provided in reference 6.

First and foremost, it is essential to read and understand the manufacturer's documentation. Prior to installation, the adequacy of the utilities, darkroom and work space should be reviewed. Simple checks include determining if the processor is physically level when installed. The temperature stability should be checked using a chart-recording thermometer. The recirculation system should be checked along with the agitation of the developer solution. Water flow rates should be verified. Developer immersion time, dryer temperature and function, and standby function should be checked. All indicator lights should be checked to verify proper functioning and, most importantly, to assure that the indicator lights on the darkroom side of the processor do not fog film. Possible film fog due to the indicator lights should be tested for all types of film which will be used in the darkroom, including blue-, green-, red-, and infrared-sensitive films. Last but not least, films should be uniformly exposed and processed to determine if the processing is uniform and to detect the presence of any processing artifacts.

A frequent problem in film processor installation is the venting of the dryer. The dryer vent should be installed according to the manufacturer's specifications. In some cases, this includes a connection to the building venting system with a special connector which is not completely sealed. The purpose of this connection is to assure that adequate airflow occurs in the correct direction so that too much air is not drawn through the processor (making temperature control a problem) and that air is not forced back through the processor from the building venting system.

Once proper installation has been verified, it is time to check the total processing system sensitometrically. In addition, a regularly scheduled program of preventive maintenance should be established. Procedures should also be developed to assure that the cross-over racks are cleaned when the processor is shut off each day and that clean-up films are run each morning after the processor has reached operating temperatures. The clean-up films should be inspected for processing artifacts or other obvious problems.

## Silver Recovery and Pollution Control

Silver, discharged in the fixer overflow, is considered a pollutant by today's environmental standards. Even though the price of silver is relatively low, the recovery of silver is cost effective and is essential as part of a pollution control program. Federal and state standards are rapidly changing relatively to the amount of silver which may be allowed in the effluent. Typically 5 milligrams of silver per liter of solution (5 parts per million, or ppm) is considered acceptable, although some states are considering lower levels such as 0.5 ppm or 0.05 ppm – that's 50 parts per billion! (It has been suggested that the city water supplied to a building may contain this amount of silver, or more!)

The abatement of silver pollution should be done actively and prospectively, before pollution control agencies decide to inspect a facility. For example, a sampling point should be located where one can easily sample the effluent. This should not be at the point where the silver recovery equipment empties into the building drain. The sampling point should be located such that it can take advantage of the dilution of the photographic chemicals by all of the other solutions discharged by the facility, i.e., at the property line.

In addition to the recovery of silver, other points should be considered in the design or remodeling of photographic processing facilities. Separate returns should be provided to a central location from the photographic processor. The overflow fixer should be returned in a separate pipe; the developer overflow should be returned separately; and the overflow wash water should be returned separately. This redundant plumbing may prove useful in the future when stricter standards are implemented. For example, the overflow fixer should be processed to remove as much silver as possible. In the future it may be necessary to mix the overflow developer with the used fixer (after removal of the silver) to help neutralize the basic developer and acidic fixer, and it may be necessary to recover silver from the wash water. In addition, the wash water stream can be used to further dilute the processed, used fixer solution.

There are three basic processes which can be used to recover silver from the fixer solution – ion exchange, metallic replacement, and electrolytic recovery. Ion exchange systems can recover silver down to the 1 ppm level or less and can recover silver from the wash water. However, they are relatively complex, space consuming, and costly. Ion exchange systems require some sophistication to operate properly.

Metallic replacement uses a cell in which iron (in the form of steel wool) is replaced by metallic silver. If these are not used properly, channeling may occur which allows the silver-laden fixer to flow directly through the cells. The efficiency of this process is quite low. It is necessary to ship the containers for recovery; this may have implications with regard to hazardous material transportation. Finally, the silver compounds in the container must go through a costly refining process, thereby reducing the financial benefits of silver recovery.

Electrolytic silver recovery uses a process whereby nearly pure metallic silver is electrolytically plated onto metallic plates in the recovery cell. This is a relatively efficient process which results in high purity silver, not requiring extensive refining. These systems can be operated in "flow through" or "batch" mode, with the batch processing systems providing the highest recovery efficiency. Automated batch recovery systems are available. For most facilities, batch electrolytic silver recovery systems should be the system of choice.

Fixer solutions overflowing from the fixer tank in the processor contain between 1 and 5 grams of silver per liter. Flow-through electrolytic recovery systems are capable of recovering silver down to 250 to 500 milligrams per liter. Batch mode electrolytic systems can recover down to 50 to 100 milligrams of silver per liter. If the pH of the fixer is adjusted prior to electrolytic recovery, it is possible to recover down to 2 to 10 milligrams of silver per liter.

The measurement of these low silver concentrations is not easy. Commercially available test papers are capable of making rough measurements only prior to silver recovery, i.e., they can measure down to about one gram per liter. Metallic test strips are available which can estimate silver content down to about 5 to 10 milligrams per liter. However, it is necessary to use sophisticated analytic chemistry techniques to reliably measure silver concentrations at the part-per-million level. Even analytical chemistry techniques may not be accurate if the appropriate reagents are not used.

## Summary

In summary, film processing is the last link in the diagnostic imaging chain. Unfortunately, it is often the most neglected element, and the one upon which all other links depend on the production of high quality diagnostic images. QC really means more than quality control.

QC MEANS QUALITY CULTURE

If one...

| | |
|---|---|
| Thinks | QUALITY |
| Plans for | QUALITY |
| And makes | QUALITY |
| | |
| Then you will get | QUALITY |

## References


1. American College of Radiology Committee on Quality Assurance in Mammography, Mammography Quality Control for RadiologicTechnologists, American College of Radiology, Reston, Virginia, 1990.

2. Frank ED, Gray JE, Wilken DA. Flood Replenishment: A New Method of Processor Control. *Radiologic Technology* 1980, 52:271-275.

3. Kofler JM Jr, Gray JE. Sensitometric Responses of Selected Medical Radio-graphic Films. *Radiology* 1991; 181:879-883.

4. American National Standards Institute. Photographic Density Measurements Geometric Conditions for Transmission Density, ANSI PH2. 19-1986. American National Standards Institute, 1430 Broadway, New York, NY 10018.

5. Stears JG, Gray JE, Winkler NT. Evaluation of pH Monitoring as a Method of Processor Control. *Radiologic Technology* 1979, 50:657-663.

6. Wagner LK. Acceptance Testing and QC of Film Transport and Processing Systems. Proceedings of the AAPM 1991 Summer School "Specification, Acceptance Testing, and Quality Control of Diagnostic X-ray Imaging Equipment," University of California – Santa Cruz, July, 1991, In Press, American Institute of Physics, New York.

# The Role of the Technologist in Film Processing

**Kathleen M. Willison**
Elizabeth Wende Breast Clinic of Rochester
Rochester, New York

The radiologic technologist plays a major role in film processing to produce quality images. Diagnostic quality guarantees that images are being attained at minimal dose and cost. Critical to diagnostic quality is understanding that even with the best radiographic equipment, screen/film combinations, positioning methods and technical application, all is lost if the processing system fails for any reason. The technologist, as the prime user of the processor, has a great responsibility.

To have confidence that the best a processing system has to offer is being achieved, comprehensive knowledge of the processor and its part in the imaging chain is essential. The key word is best – for many processing systems are set up, used or maintained inadequately, sometimes unbeknownst to the users. Expertise or at least a working knowledge in the areas described below is crucial to developing confidence in the processing system – a system with fewer problems and one requiring less effort to diagnose problems. Finally, while there always seems to be one technologist in every department who has a wealth of information about processing, it is every technologist's responsibility to be informed.

## Manufacturer, Dealer and Servicing Organization

The technologist should be aware of the responsibilities and limitations of the processor manufacturer, the film manufacturer, the equipment manufacturer, the dealer and the servicing organization. The support personnel connected with these organizations (if reputable) are an excellent source of information for new products, product applications and troubleshooting. Do not hesitate to call upon them, but be aware of their limitations and, also, of your responsibility to be informed. When severe or seemingly unsolvable problems occur, it is helpful to involve all simultaneously in order to arrive at a workable solution.

## Intended Application and Compatibility

When choosing a processor, consider the type of film as determined by the type of radiographic study to be processed. Daily throughput will also be a consideration.

Finally, purchase film, photochemicals and the processor from the same manufacturer who has developed the components as a compatible system.

If a processing system is chosen with the above in mind, many problems that occur due to incompatibility will be avoided.

## Proper Installation

Processing difficulties related to poor installation can develop immediately after installation, but they can also have a cumulative effect, not identified until many months later. While the technologist may not have indepth knowledge of the following areas, he or she can at least follow the recommendations of the manufacturer. Also take into account the dealership installing the processor: are they reputable; are they authorized dealers for the manufacturer; and are they familiar with the application for which the processor is being used?

The technologist should be aware of the following elements involved in processor installation.

1.  Plumbing requirements (into and out of the processor)
2.  Electrical requirements
3.  Ventilation of the Processor
4.  Darkroom Integrity

The final two elements are often overlooked. Ventilation of the processor is critical to maintaining image quality. Without proper ventilation, unpleasant fumes can build up. Also, chemicals in an unvented or poorly vented processor will evaporate and cause condensation, contamination of chemicals, and streaking artifacts. Follow the manufacturer's recommendations. Additionally, ventilation is used for the removal of a portion of the processors heat output. High humidity and high temperature will make the workplace most unpleasant.

Every technologist should be concerned about darkroom integrity:

•   Air quality - this includes the temperature, the amount of humidity in the air, airflow through the darkroom, and air "cleaning." All darkroom's air systems should be equipped with a thermometer, hygrometer (Figure 1), a humidifier, dehumidifier, and an air purifier. (Table 1)

•   Lighting - use appropriate safelights with the correct bulb wattage. A 15-watt bulb is recommended for safelights 4 feet above the working surface; use a 7-watt bulb for closer distances. A darkroom fog test should be done semiannually to check the integrity of the safelights and the light tightness of the darkroom.

•   Cleanliness and storage - clean the darkroom daily to maintain as dust-free an environment as possible. Storage should be kept to a minimum. Film should always be stored upright (not flat) to avoid pressure marks and pick-off. Open shelves, carpeting and unpacking of boxes, all create dust in the darkroom and dirt artifacts on film, and should be avoided.

**Table 1**

| Recommended equipment | Purpose | When to use |
|---|---|---|
| Thermometer | Monitors temperature | 24 hours a day. Keep temperatures at or below 70°F (temperatures above 70°F can affect how well a film keeps). |
| Hygrometer | Monitors humidity | 24 hours a day. |
| Humidifier | Moistens the air | When hygrometer reads below 50% RH to eliminate chance of static artifact. Filter must be cleaned periodically. |
| Dehumidifier | Removes moisture from the air. | When hygrometer reads above 50% RH to eliminate clumping artifacts due to moisture. Filter must be cleaned periodically. |
| Air Purifier | Cleans the air | 24 hours a day to combat dust. Filters must be cleaned periodically. |

## Processor Components and Functions

While it is not within the scope of this paper to detail the internal subsystems of the processor, it is at least important to mention them. The technologist should have an understanding and, if possible, a "working" knowledge of:

1. The transport system (which includes the feed tray, roller racks, guide shoes, crossovers and the dryer) that moves the film through the processor. Additionally, this film movement provides agitation for even chemical distribution, developing and fixing. The roller racks are also responsible for agitation of the chemicals at the films surfaces and also act as a squeegee to remove chemicals from the film.

2.   The recirculation and replenishment systems (which include pumps, heaters and filters) keep the chemicals at recommended temperatures while also providing even mixing and distribution.

The replenishment system (and replenishment rate) is often overlooked, but is often the culprit in processing dilemmas.  (See later discussion under principles of film processing.)

3.   Processing stages (developer, fixer, wash and dryer).  Knowing what takes place in each of the processing stages will help in sorting out processing problems.

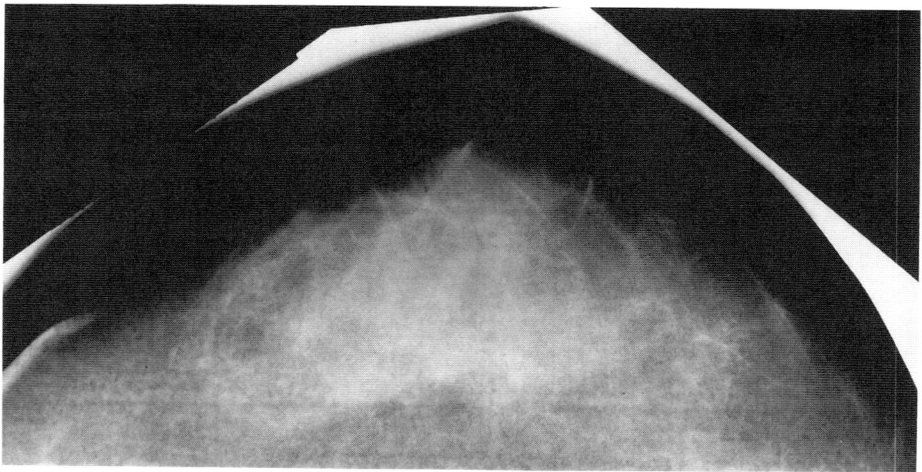

**Figure 1. An hygrometer to monitor humidity in the darkroom will help prevent this type of plus-density artifact, due to silver clumps caused by excessive humidity.**

## Film Travel through the Processor

Knowing the path of film travel through the processor will help in solving artifact problems (Figure 2).  It is helpful to know what parts of the transport system come into contact with the film, especially for single-emulsion films where artifacts are more readily noticed.  Films run emulsion side up have more roller contact, while films run emulsion side down have more contact with guide shoes.  Plus-density artifacts occur in the developer; minus-density artifacts occur in the fixer.  Always consider handling problems when trying to get at the source of artifacts.  Arthur Haus and Edward Hendrick suggest that two films be run perpendicular to one another; the artifact is caused by the processor if it is in the same direction on both films. Handling artifacts can confuse the issue of where the artifact originated (Figures 3, 4, 5, 6). Handling artifacts that occur before the exposure are minus-density; those occurring after the exposure are plus-density. Most processing artifacts tend to be linear in one direction whereas handling artifacts rarely are.

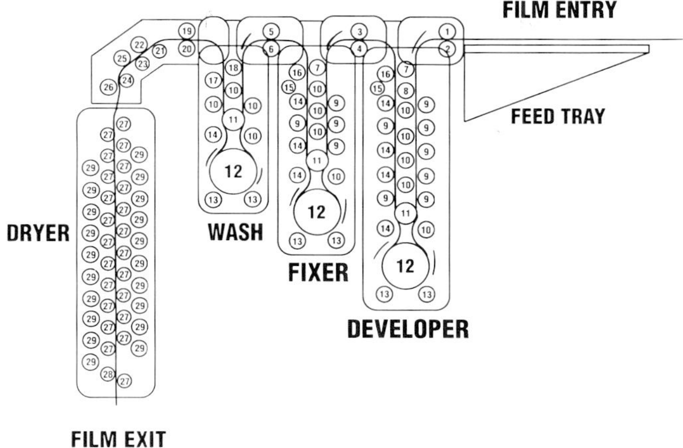


Figure 2. Be acquainted with the path that a film travels in the processor and where contact is made with various parts. (Reprinted with permission from Haus, A.G., Batz, T.A., Dickerson, R.E., Lillie, R.F., Oemcke, K.W., and Lanphear, J.D: Automating film processing in medical imaging. In Siebert, J.A., Barnes, G.T., and Gould, R.G: Specification, Acceptance Testing and Quality Control of Diagnostic X-Ray Imaging Equipment. American Institute of Physics, New York, NY, 1992.)

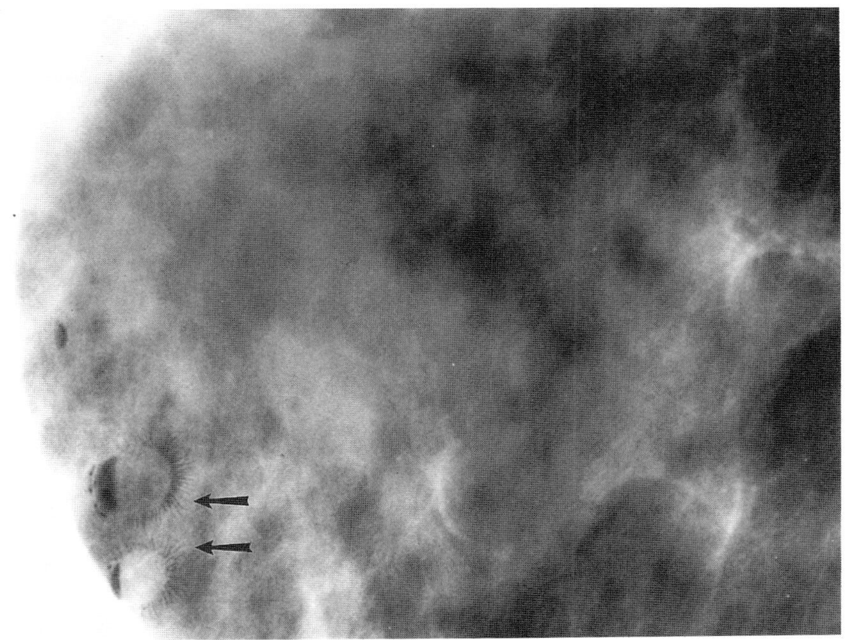

Figure 3. Handle films by the corners. Finger prints (arrows) imposed after exposure can leave these static type of plus-density artifacts.

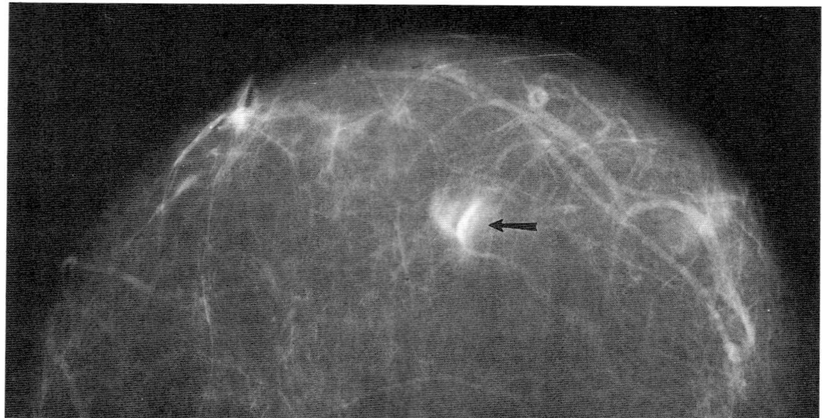

Figure 4. Handling artifacts can be easily avoided.  This minus-density artifact is a fingernail crimp imposed before exposure during cassette loading.

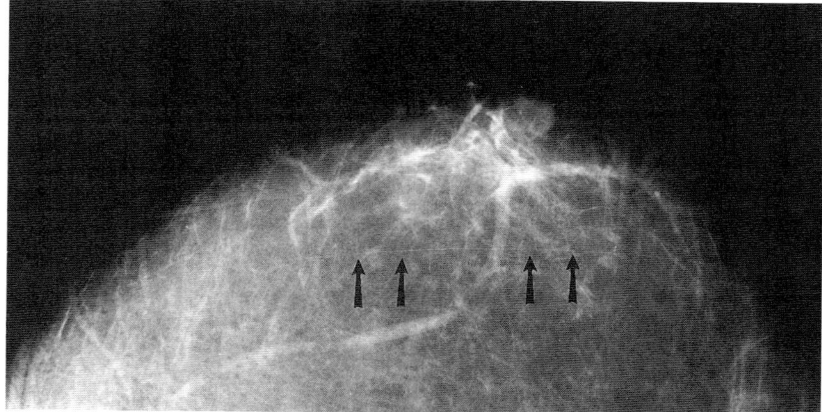

Figure 5. This arbitrary minus-density artifact was caused by nail polish on the intensifying screen.

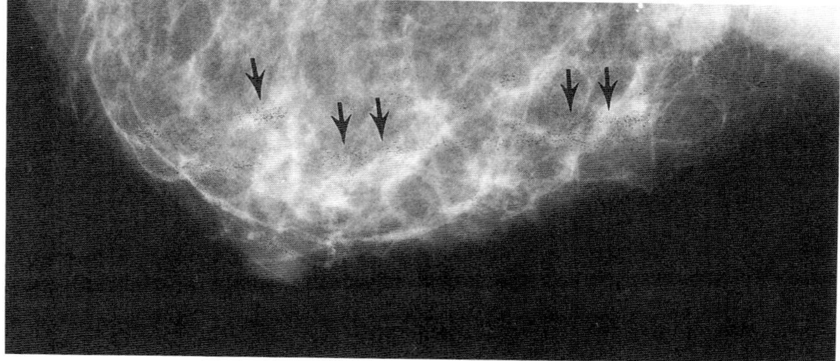

Figure 6. This plus-density was due to insufficient drying of the intensifying screen after cleaning.

## Maintenance and Care Procedures

Maintenance and processor care include not only daily, weekly and monthly cleaning of various components, but also testing of the processor (Figures 7, 8, 9, 10). The technologist should know these responsibilities, outlined in Table 2, regardless of who is responsible for them. Proper maintenance and care not only assure proper processing, but also increase the life of some processor components. Sensitometry should be carried out prior to processing any patient films so that any dilemmas can be resolved. The most sensitive film in the darkroom (usually single-emulsion film for mammography) should be used for sensitometry. Consistency in method is critical so one person should be responsible for this task. While sensitometry guarantees that a certain level of consistency is maintained, it does not guarantee that the level is the best the processing system has to offer.

**Table 2. Maintenance & Care Procedures for the Processor**

|  | **Technologist** | **Servicing Organization** |
|---|---|---|
| **Daily** | **Beginning of Day:**<br>• Roller transport cleanup film<br>• (never reuse film) to remove<br>• buildup of chemicals, dirt, etc.<br>• Sensitometry - carrying it out<br>• interpretation and recording.<br><br>**End of day:**<br>• Wash both developer and fixer crossovers<br>• with a soft cloth and warm water.<br>• Clean darkroom.<br>• When turned off at the end of the day,<br>• vent processor by leaving lid ajar, but do<br>• not completely uncover. |  |
| **Weekly** | • Remove, wash and dry developer and<br>• fixer racks to clear away chemical buildup.<br>• Clean intensifying screens. |  |
| **Monthly** |  | • Check replenishment rates<br>• Change chemical (with starter)<br>• Clean processor tanks, racks<br>• Change developer filter cartridge<br>• Replace worn parts<br>• Other |
| **Quarterly** | Fixer retention analysis |  |

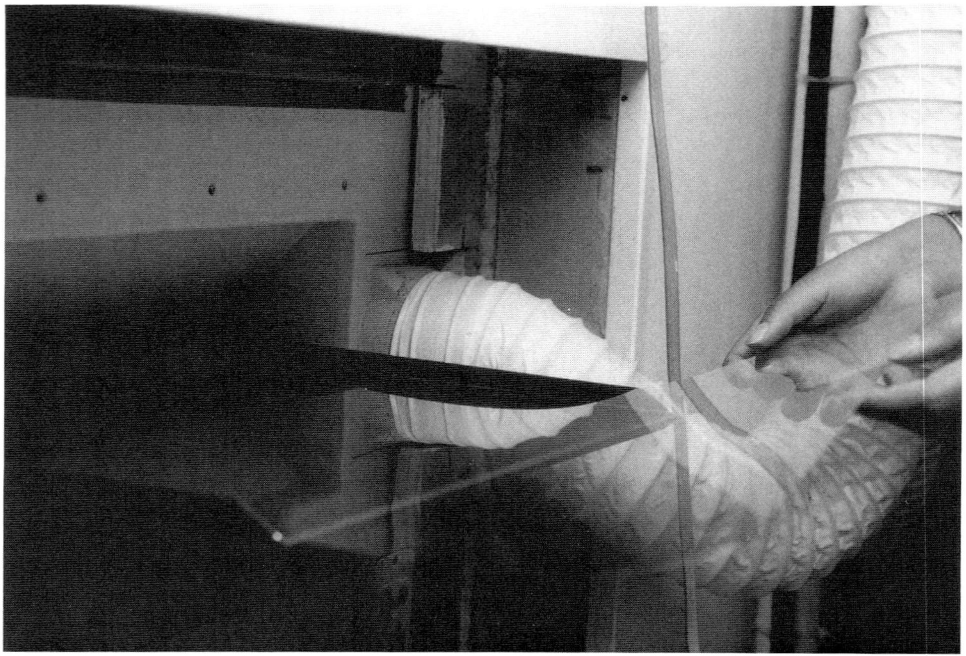

Figure 7. Use of roller transport cleanup film (Eastman Kodak Company) in the morning prior to processing patients' films to remove sediment that might have built up overnight. Roller transport cleanup film is also useful after a processor jam has been cleared.

## Principles of Film Processing

In order to insure that the processor is producing an optimal image, it is important to understand screen/film combinations and processing options. The effects of various processing chemistries and processing parameters, including development time, temperature and replenishment rates, must be taken into consideration. It is necessary to know how these elements work together to form the resulting image.

Each film is designed with a specific H&D curve (the relationship between exposure and the resulting image) and average gradient (contrast property of the film). These values are derived from the sensitometric strip and describe a film's characteristics with optimum processing. How close a processing system can come to producing these same characteristics depends on how the following parameters are chosen and how well they work together. Unfortunately, cost is often the deciding factor in choosing a certain element in a system; however, initial cost must be compared to the overall cost of problem solving when incompatibility occurs.

• Intensifying screen - the screen chosen must be compatible with the film. Often a screen/film combination is chosen based on dose or speed. While these may be positive attributes, they are usually selected at the risk of losing detail and/or contrast.

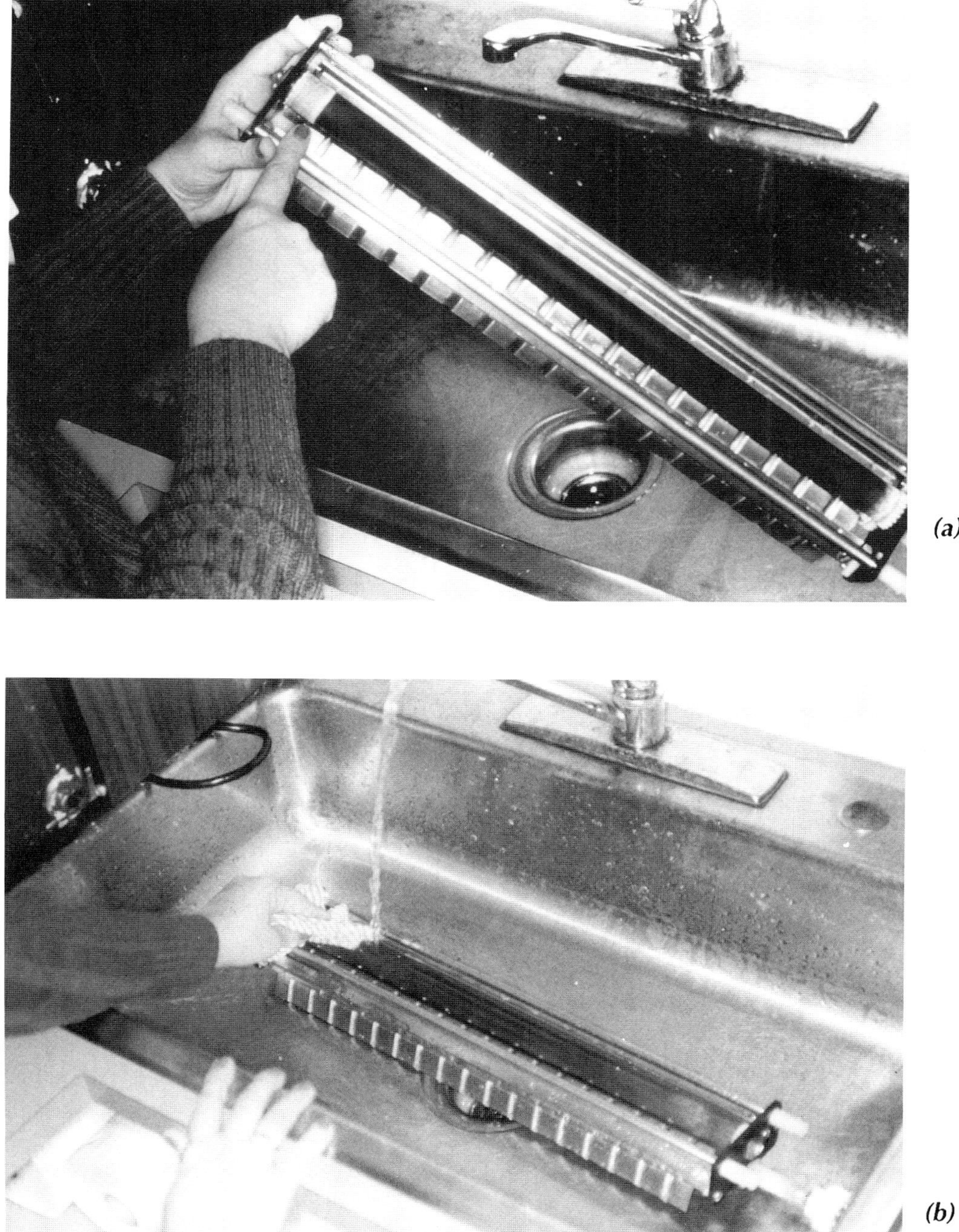

Figure 8. Oxidation of chemicals that occurs on the crossover rollers, must be removed daily with a soft cloth to avoid buildup and artifacts.

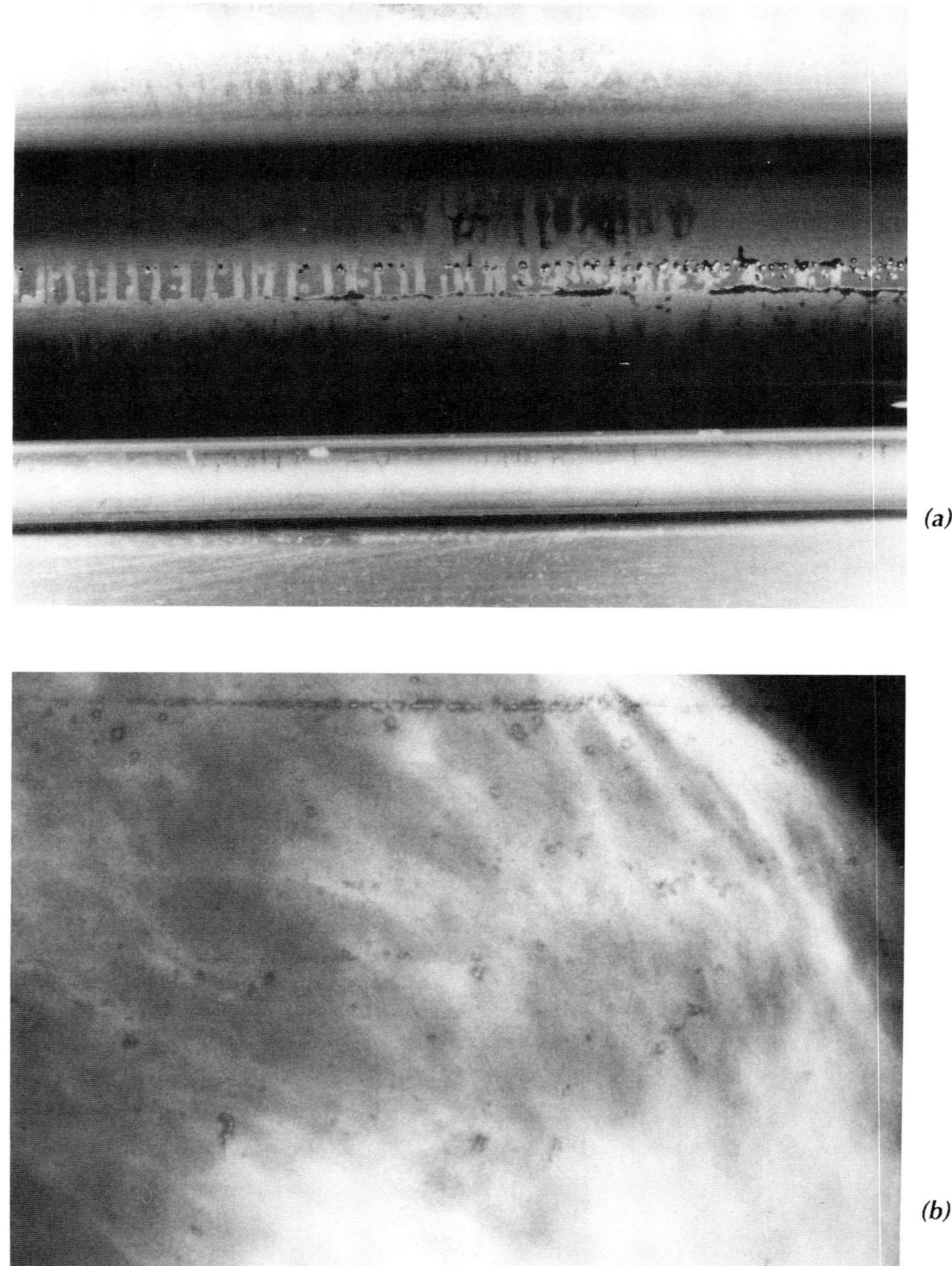

Figure 9. One week's buildup of chemical on the developer rollers (a) caused the plus-density artifacts on this patient's film (b).

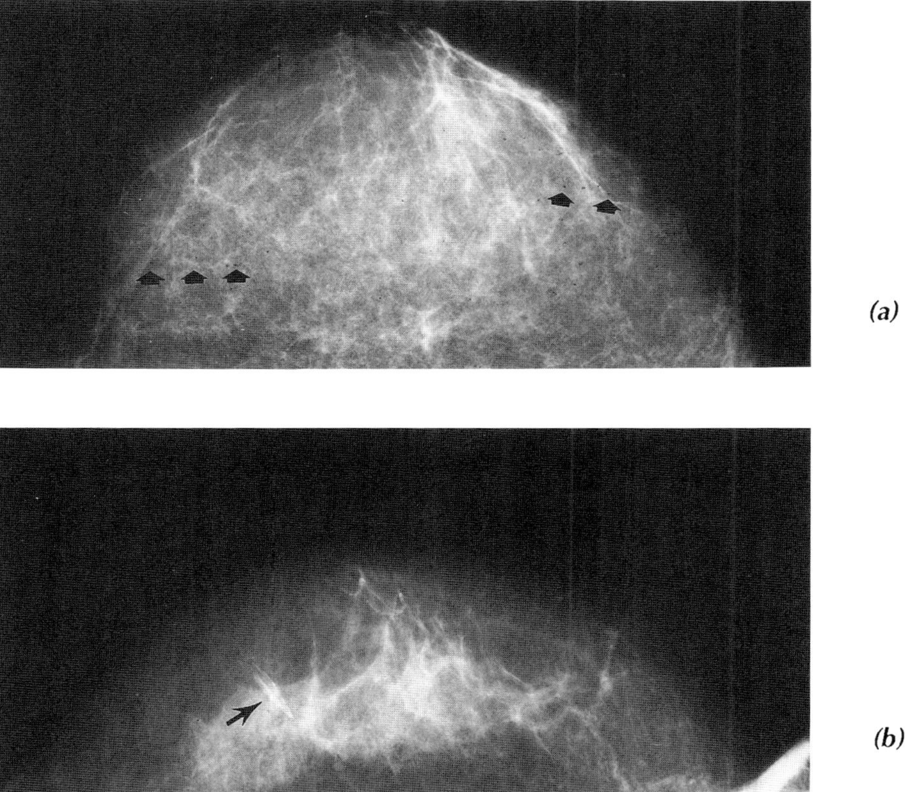



**Figure 10. Daily cleaning of the crossovers is critical. This artifact was caused by bubbles of oxidized chemical bursting on the film at contact (a), and (b) buildup of hardened oxidized chemical that broke off and fell into the developer, causing scratching of the emulsion. These types of artifacts are often intermittent and hard to track down.**

• Processing option - available now is the choice of standard or extended processing. Standard processing has a development time of 19-23 seconds, where extended processing has a development time of approximately 43 seconds. Many people have the misconception that a long run time of 2 1/2 or 3 minutes indicates extended processing; however, it is developer time or a combination of developer time and temperature that denotes the extended cycle. When choosing a processing option, be sure the film is compatible with that type of processing.

• Chemistry - the brand of chemistry used will affect the resulting image. A "systems" approach is recommended whenever possible. This means that a specific manufacturer's film should be used with the same manufacturer's chemistry (Figure 11). This not only produces the best a film can offer, but also makes problem-solving less complicated. Matching chemistry is especially critical for single-emulsion films

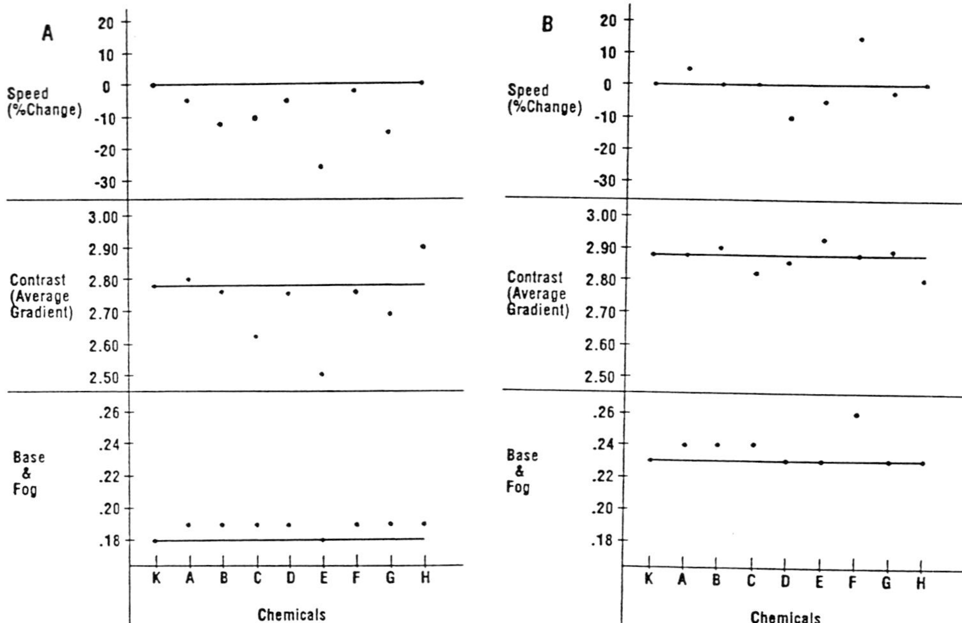


Figure 11. Charts produced from film processing survey data charts which show film processing variations due to use of different chemicals; data shown are for Kodak ortho M film SO-177 (Figure 11A) and Kodak T-Mat G film (Figure 11B). The letter K indicates processing data (and expected values) using Kodak processor and Kodak chemicals. A horizontal line is drawn through the letter K. Letters A through H are data for different brands of chemicals. Data were obtained using film strips which were sensitometrically pre-exposed to light that simulates the light spectrum from Kodak Lanex screens. Film speed differences, film contrast (average gradient) and base plus fog values were determined from the sensitometry data. (Reprinted with permission from Haus, A.G., Batz, T.A., Dickerson, R.E., Lillie, R.F., Oemcke, K.W., and Lanphear, J.D: Automating film processing in medical imaging. In Siebert, J.A., Barnes, G.T., and Gould, R.G: Specification, Acceptance Testing and Quality Control of Diagnostic X-Ray Imaging Equipment. American Institute of Physics, New York, NY, 1992.)

in those studies where detail is critical. In addition, conscientious chemistry mixing and replenishment rate checks will ultimately determine how well the chemistry works. If there is concern that chemistry has been incorrectly mixed, then both pH and specific gravity measurements can be determined. These values should be compared to the manufacturer's recommended levels and corrective action taken if necessary.

• Processing parameters - attention to development time, temperature, and replenishment rate is critical to producing a consistent quality image. Manufacturer's recommendations should be followed for development cycle and temperature setting. Replenishment rates are set according to film size, the orientation of the film, type of film (single- or double-emulsion), type of examination and the number of films processed in a specific time period. For low volumes, flooded replenishment (where the developer and fixer replenish automatically at regular time intervals) is recommended to maintain consistent sensitometric levels.

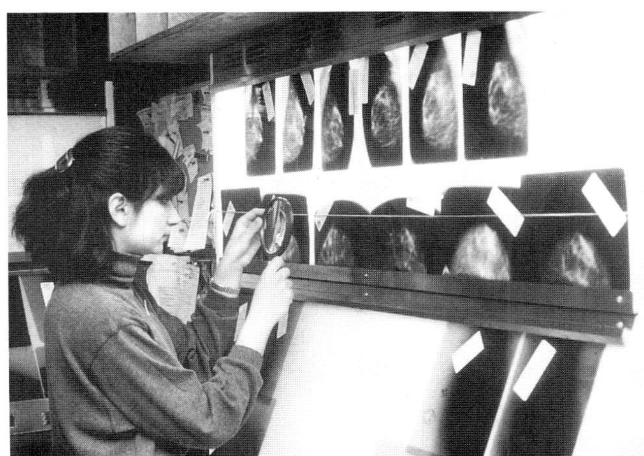

**Figure 12. Daily use of a magnifying glass to examine the image helps to identify artifacts that would otherwise go unrecognized.**

Lastly and most important according to Kimme-Smith, Basset & Gold is the technologist's critical eye (Figure 12). The technologist must give special attention to the image emerging from the processor. The use of a magnifying glass is critical to identifying a processing artifact: for example, what was attributed to a decrease in film contrast might actually be a processing artifact that obscures the film.

It is the technologist's responsibility to deliver quality images which are artifact-free for interpretation. When this is not accomplished, it is also the technologist's responsibility to find out why and then to solve the problem. The best way for the technologist to insure that the processing system is operating optimally is to be well-informed about the areas just described.

## References

1. Workbook for Quality Mammography, Kimme-Smith, Basset, Gold, Williams &Wilkins 1992.

2. Haus AG, Batz TA, Dickerson RE, Lillie RF, Oemcke KW, and Lanphear JD: Automating film processing in medical imaging. In Siebert JA, Barnes GT, and Gould RG: Specification, Acceptance Testing and Quality Control of Diagnostic X-Ray

Imaging Equipment. American Institute of Physics, New York, NY, 1992.

3. Mammographic Imaging: A Practical Guide. Andolina, Lille, Willison, J. B. Lippincott, Co. 1992.

4. Committee on Quality Assurance in Mammography: Mammography Quality Control for Radiologic Technologists. Reston, Virginia, American College of Radiology, 1992.

5. Haus, A.G: Screen-Film Processing Systems and Quality Control in Mammography, Presented at the Symposium on the Physics of Clinical Mammography, St. Louis, 1990.

6. Processing Mammographic Films: Technical and Clinical Considerations, Tabar L, Haus AG, *Radiology* 173:65-69, 1989.

# Chemical Compliance Issues

**A. David Charlton**
Eastman Kodak Company
Rochester, New York

## Introduction

Its no secret that there are many compliance issues confronting the hospital administrator today. There's the ubiquitous red-bag waste, and concerns about radiation equipment and low-level radioactive waste. And if you are involved with processing radiographic film, you're probably aware of silver restrictions for the processing effluent going down the floor drain to a waste treatment facility.

The focus of this paper is several compliance issues concerning the chemicals used to process x-ray films. Three items will be addressed:

1) OSHA compliance
2) sewer use codes
3) regulations governing the storage and shipment of the recovered silver

Violations can result in substantial fines for non-compliance, including criminal prosecution of facility managers. Because of this, neither Eastman Kodak Company nor the author are providing regulatory or legal advice in this paper. Compliance responsibility lies with the concerned individual, either customer or reader, and they should seek professional counsel when deciding their course of action.

## Occupational Safety and Health Act

One regulation of the Occupational Safety and Health Act (OSHA) is known as the "Employee Right-to-Know Law". It requires that an employer train employees and keep them informed about the hazards they may encounter in their workplace.

The first item an inspector will look for is OSHA poster #2203. It must be prominently displayed in the work area. It describes specific rights of the worker, and its absence can result in a $1,000 fine.

At first glance, the typical chemical mixing scene in Figure 1 looks like a good one. The area is clean and well lighted, and the technician is even following the mixing instructions. But an OSHA inspector is looking for four specific things that could result in fines up to $7000 each if not present.

Three citations could be issued if the employee was not wearing personal protective equipment when handling chemicals. Proper eye protection, gloves and an apron made of a chemically impervious material are required.

The fourth item involves labels on the chemical replenisher tanks. Labels are required to identify the chemical components in the tanks, to include brief comments on the hazards presented, to indicate the source of their manufacture and to relate the product to a Material Safety Data Sheet.

If you use an automatic mixer that stores the working solutions for longer than one shift, the tanks holding the chemicals must have the warning labels.

These same chemicals are in the film processor tanks, so they, too, must be labelled. Furthermore, the regulations require that labels be placed on the side panels of equipment if these panels obscure the tanks.

Don't forget about the fixer in the silver recovery system. Both electrolytic recovery units and steel wool canisters require OSHA warning labels. Note that these labels are different from the Hazardous Waste labels required by other regulations covering storing and shipping metallic replacement recovery cartridges.

OSHA requires a listing of any products in use at the workplace which contain hazardous chemicals. The list makes reference to Material Safety Data Sheets which you are required to have for each chemical in use in the area. Employees must have easy access to them, and most important, be trained to have a working knowledge of how to cope with the hazards described in them. Material Safety Data Sheets are available from the manufacturers of the products you use, or the dealer who sells them.

During an inspection, the OSHA inspector often asks that an employee share in the inspection tour to determine how well informed the employee is about these chemical hazards. The Inspector may ask the employee to find the MSDS for a specific chemical and explain what the information means as it relates to the job.

If you haven't picked up any citations on that exercise, it's probably because you have a well-defined and properly executed Hazard Communication Program in place.

OSHA requires a written plan that describes where the responsibility lies for training employees, who the trainer is, what the content of the training program is, which employees received the training and when. It is critical that each employee working with chemicals be trained before being exposed to them on the job. Failure to meet this requirement can mean a $7,000 fine for each day each employee was on the job without appropriate training. Furthermore, having a training program in place but not in use could be interpreted as a "willful" violation which can increase the fine to a maximum of $70,000 per employee, per day.

The Inspector will ask for documentation that employees have been trained in handling chemicals safely. Documentation can be a formal statement signed by the employee, or simply a test paper on the subject showing the grade attained and the signature of the employee.

When it comes to the eye-wash station, OSHA mandates unrestricted access to the area. It is likely that when it is needed in an emergency, the worker probably will be unable to see any obstacles. It can be a costly mistake to use that space as a temporary storage area for mop pails or a wastebasket.

Another area of concern is adequate ventilation in the darkroom to minimize chemical odors. This requires a correctly installed exhaust system for each processor.

Kodak's "Processor Installation Site Specifications" call for an air exchange rate of ten room volumes per hour. The specifications also require positive air pressure on the darkroom side of the processor. This moves the air into the feed slot of the processor and across the tops of the chemical tanks. It is then carried out by the exhaust duct of the processor and through the building exhausxt system to outside air.

It's recommended to have an adjustable slot at the entry point of the processor exhaust duct with the building exhaust system in order to control the effect of the building exhaust's drawing cold air through the processor. This may cause changes in the developer temperature which can produce variations in film quality.

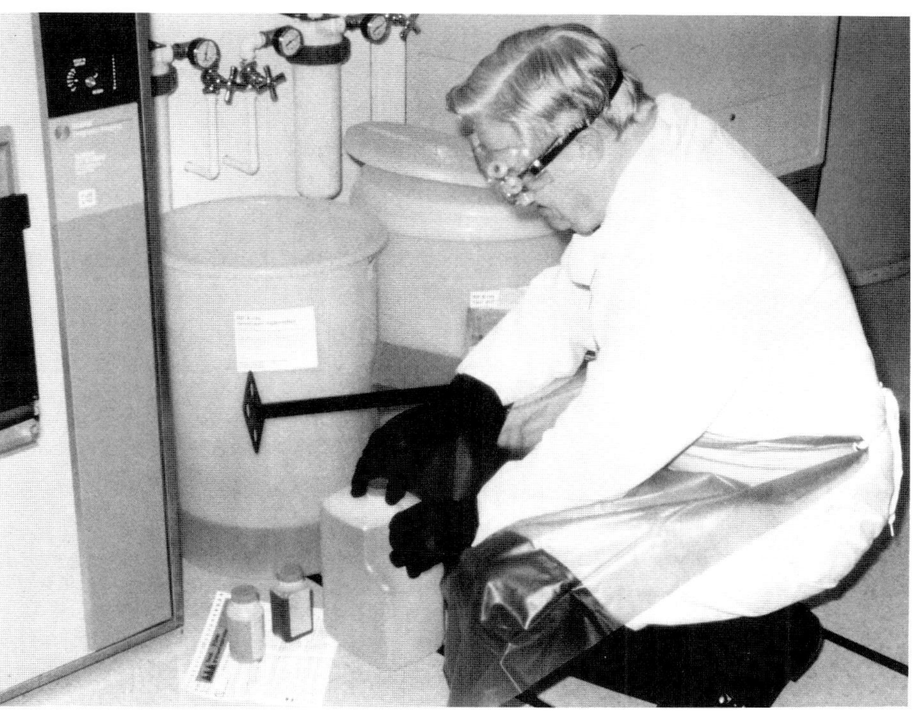

**Figure 1. OSHA requires that employee wear personal protective equipment and that chemical tanks be labeled to detail their contents.**

## Sewer Use Codes

When disposing of the chemicals themselves, there are two basic options:

    1) Pre-treat and discharge them to the sewer;

    2) Collect them for removal by a service company.

There are regulations governing both options.

Federal legislation passed in 1972 amended the earlier "Water Pollution Control Act" and established minimum standards for the quality of water being discharged to the environment. States also may legislate standards, but these must be the same or tighter restrictions.

It is the responsibility of the waste treatment plant operator to meet the federal or state requirements under which the treatment plant may discharge its treated effluent to the environment, usually a lake or river.

The federal legislation makes provision for waste treatment plants to establish their own codes for their customers to meet in order that the treatment plant effluent will not violate the National Pollutant Discharge Elimination System Permit under which it must operate.

So your first step is to get a copy of the sewer use regulations that pertain to your facility. Contact the local waste treatment authority to obtain a copy, and become familiar with them. Among many pages of numbered paragraphs, there are two critical subjects.

First, of course, is the listing of the parameters describing effluent characteristics that are acceptable for discharge to the sewer.

Conventional photographic processing effluents are within most sewer codes. for physical characteristics such as pH, temperature, suspended solids, color, odor, oils and flammable materials.

Chemical characteristics include items such as biochemical oxygen demand. This is a measure of the amount of dissolved oxygen in the waste stream that the effluent will consume through biological degradation over a 5-day period. The dissolved oxygen is required by the microorganisms in the waste treatment plant that do the real work in breaking down the waste and producing a clean effluent. Without oxygen the microorganisms die and the treatment of the waste stops.

Also included will be a list of chemicals and the concentration of each that is the permissible limit for your waste stream. The way this limit is most frequently expressed is miiligrams of silver per liter of effluent (mg/L). It is sometimes expressed as parts of silver per milliom (PPM). Milligrams per liter and parts per million are equivalent units of measure.

The second factor that is important to your compliance effort is the procedure by which the authority evaluates your facility effluent. Sampling and analysis is the method most frequently used.

There will be a section in the code that describes the sampling point, where it is to be located, and the reasonableness of access to it. The construction of the site, and any special plumbing or permanent sampling equipment required by the code will be installed and maintained at your expense.

It is vital to establish the most favorable but acceptable sampling point that the code allows. The most favorable sampling point is a manhole access where the building sewer lateral joins the city sewer main. The most stringent case, and the one most difficult for you to meet, is where the sample is taken at the outlet of the silver recovery system before the effluent enters the floor drain.

Many recovery systems are plumbed with the recovery system drain line separate from the processor drain line. However, if you read the code carefully, you may find words such as "sample at the end of the process." The photographic process is develop, fix and wash. So it is advisable to plumb the recovery system effluent into the developer and wash drain line from the processor before it enters the floor drain, so as to take advantage of some legitimate dilution. (See Figure 2).

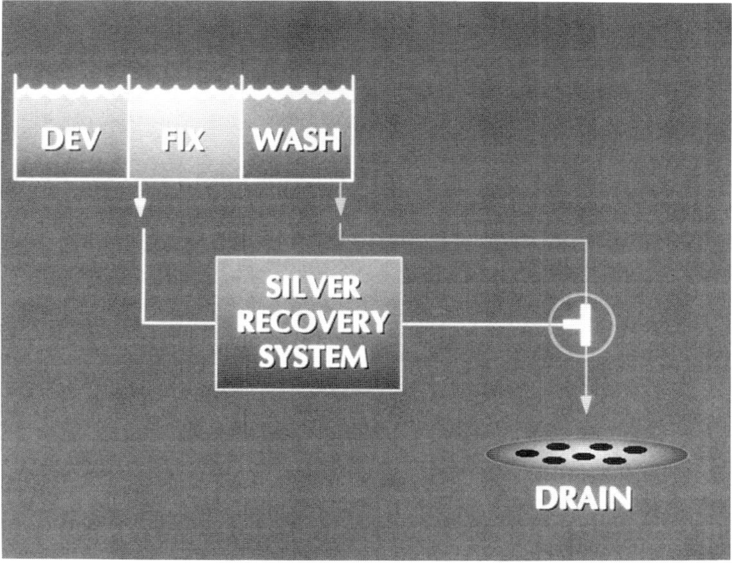


**Figure 2. Include all process streams if the sample point is specified as "the end of the process."**

Another important factor is whether the sample is representative of the total effluent being evaluated. There are two popular methods of sampling:

1) Grab sampling; (Figure 3)
2) Composite sampling. (Figure 4)

A grab sample is collected by use of a hand pump or by simply dipping out a bottle full of whatever waste stream the inspector considers representative or convenient. This is why it is prudent to make the drain line modification mentioned earlier.

A more representative sample is a composite sample. This consists of a pump that withdraws a predetermined volume of solution from the waste stream on a regular timed-cycle and discharges it into a container. At the end of a representative period of time, the contents of the container are well mixed, a sample is taken from the mixture and sent to an EPA or state-accredited lab for analysis.

Another potential problem is the credibility of the results of the chemical analysis.

This may be due to some of the unusual chemical compounds found in photographic processing effluent. Call your chemical manufacturer if the analytical lab you use has problems obtaining valid analytical data because of unfamiliar photochemical interferences. The manufacturer's analytical chemists should be able to resolve the problems.

It should be clear now that the sampling point, sampling method and analytical laboratory are very important when demonstrating your compliance with a sewer code. If you have been cited by an environmental authority, you should evaluate the sampling point requirements, the sampling procedure, and verify the analytical results before buying new silver recovery or waste treatment equipment.

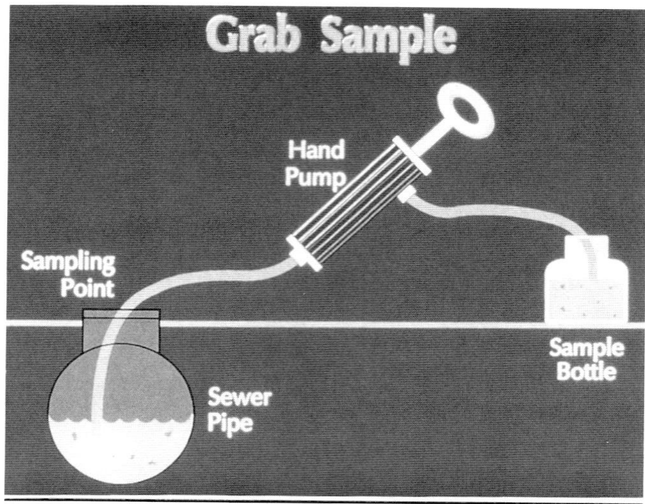


Figure 3. A grab sample is a single sample taken at random in the processing day.

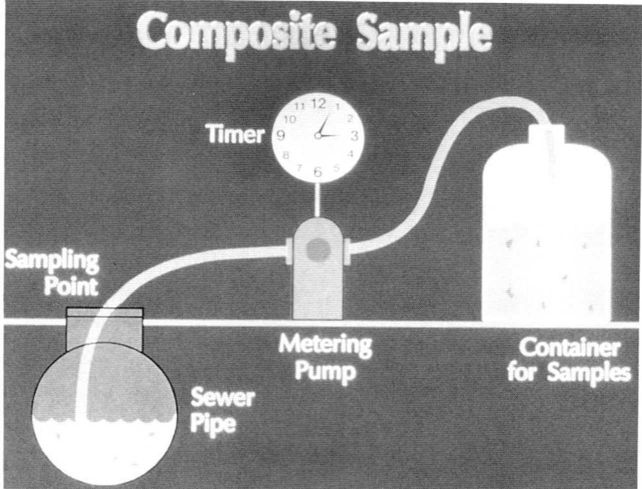


Figure 4. A composite sample is taken from a mixture of many small samples collected on a timed basis over a specified period.

## Collect-and-Haul Option

If you find that you still have a sewer code compliance problem, an alternative is to collect the fixer which contains the silver, and have it hauled away by a solution disposal service. This doesn't necessarily mean they have also hauled away your problems.

Another piece of federal legislation, the "Resource Conservation and Recovery Act," established definitions for hazardous materials and procedures governing their treatment, storage, transport, and disposal. Of concern is the definition of hazardous materials.

One definition describes solutions containing more than 5 milligrams per liter of silver as hazardous waste. Seasoned photographic fixer is regulated under this legislation.

Collecting the fixer in a container is simple enough. Just remember to put an OSHA warning label on it. As for the storage regulations, they vary with how much "hazardous waste" you generate per month. For example, if you generate less than 100 kilograms per month, (about 27 gallons of fixer), you may store up to 1000 kilograms for 180 days before labeling and disposal requirements apply. Corresponding constraints apply as the amounts generated on a monthly basis increase.

*Note: Additional information may be found in the Code of Federal Regulations, Title 40, Parts 260-262.*

When the solution is picked up by a service company, it must be accompanied by a "Uniform Hazardous Waste Manifest." You must specify delivery to a permitted hazardous waste recycler or disposer, and the solution must be transported only by a licensed hazardous waste hauler.

Your facility, the transporter and the receiver of the solutions must have EPA ID numbers which you are required to insert on the top part of the manifest. The manifest has several copies, one of which is returned to you by the disposal facility within 30 days. This copy must indicate in section K how your material was disposed. This is important, as you have "cradle to grave" responsibility for the hazardous material you generated. If your material is later identified in a Superfund cleanup site, you will share in the cleanup cost. It is best to assure that your material goes to a refiner or recycler who will process the silver and return it to commerce. Then you know its gone for good.

Other items caught under the umbrella definition of hazardous material include electrolytic flake silver, and steel wool recovery cartridges that have not been properly washed prior to shipment. The regulatory concern is the soluble silver in the residual fixer that could leach out of a batch of electrolytic flake silver or a steel wool cartridge – not the silver being shipped. In case of a vehicular accident, the soluble silver might reach the environment via a storm drain or roadside ditch.

In most states, however, if the material is rinsed adequately to remove the residual fixer, the residue is inert and may be shipped without using the Hazardous Waste Manifest. Information on the proper procedure for washing this material is available from your chemical supplier or silver service company.

## Miscellaneous Concerns

Though not intended as part of this discussion, it should be noted that the Department of Transportation also has regulations regarding the shipment of chemicals and hazardous materials. Generally, these requirements cover packaging, labeling and vehicle markings.

Other chemical compliance issues that confront the hospital administrator include mercury treatment and disposal, barium, lead and formaldehyde. Both employee exposure under OSHA, as well as proper disposal under RCRA, must be addressed.

And one final thought to consider: if the underground fuel storage tank used for the emergency generator at your facility is more than ten years old, there's a good chance it is corroded. It may be releasing fuel oil which can result in ground water contamination. The most likely spot is where the transmission pipe is connected to the tank. It may be prudent to have a professional environmental site assessment of the storage tank area. If you discover a problem, you can correct it on a practical schedule, rather than under the pressure of an expensive compliance citation.

## Conclusion

If there is not yet a safety or compliance officer designated in your facility, it is strongly recommended that such an appointment be made. Noncompliance with the regulatory issues covered in these remarks creates the potential for expensive citations and, perhaps litigation brought by regulators, present or former employees, or environmental organizations. Such actions affect the financial position of your operations, the morale of your employees, and the image of your institution in the community.

This is surely a prime example of the old adage, "an ounce of prevention is worth a ton of cure."

# A Method of Verifying that Film is Providing Appropriate Speed and Contrast in the Clinical Environment


**Robert Moore***
**Arthur G. Haus****
**Charles W. Baker****
**Jeff D. Johnson***
**Frederick J. Netherda***
**Ann Richards*****
Eastman Kodak Company
* Windsor, Colorado
** Rochester, New York
*** Toronto, Canada

**Perry Sprawls, Jr.**
Emory University, Atlanta, Georgia

**Carolyn Kimme-Smith**
UCLA School of Medicine, Los Angeles, California

**Martin Yaffe**
**Gordon Mawdsley**
University of Toronto, Toronto, Canada


## Introduction

In the production of a radiographic image, film processing is the step that is most susceptible to variability. Film processing that yields sensitometric results varying significantly from the manufacturer's design specifications could result in degradation of image quality and/or increased radiation dose to the patient. At the very least, the resultant radiograph will not provide the speed and contrast characteristics which it was designed to produce.

In order for film processing to contribute to reliable image characteristics, results must be precise, i.e., reproducible or consistent. Also, since the film is designed to provide certain characteristics of speed and contrast, it is important that when used in the field, similar characteristics are obtained, i.e., the results obtained at a facility are accurate.

In this paper, we report on a survey in which the variability of sensitometric film processing parameters, i.e., speed, average gradient and fog density was assessed, and we describe a method for standardizing processor sensitometry to an absolute scale for a given film product. This method establishes tolerence limits for speed, contrast and fog. Although the data described here were obtained from mammographic imaging facilities, the basic principles discussed apply to any radiographic processing.

## Definitions

For this study, using the Kodak process control sensitometer and densitometer, the following variables were defined. These definitions pertain to sensitometric factors which are determined by exposing the film under consideration with a 21-step sensitometer and measuring optical density of the processed film with a densitometer. Both instruments must have been cross referenced to a known standard to give meaningful results.

| | |
|---|---|
| Base + Fog (B+F) | The optical density of the film at Step #1 where there is no practical light exposure to the film. |
| Speed Index<br>Mid Density (MD) | The optical density as measured on Step #11 of the sensitometric image. |
| Average Gradient | The slope of the sensitometric curve between net optical density of 0.25 above B+F and 2.00 above B+F. Units are "optical density difference per difference in logarithm of exposure." |
| Contrast Index<br>Density Difference(DD) | The difference in optical density expressed as step #13 minus step #9. |
| D Max | The optical density as measured at step #21. |

## Reference Curves

Reference curves were established for three Kodak mammography films. Films were exposed emulsion side down by a Kodak process control sensitometer, set for green-sensitive, single-emulsion films. The sensitometer has settings to adjust the light output to the class of films being tested. For reference curves, the settings on the sensitometer were number 4 for Min-R M film, number 3 for Min-R E film and number 2 for Min-R H film. For each product, the manufacturer's recommended processing conditions were used. Min-R M and Min-R H films were processed in an

M6A-N processor with Kodak RP X-Omat developer and fixer. For Min-R E film, extended cycle processing was used. Processing parameters to generate the reference curves are given in Table1. Fresh chemistry with starter was used. Sensitometric reference curves for Min-R M, Min-R H and Min-R E films are given in Figures 1, 2 and 3.

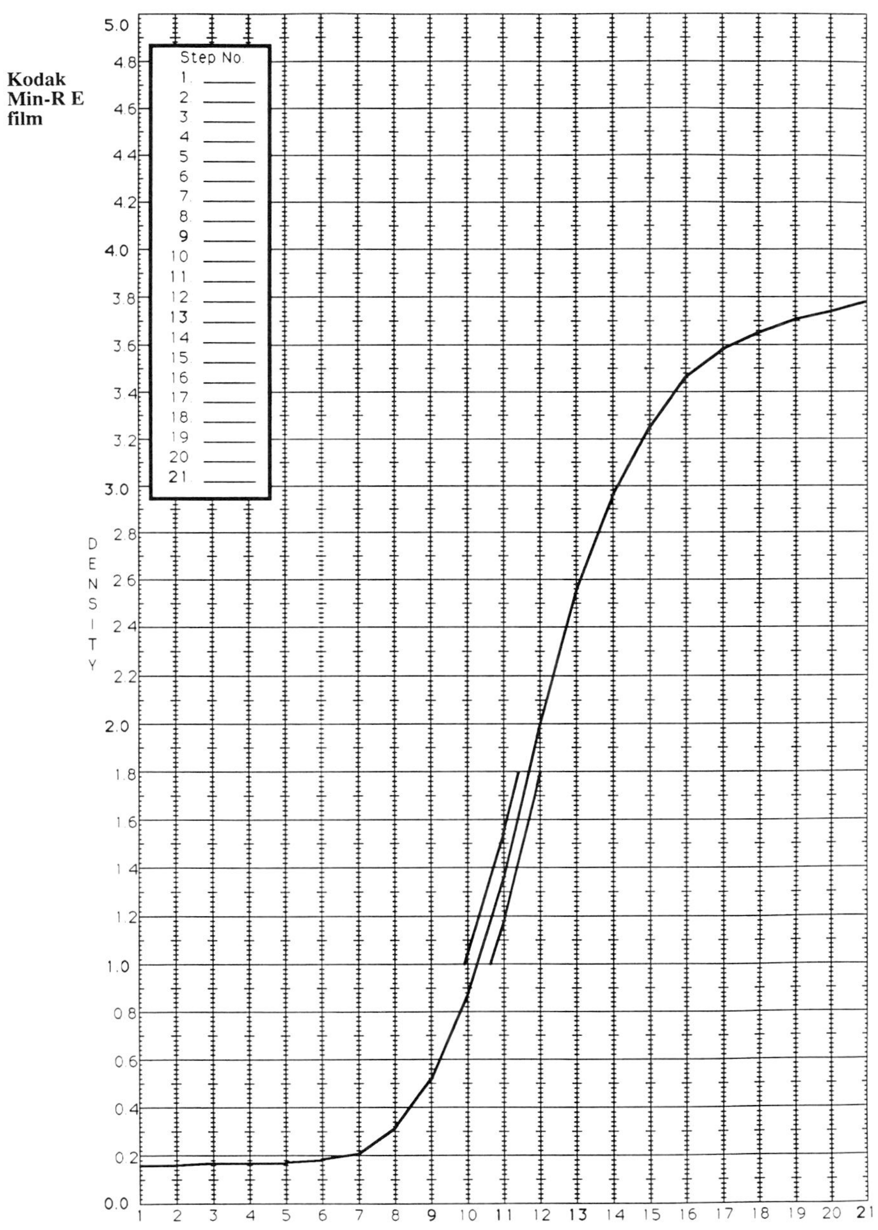



**Figure 1. Example of Min-R E film process verification curve**

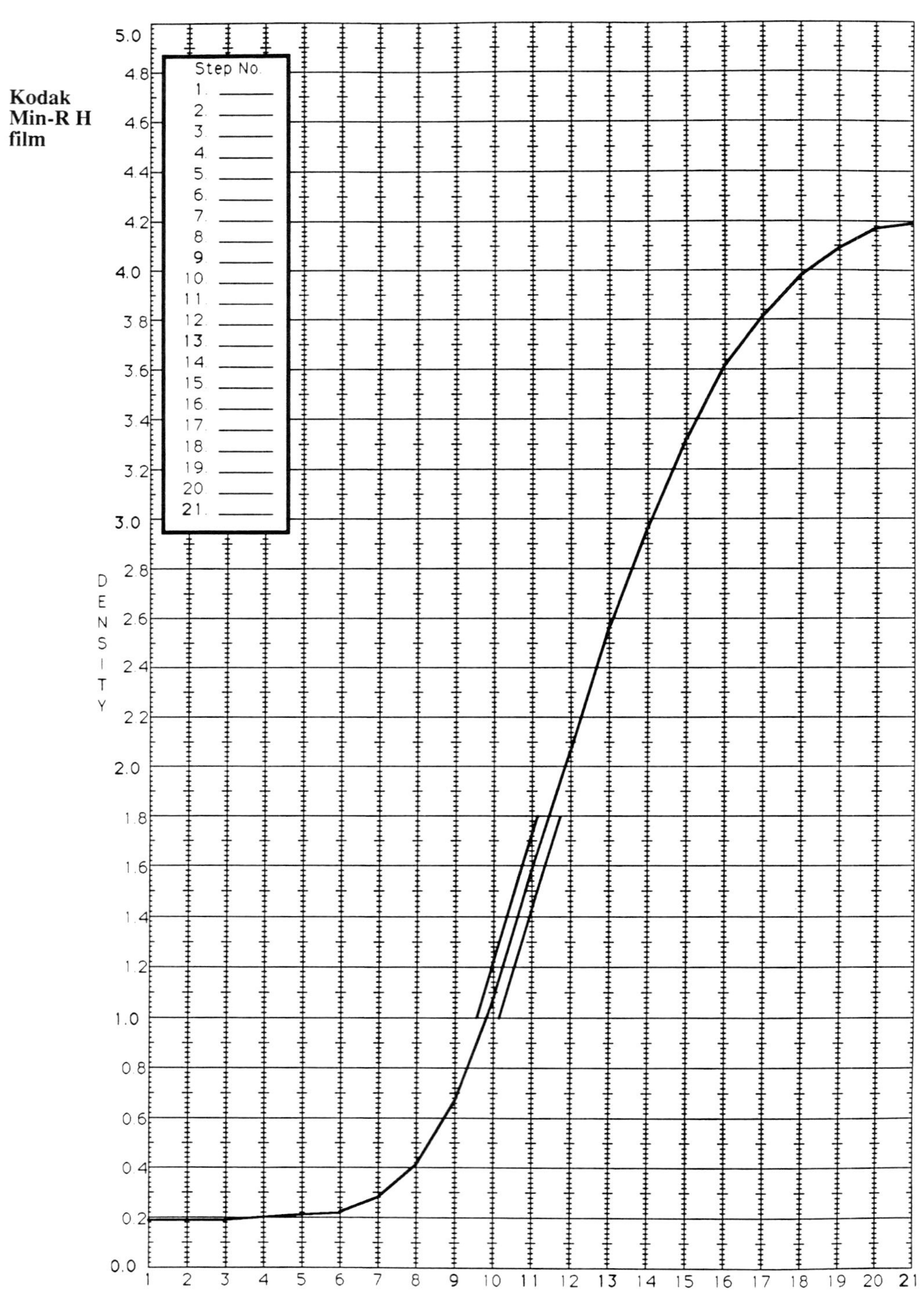



Figure 2. Example of Min-R H film process verification curve

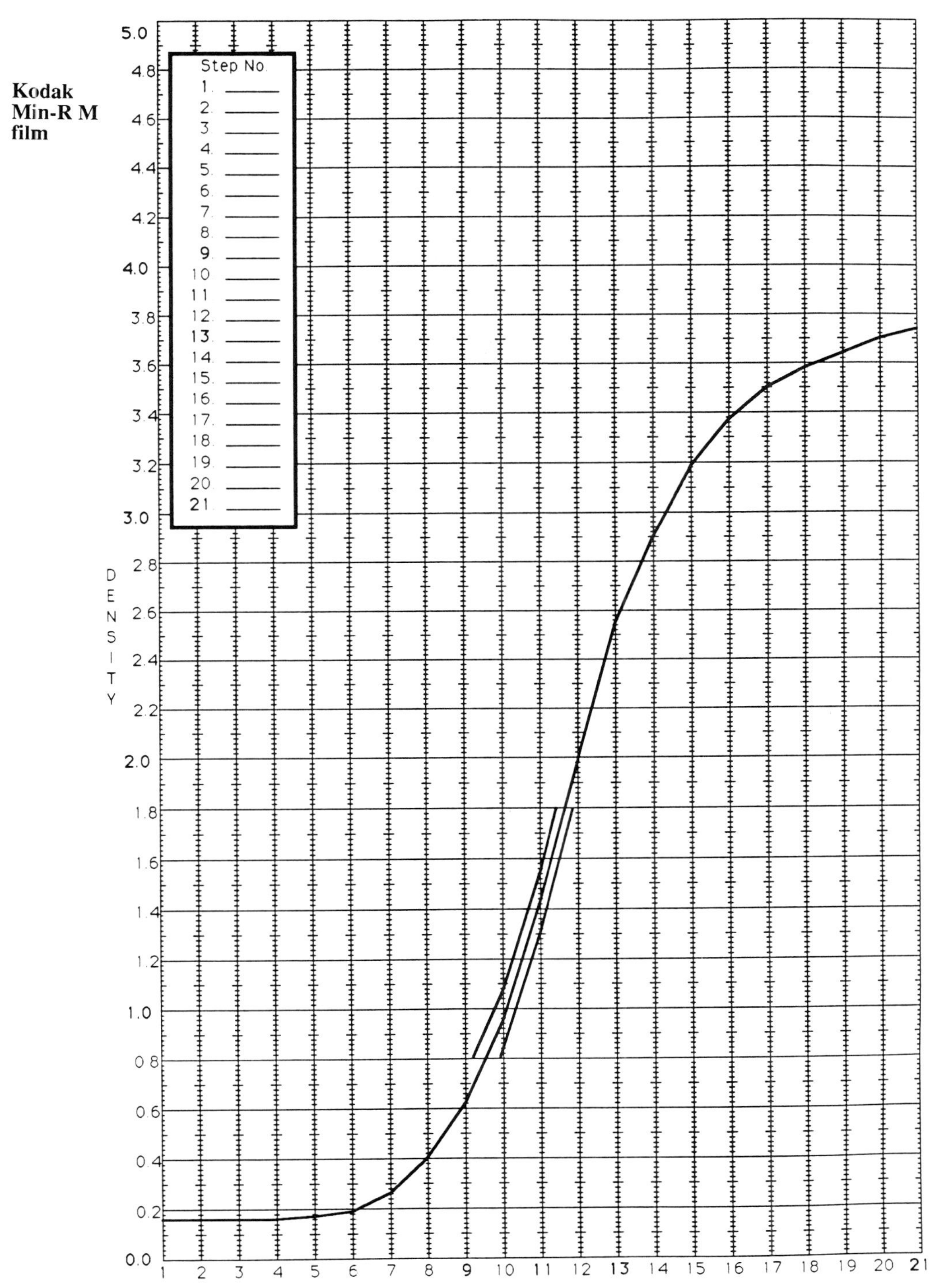



Figure 3. Example of Min-R M film process verification curve

## Table 1. Reference Curve Generation for KODAK Mammography Films

| Parameter | Units | Min-R M | Min-R H | Min-R E |
|---|---|---|---|---|
| Developer Temp. | Degrees F | 95 | 95 | 95 |
| Process cycle time | Std./Ext. | Standard | Standard | Extended |
| Base + Fog | Optical density | 0.16 | 0.19 | 0.16 |
| Speed Index | Optical density | 1.43 | 1.58 | 1.36 |
| Average Gradient | Delta optical density/delta fog exposure | 2.76 | 2.86 | 3.13 |
| Contrast Index | Delta optical density | 1.92 | 1.91 | 2.04 |
| D Max | Optical density | 3.74 | 4.19 | 3.78 |

## Data Acquisition

Independent surveys of film processing were carried out at a total of eighty-six clinical mammography sites in the vicinities of three North American cities: Los Angeles, Atlanta and Toronto. Information on key process parameters (physical, chemical and sensitometric) was gathered from each site.

All Kodak process control sensitometers and densitometers used in this study were cross-referenced to devices traceable to National Institute of Standards and Technology (NIST) standards, In the case of chemical analysis, reagent grade buffers were mixed according to scientifically accepted formulae and used in test instruments which were calibrated according to manufacturers' specifications.

All of the sensitometric data were compared to the reference curves.

Tolerances were defined as follows:

| | |
|---|---|
| Base + Fog | 0.02 OD above the reference curve |
| Speed Index | ± 0.18 about the reference curve |
| Average Gradient | ± 0.15 about the reference curve |

Measures of the following fifteen process parameters were made:

## Table 2. Processing Parameters

| | |
|---|---|
| Developer temperature | Hydroquinone |
| Base + Fog | Phenidone |
| Speed Index | Sulphite |
| Average gradient | Bromide |
| Contrast index | Total alkalinity |
| Maximum density | Solution density |

**Table 2 (continued) Processing Parameters**

Specific gravity *                  Process cycle
pH

* Specific gravity and solution density are two methods of measuring the same parameter. Both were considered since specific gravity is a test which is easy to perform in the field but less accurate than solution density which requires more sophisticated equipment to perform. A similar case can be made for total alkalinity and pH with pH being the more accurate of the two measures.

Although concentrations of the key chemical parameters were measured, their ranges and effects will be examined in a separate laboratory study.

## Data Evaluation

A correlation analysis was performed on the 15 identified parameters to examine any linear relationships between them. It indicated that no single parameter could be described as having a significant effect on any other. For future studies involving chemical analysis, replicate testing or some other statistical methodology may be required to accurately characterize their effect. Internal studies done at Kodak have indicated that developer temperature has approximately a 0.02 logE (5%) per degree F effect on speed for mammography films. Approximately 10% of the sites surveyed were processing more than 1.8 degree F from manufacturers' specifications.

Results of this study indicate considerable variability and there is significant opportunity for process improvement. In the 86 sites audited, 6% were producing results with high fog, 42% were producing results out of specification for average gradient. Of the 86 total sites, only 31% were producing results within tolerance for all three parameters. It is interesting to note that even for one of the least complicated and best understood physical parameters, developer temperature, 26% were processing more or less than 0.5 degree F from the manufacturer's specified developer temperature, with an additional 11% processing at the specification limit (± 0.5 degree F). Figure 4 illustrates the frequency and range of temperature variability.

The histograms provided in Figures 5-10 show the range of the data for each sensitometric parameter; the arrows represent the reference aim and tolerances. All data was normalized by film type so that it would be relative regardless of the exposure setting used on the sensitometer. Clearly there is significant opportunity to bring these processes up to some standard (accuracy). Other studies have also indicated that there are often problems in maintaining day-to-day reproducibility (precision).[1-7] This paper, therefore, concentrates on a method for establishing accuracy of sensitometric performance.

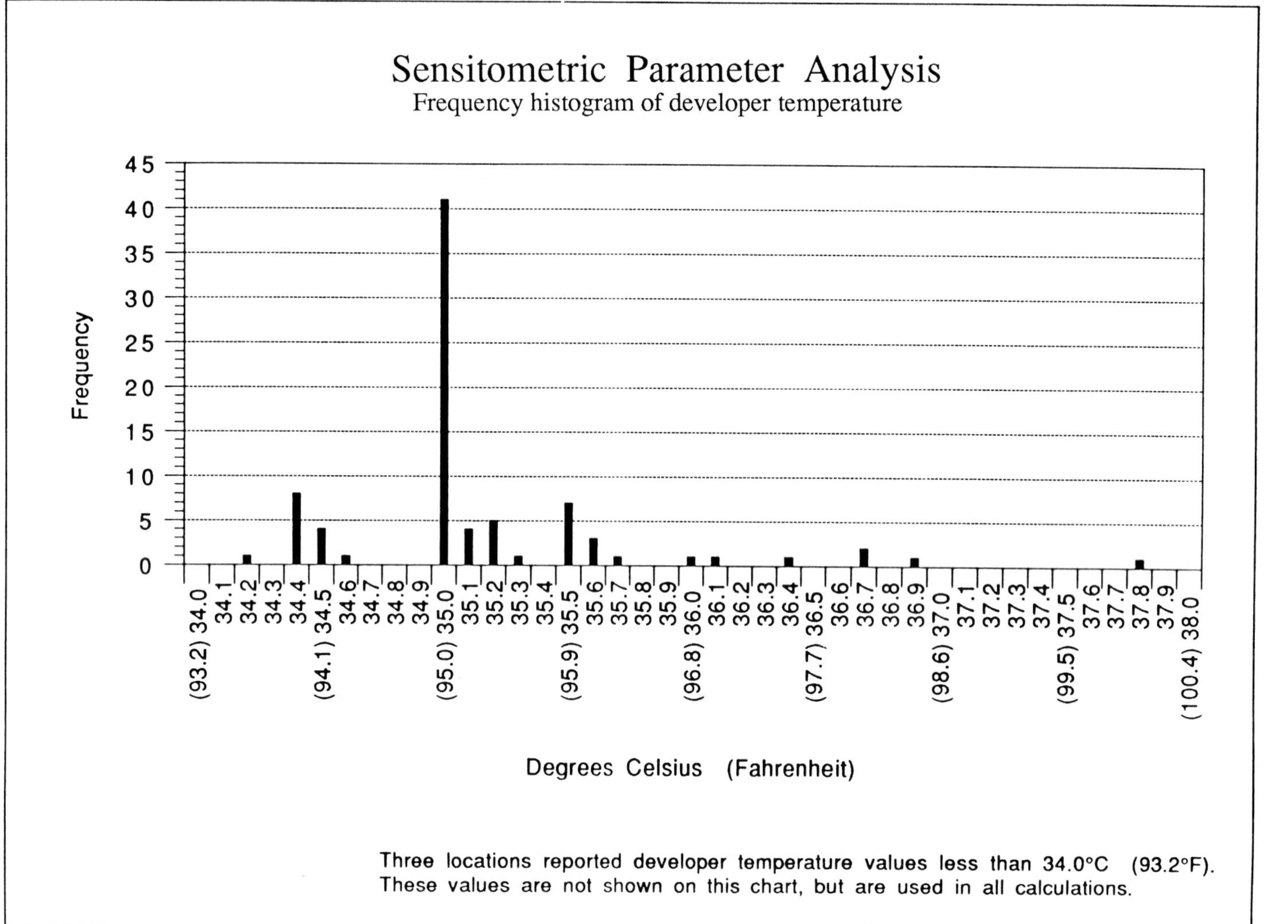


Figure 4. Frequency histogram of developer temperature measurements

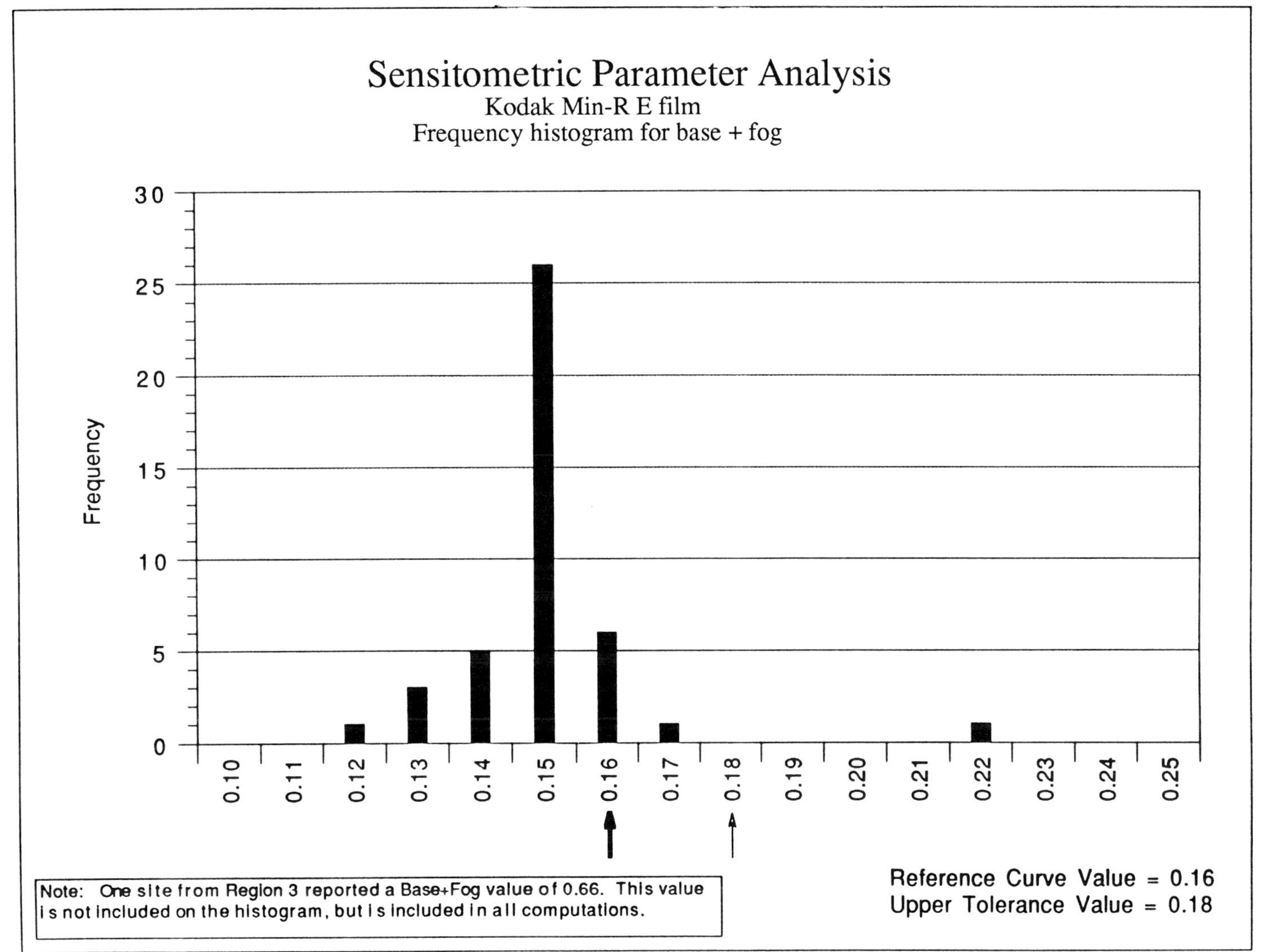



Figure 5. Kodak Min-R E film, frequency histogram of base + fog measurements

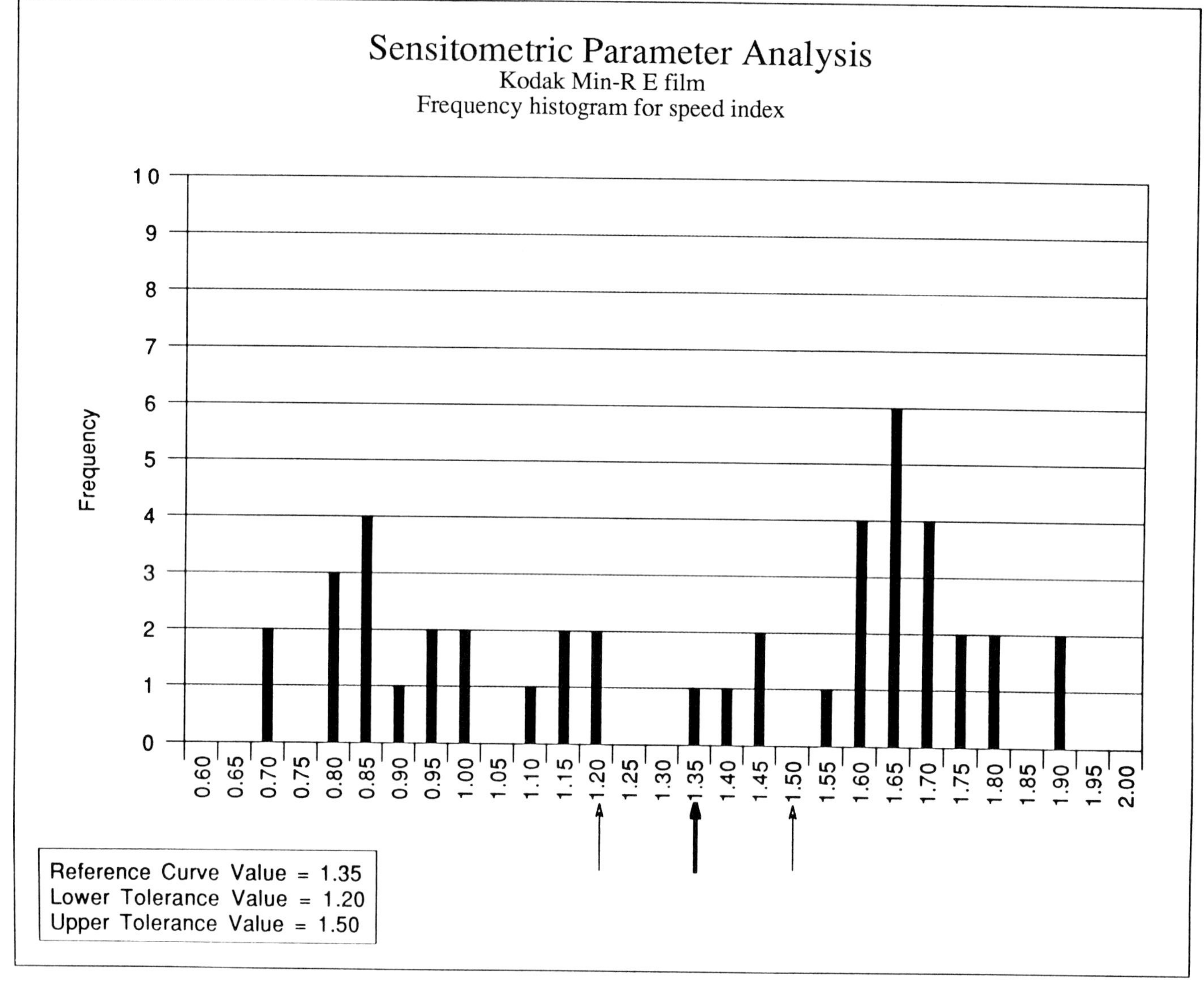


Figure 6. Kodak Min-R E film, frequency histogram of speed index measurements

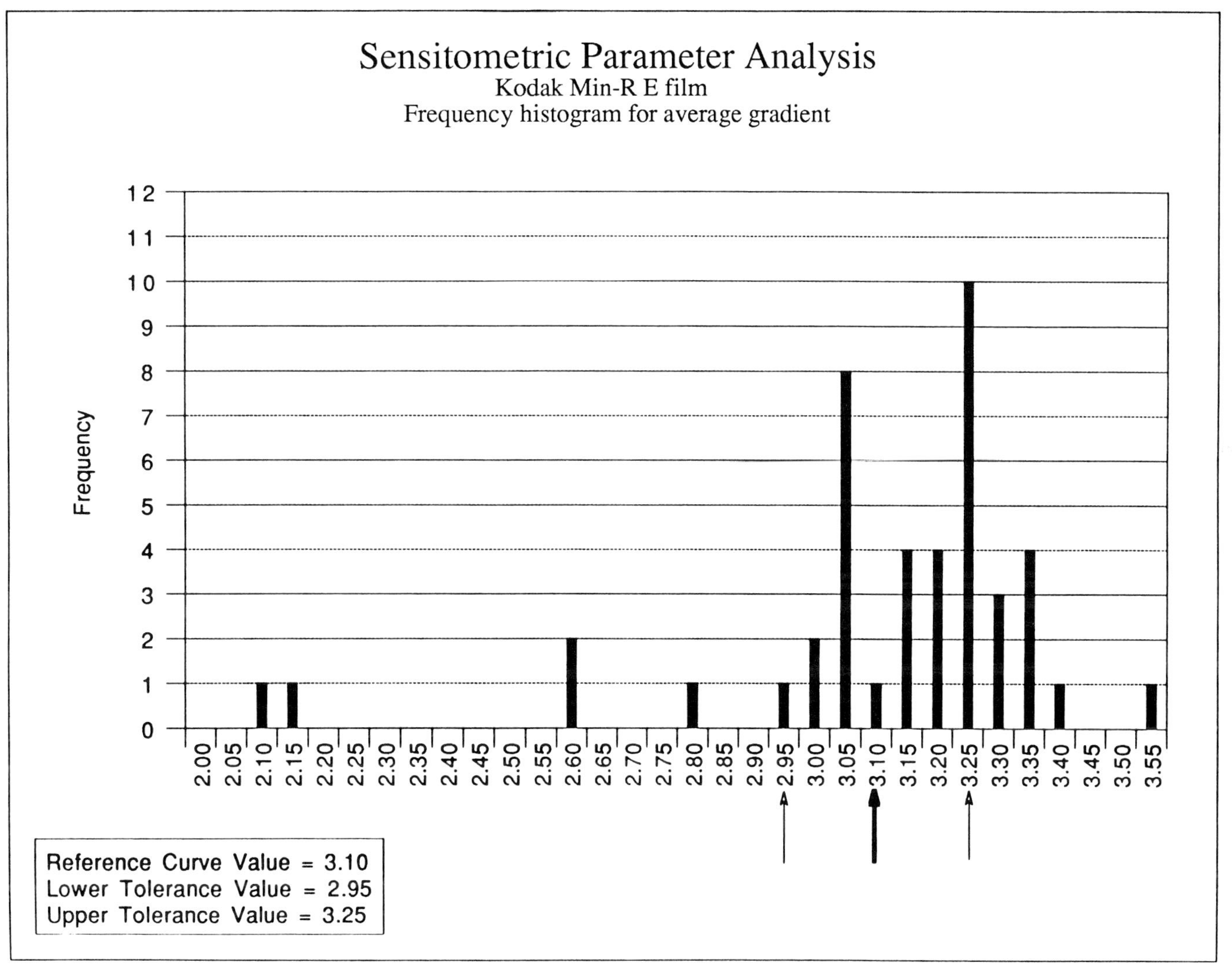


Figure 7. Kodak Min-R E film, frequency histogram of average gradient measurements

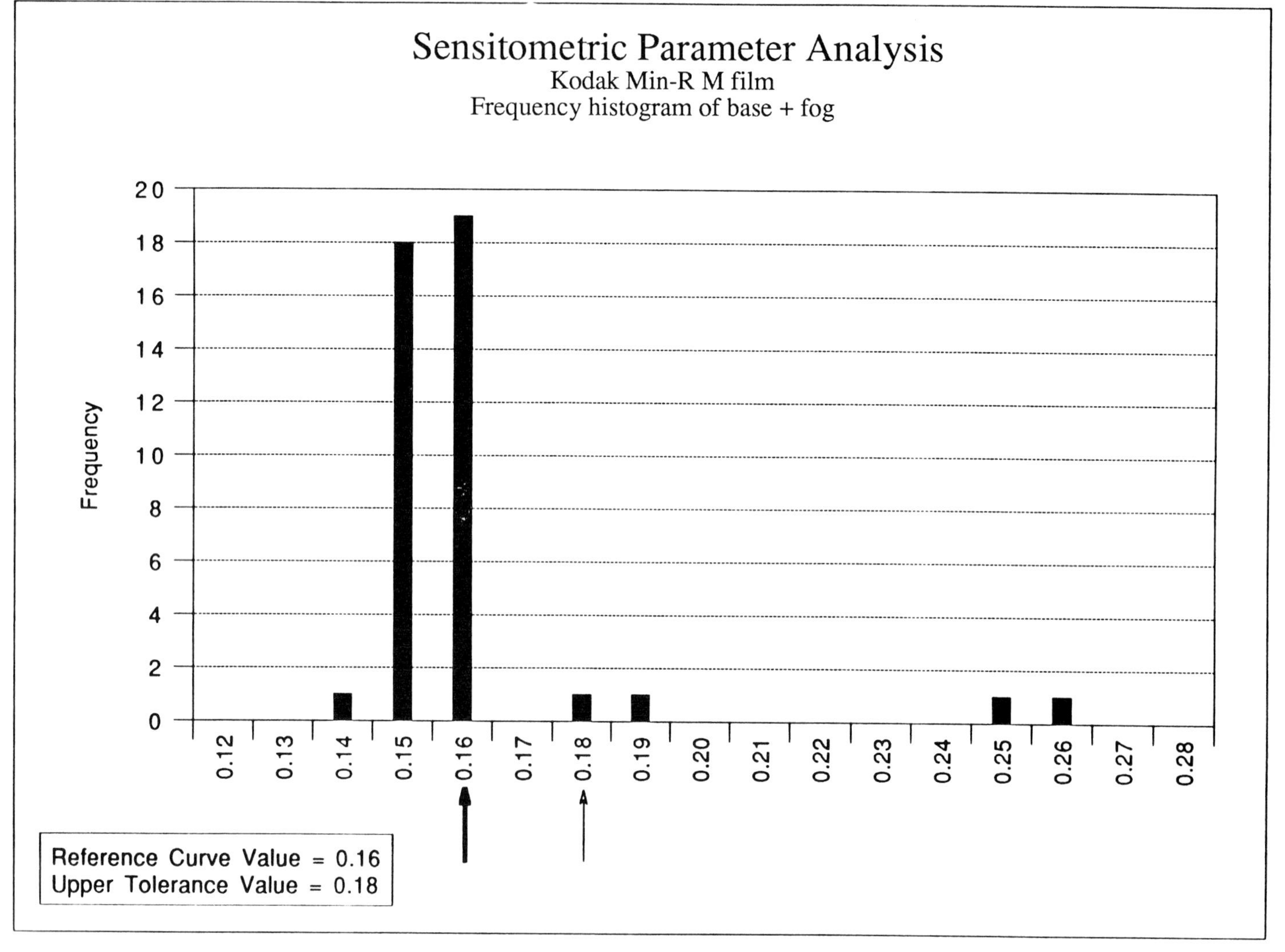



Figure 8. Kodak Min-R M film, frequency histogram of base + fog measurements

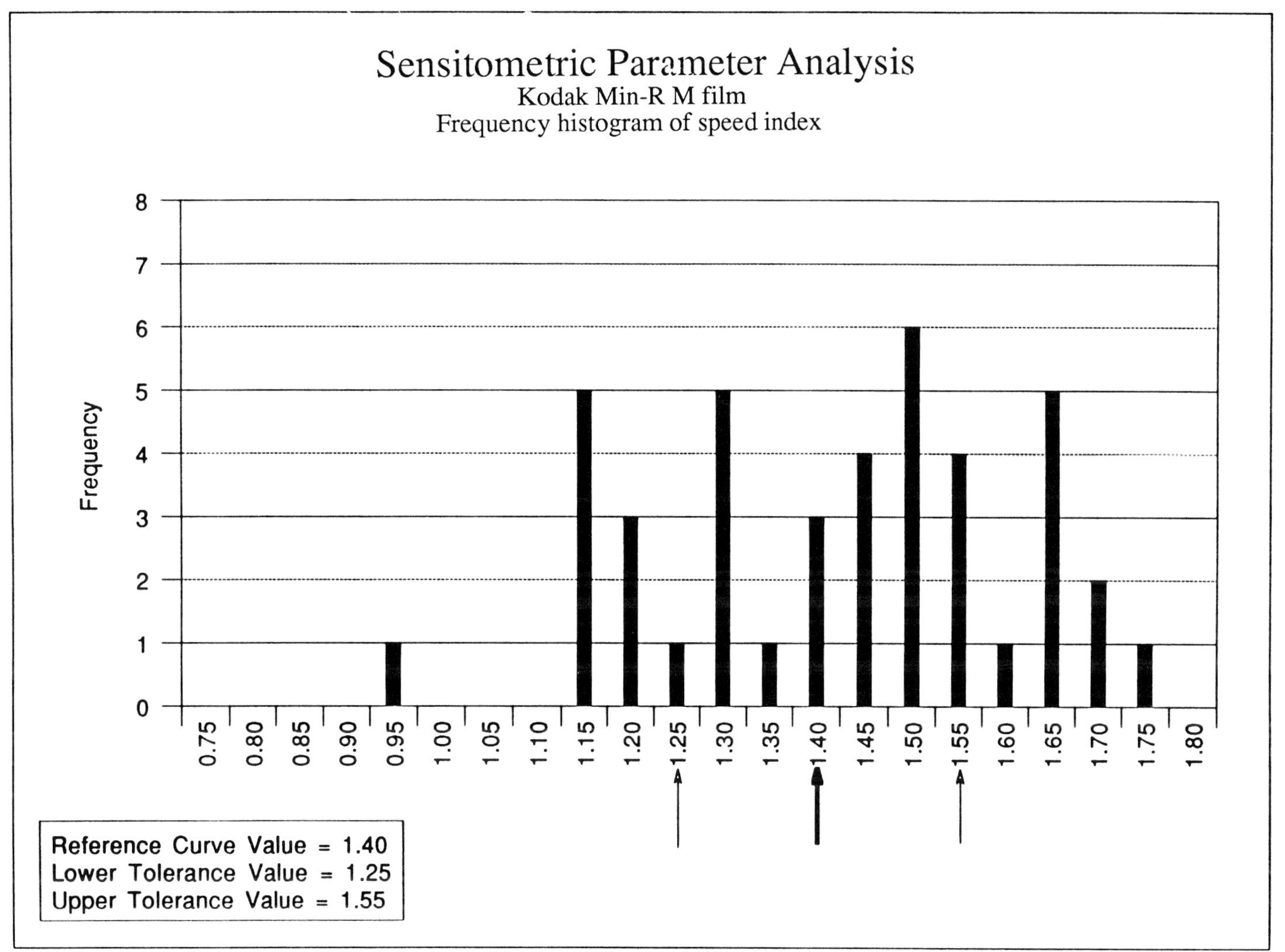


Figure 9. Kodak Min-R M film, frequency histogram of speed index measurements

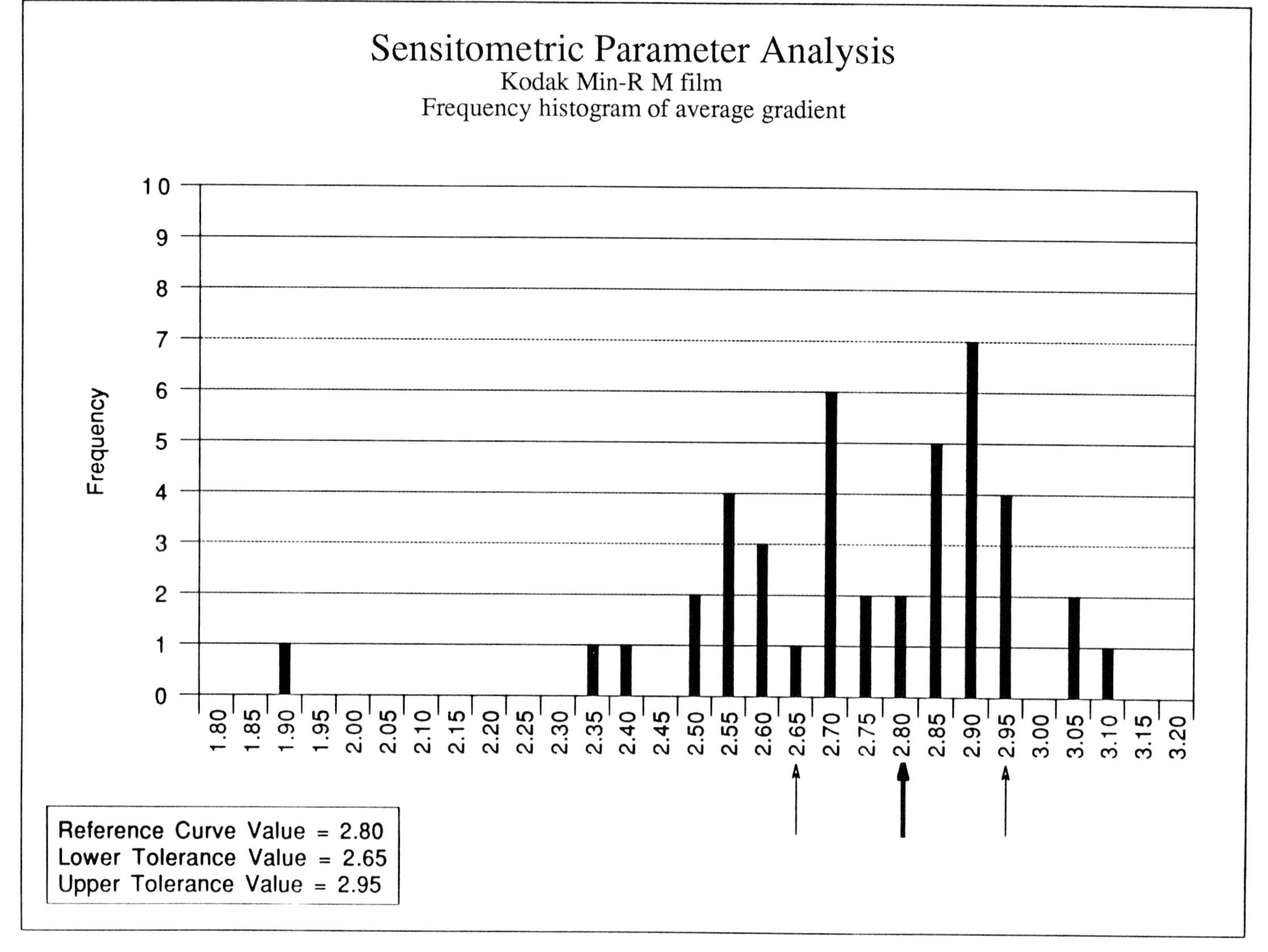


Figure 10. Kodak Min-R M film, frequency histogram of average gradient measurements

## Producing the Right Result: Accuracy

There are basically four requirements that must be met in order to obtain the manufacturers' specified photographic performance in medical imaging:

1. Processing MUST be carried out utilizing recommended development time, temperature and replenishment rates.

2. Processor maintenance MUST be performed in accordance with manufacturer's specifications.

3. Chemical mixing MUST be accomplished in accordance with the manufacturer's specifications.

4. Darkroom safelighting MUST be installed and maintained according to the manufacturer's specifications.

In the past, users in the field have not been able to evaluate how accurately their processing reflects the design sensitometric characteristic for the film. This has been due to the lack of a reference sensitometric curve. To know that a process is producing the correct result requires the technical support of film manufacturers. A sensitometric curve generated under well understood and tightly controlled conditions must be available. Such curves are provided in Figures 1-3. The data of the curve must be usable under field conditions at a clinical location. This can be accomplished if sensitometers used in the field are cross-referenced with respect to the one that generated the reference curves.

## Steps in Verifying Processing Conditions

The processor must be checked to insure that key process parameters are actually set to the manufacturer's specifications. The tools used to measure the conditions need to be calibrated, with the calibration traceable to a national or international standard.

1. A film used in clinical imaging is exposed by a sensitometer selected to perform within limits established for the process verification protocol and processed at the location being verified. The same type of film and exposure must be used as was used to generate the reference curve.

2. The film is then measured with a calibrated densitometer, and a sensitometric curve is generated. That curve and its associated densities represent how that processor was performing at that specific point in time.

The two curves are compared for both relative speed and curve shape. If the generated test curve falls within the manufacturer's tolerances for speed and the curve shapes are similar, the process will produce the desired results. If the locally generated curve meets these criteria, no further action is necessary. If it falls outside of the speed specifications or has a dissimilar curve shape, additional troubleshooting is required. Two examples of non-standard conditions are illustrated in Figures 11 and 12.

The first depicts a process that is high in fog and low in speed (curve 'B') relative to the reference curve (curve 'A'). Corrective action might be: 1) determine if darkroom safelight intensity is too bright by running a safelight test, and 2) check the developer temperature to ensure that it is set to the manufacturer's specifications.

Figure 12 gives "before" and "after" curves with curve 'B' representing a condition where incorrect replenishment rates were being used for a period of time, and curve 'C' showing sensitometric performance after the rates were set to the manufacturer's specifications. Note that curve 'C' does not perfectly align with curve 'A'; this offset is within acceptable limits.

It is important to note that the achievement of good agreement with these reference curves in the field can depend significantly on the "system" being used in the imaging chain. A mixture of processors, chemical and films from different manufacturers can greatly complicate this activity and might, under certain circumstances, make good agreement impossible.

Note also, that in the analysis of processing histograms, processes that were providing results higher in speed and average gradient were characterized as "sub-optimal" because they were outside the tolerances for recommended processing. While they may fall into that category from a purist's viewpoint, in some cases they may provide a more diagnostically useful image. While alternative processing techniques to achieve higher speed and contrast should not be encouraged, they must be evaluated carefully and impose additional effort in quality control to maintain stability.

If one set of conditions had to be described as less desirable, it would be those representing low speed and/or average gradient which will result in increased patient dose and image characteristics which most radiologists would consider sub-optimal.

## Conclusion

When process verification is correctly applied and followed up with daily process control, the process will yield consistant, high-quality results, in accordance with the sensitometric curve for which the film is designed.

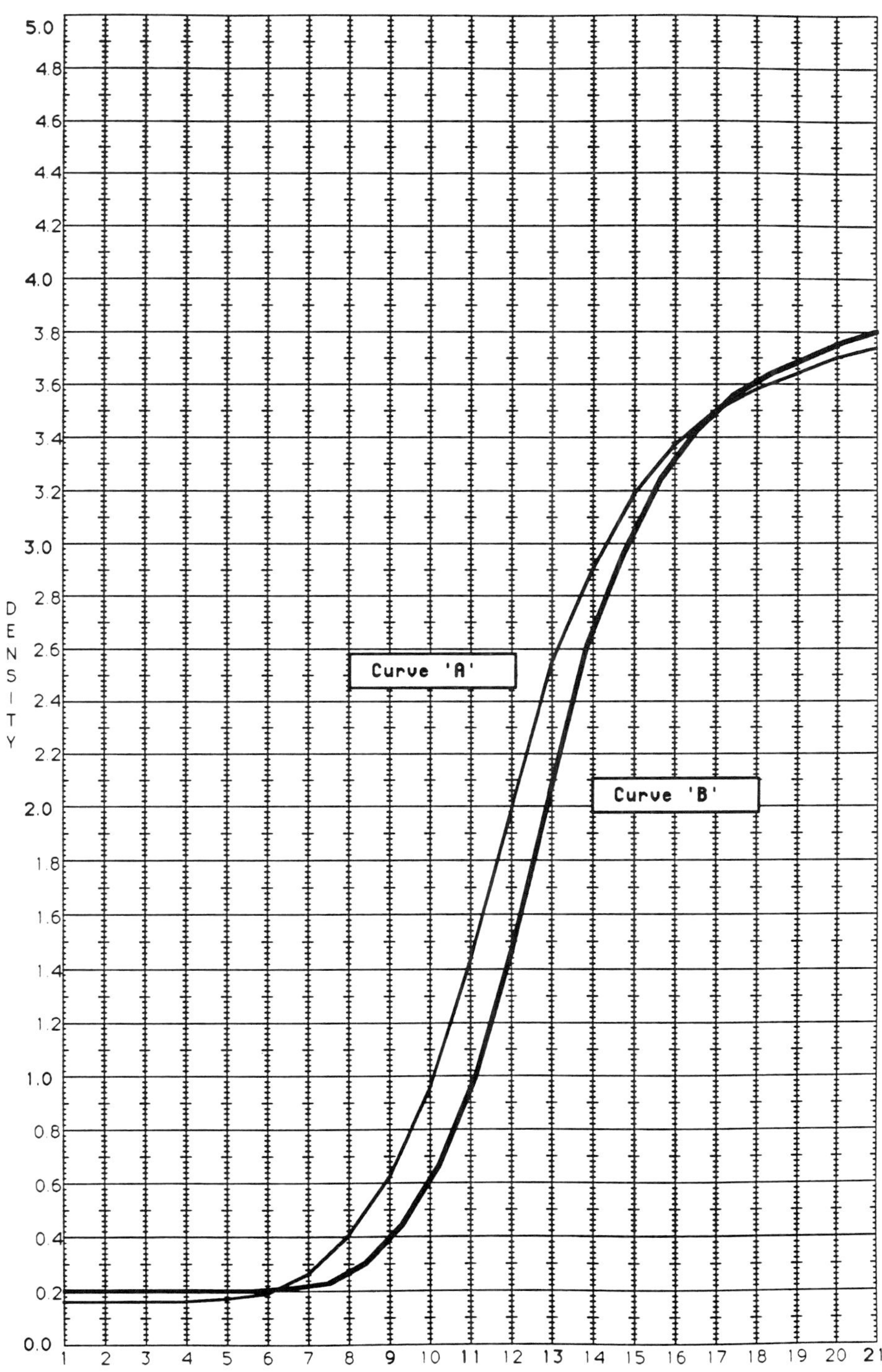



Figure 11. Example of non-standard processing conditions (high base + fog and low speed)

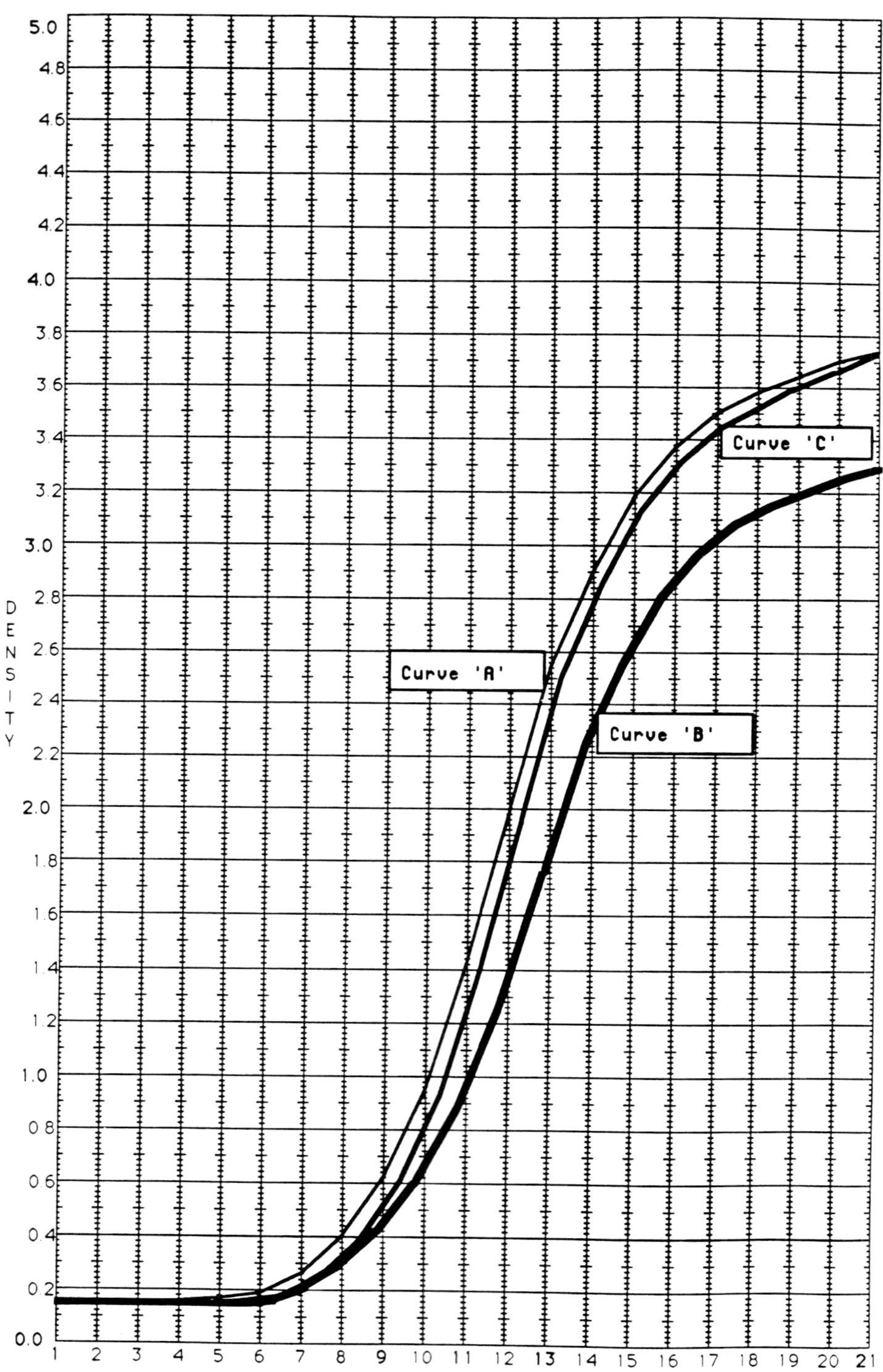


Figure 12. Example of non-standard processing conditions (incorrect replenishment rates)

## References

1. Kimme-Smith K, Rothchild PA, Bassett LW, Gold RH, Moler C: Mammographic film processor developer temperature, development time, and chemistry: effect on dose, contrast and noise. *AJR* 152:35-40, 1989.

2. Tabar L, Haus AG, Processing mammographic films: technical and clinical considerations. *Radiology* 173: 65-69, 1989.

3. Suleiman OH, Slayton RJ, Conway BJ, Rueter FG. Effects of temperature, chemistry, and immersion time on x-ray film. *Radiology* 177P, 132, 1990.

4. Conway BJ, McCrohan JL, Rueter FG, Slayton RJ, Suleiman OH. Processing trends: Observation from 8 years national automatic film processing data (1982-1989). *Radiology* 177P, 173, 1990.

5. Haus AG, Kimme-Smith C, Baker CW, Jones CD. A Sensitometric method of on-site evaluation of film processing compared to manufacturers' expectation. *Medical Physics* (abstract) 18(4):851, 1992.

6. Sprawls P, Moore RG. Improving mammographic film processing accuracy. *Radiology* (abstract) 181(P): 271, 1991.

7. Haus AG, Batz TA, Dickerson RE, Lillie RF, Oemcke KW, and Lanphear JD: Automatic film processing in medical imaging. In Seibert, J.A., Barns, G.T., and Gould, R.G: Specification, Acceptance Testing and Quality Control of Diagnostic X-Ray Imaging Equipment. American Institute of Physics, New York, NY, 1992.

# Procedure For Processor Quality Control: A Step-By-Step Approach

**Susan M. Jaskulski**
Health Sciences Division
Eastman Kodak Company
Rochester, New York

Daily processor quality control by mammography facilities is required by the American College of Radiology (ACR) as part of the accreditation process, by Medicare as a condition for reimbursement, and by some states. These QC tests are usually performed by the radiologic technologist for whom quality control is a primary responsibility. The purpose of processor quality control is the monitoring and maintenance of a controlled processing environment, a critical requirement for high-quality mammographic images.

## Tools Required

The proper tools must first be obtained; these include a sensitometer; a densitometer; a digital, clinical, fever thermometer; processing control charts; and a box of mammography film.

The sensitometer is the instrument used to expose the sensitometric strip from which measurements will be taken. A sensitometer which exposes 21 density steps and allows single- or double-emulsion film to be exposed by green light should be used. The single and green settings on the sensitometer must be selected if using single-emulsion film. Double-emulsion mammography film requires the dual and green settings. The settings should be verified prior to each use, especially if the sensitometer is carried between several darkrooms and utilized for general radiology as well as mammography.

A densitometer is used to take several optical density readings from the sensitometric strip. Either a spot reading or automated scanning type of densitometer may be used.

An inexpensive digital, clinical, fever thermometer, commonly available from local pharmacies, can be used to measure the temperature of the developer solution. The typical range is from 92 to 96 degrees Fahrenheit, depending on the type of processor. A digital, clinical, fever thermometer registers temperatures between approximately 90 and 108 degrees Fahrenheit.

Of greater importance is the reading accuracy, precision and repeatability of the thermometer. The ACR recommends that the developer temperature be maintained within ± 0.5 degrees Fahrenheit. The thermometer used should have at least an equivalent accuracy. It should be compared to a calibrated or reference thermometer. The accuracy of a digital, clinical, fever thermometer is approximately ±0.2 degrees Fahrenheit. Thermometers containing mercury or made of glass should not be used because of the possibility of contamination should the thermometer break and because of the ease of breakage.

Processing control charts are needed to record all processing parameters and to make comparisons of the data. Medium density (MD), density difference (DD), base + fog (B+F), and temperature are recorded. In addition, information related to the type of film, processor and all actions associated with maintaining a controlled processor should be recorded on the chart.

Finally, a fresh, unopened box of 18 x 24 cm mammography film of the same type used for clinical images (full breast or screening) must be selected and labeled for quality control purposes. The emulsion number, usually located on the outside of the box, should be recorded on the control chart. It is important to use only film from the designated box in order to exclude film variability from evaluation of the processing environment. A box of 100 sheets will last up to four or five months when monitoring a single processor. To avoid affecting quality control results from prolonged safelight exposure and suboptimal storage conditions, quality control film should not be cut in half to economize.

## Prior to Establishing a Quality Control Program

Before establishing a quality control program, the darkroom and processing environment must first be thoroughly evaluated and any deficiencies corrected. For example, the darkroom must be lighttight and have adequate ventilation. The processor must be filled with fresh, high-quality chemicals. The correct amount of the chemical manufacturer's developer starter must be added after each preventive maintenance procedure is completed. The processor and film manufacturers should be consulted for the recommended developer temperature for the processor, and for the replenishment rates recommended for the volume of film processed daily; both are critically important for achieving proper processing results.

While ensuring the proper developer temperature is relatively easy, the proper replenishment rate is often difficult to establish. The effects of fluctuating film volumes, low film volume, and processors not dedicated to single-emulsion film must be considered. Daily patient volumes should be managed so to be as consistent as possible; all films should be positioned consistently on the film feed tray to help maintain the stability of the processing environment. Low film volume, zero to thirty 18 x 24 cm sheets of mammography film per day, requires flooded replenishment. Flooded replenishment uses a timer on the processor to automatically pump fresh replenisher periodically into the developer and fixer tanks of the processor. This helps maintain the chemical activity of the processing solutions.

Replenishment information for processors dedicated to mammography for low, medium and high volume is usually available from film manufacturers. The need for attention to the above considerations can be minimized through the use of new-technology processors which control replenishment rates and maintain chemical activity by replenishing according to the area of film processed.

## Establishing a Quality Control Program

Each morning, after the processor has reached the normal operating temperature, the temperature of the developer should be checked by inserting the thermometer probe into the developer tank. The reading should be within $\pm 0.5$ degrees Fahrenheit of the temperature recommended by the film manufacturer.

Consistent placement of the thermometer probe in the developer tank is important. The best location is toward the non-drive side of the tank. Afterwards, the probe should be rinsed with tepid water and wiped dry before storing.

After checking the settings on the sensitometer, insert a sheet of film from the box of quality control film into the sensitometer so the emulsion side of the film is toward the light source (Figure 1). Process the film immediately after exposure; position the film on the feed tray so that the less exposed density step is fed first into the processor. Proper safelight illumination in the darkroom is generally used when generating a sensitometric strip, but total darkness may give even more consistent results.

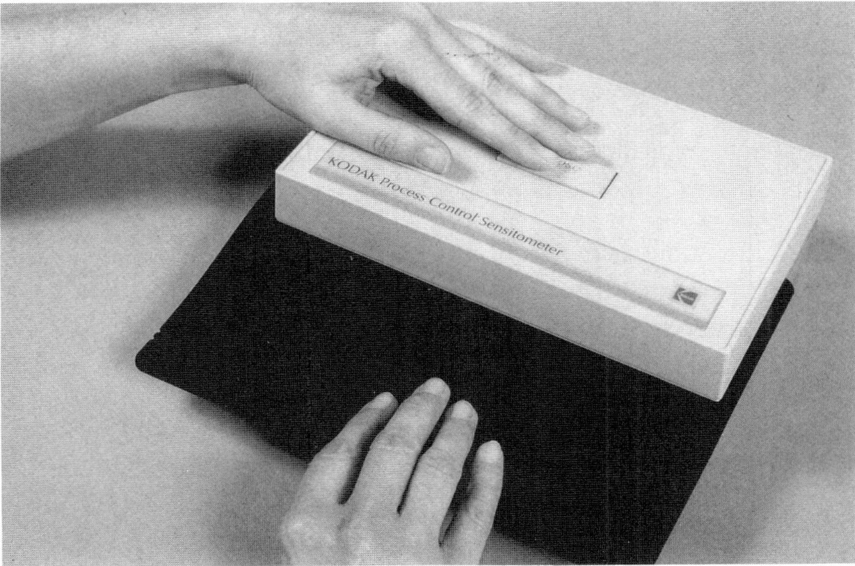


**Figure 1. A single-emulsion film inserted into the sensitometer so the emulsion is toward the light source (down) and the film identification notches are away from the sensitometer and toward the operator.**

Consistent methodology throughout the entire quality control procedure is essential. The sensitometric strip should always be generated and processed the same way and at the same time each morning following the facility protocol. Such a protocol might be, for example: 1) insert the film, emulsion side down, into the sensitometer so that the film identification notch(es) are away from the sensitometer and toward the operator (Figure 1); 2) expose the film; 3) process the film immediately after exposure by placing the film emulsion side up on the righthand side of the feed tray so that the notched edge is the leading edge (Figure 2).

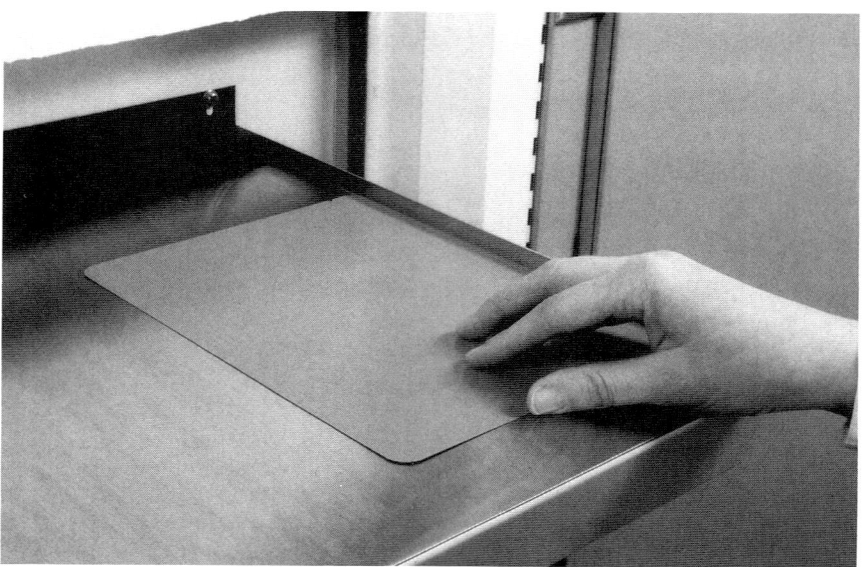

**Figure 2. A single-emulsion film placed on the right hand side of the feed tray, emulsion side up and with the notched edge as the leading edge.**

This example resulted in the less exposed end of the 21 steps being processed first. The exposed portion of the film was also positioned toward the center of the processor and away from the edges of the rollers, usually the first area to show signs of wear and possibly cause artifacts.

When establishing a quality control program, a sensitometric strip should be generated for five consecutive days. On the fifth day, the optical densities of all 21 steps from each of the five days should be read using the densitometer and the averages of the steps should be determined.

The average value of step 1, the step with no light exposure, becomes the aim value for base + fog (B+F). B+F reflects the optical density of the film support and any negligible exposure to the silver in the emulsion. An unexposed area of the film may also be measured for the B+F value instead of step 1, provided the same area is consistently measured on each sensitometric strip. The B+F aim value is transferred to the middle line of that area on the processing control chart. The upper limit of +0.03 should be calculated and noted on the chart.

The mid-density (MD) step, also called speed, speed point, or speed index, is the point with an average value closest to 1.20. This falls approximately in the middle of the straight line portion of the H&D curve, as shown in Figure 3. The MD aim value is recorded on the middle line of that area on the processing control chart and the step to be measured daily for MD recorded beside it.

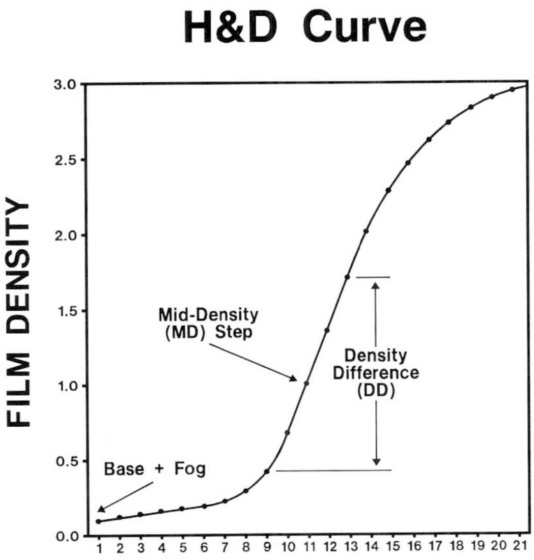

## H&D Curve



Figure 3. A typical mammographic H&D curve showing Base + Fog at step 1, the Mid-Density (MD) step in the middle of the straight line portion of the curve, and the two points used to calculate the Density Difference (DD) at either end of the straight line portion of the curve.

For mammography, MD has preferred minimum and maximum operating limits of ±0.10 and ±0.15. These values should be calculated and recorded on the chart. Daily values should never exceed the limits. Data plotted between the preferred and operating limits indicate a need to closely monitor the processor to make sure it does not exceed the limits.

The contrast index, also known as the density difference (DD), must be calculated by utilizing two steps. The average value of the step closest to, but not less than 0.45, is subtracted from the average value of the step closest to 2.20. The difference in density is recorded as the value for DD. The steps used for the calculation should also be noted. The same preferred minimum and maximum limits of ±0.10 and ±0.15 apply for DD as for MD. The particular steps for MD and DD, once chosen, should be measured consistently thereafter.

Finally, the developer temperature recommended by the manufacturer should be recorded on the processing control chart. Developer temperature should be maintained within ± 0.5 degrees Fahrenheit.

Figures 3 through 5 show a typical mammographic H&D curve, an example of the calculation of the aims for B+F, MD and DD (using only the pertinent density steps) and a mammography processing control chart with the aim values and limits recorded.

After defining the aims on the control chart, the values for B+F, MD, DD, and temperature should be plotted as part of the daily procedure.

$$\frac{\text{1st}}{\text{Day}} + \frac{\text{2nd}}{\text{Day}} + \frac{\text{3rd}}{\text{Day}} + \frac{\text{4th}}{\text{Day}} + \frac{\text{5th}}{\text{Day}} \div 5 = \text{Average}$$

Step 1     0.16 + 0.17 + 0.17 + 0.18 + 0.17 ÷ 5 = 0.17     Base + Fog Aim

Step 11    1.05 + 1.21 + 1.12 + 1.23 + 1.21 ÷ 5 = 1.16     Medium Density Aim

Step 13    2.20 + 2.16 + 2.21 + 2.14 + 2.10 ÷ 5 = 2.16
Step 9      .49 +  .46 +  .48 +  .45 +  .43 ÷ 5 = −.46
                                                    1.70     Density Difference Aim

**Figure 4a. Calculation of aims for Base + Fog, Medium Density, and Density Difference.**

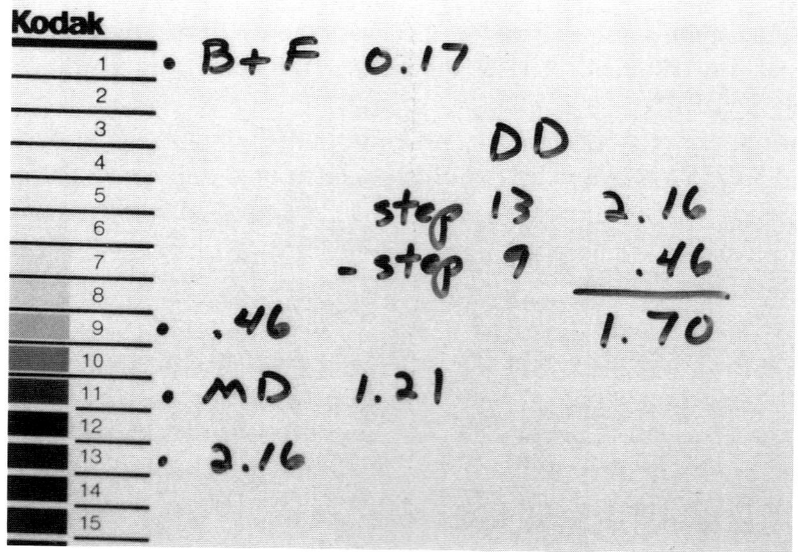


**Figure - 4b. B+F, MD, and DD aims shown on a sensitometric strip.**

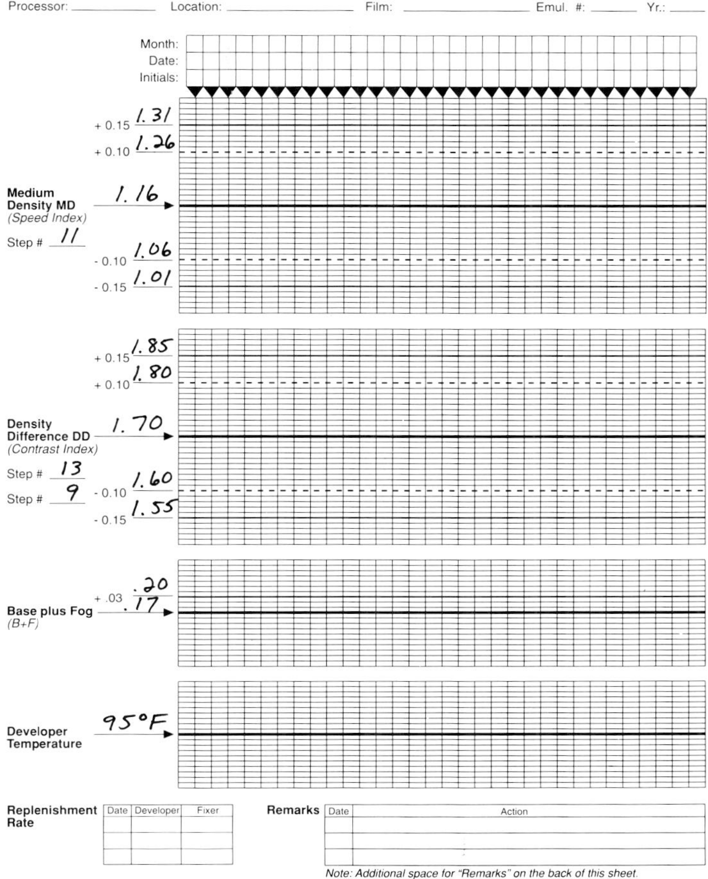


**Figure 5. Mammography processing control chart showing aims, upper and lower limits, and steps to be read daily.**

## Table 1.   Processor quality control data for three days.

|  | Day 1 | Day 2 | Day 3 |
|---|---|---|---|
| B+F | 0.17 | 0.18 | 0.18 |
| MD | 1.21 | 1.27 | 1.32 |
| DD | 1.67 | 1.74 | 1.76 |
| Temperature (degrees F) | 95.0 | 95.2 | 95.8 |

Table 1 shows typical values for the first three days. Figure 6 shows the values plotted on the control chart.  The MD value for Day 3 has exceeded the upper limit, indicating the processor is out-of-control.  Whenever an out-of-control situation occurs, the processor quality control procedure should be repeated to verify the condition and to confirm that the procedure was performed properly. Mammography films should not be processed until the problem has been determined and corrected. In this example, the water had not been turned on, thereby allowing the developer temperature to increase and causing the MD value to exceed the upper limit.  With the problem found and corrected (water turned on), the processor was brought back into control. (Figure 6).

There are many variables which contribute to an out-of-control processor. Detailed information to help bring the processor back to the desired operating level is available in published troubleshooting manuals.

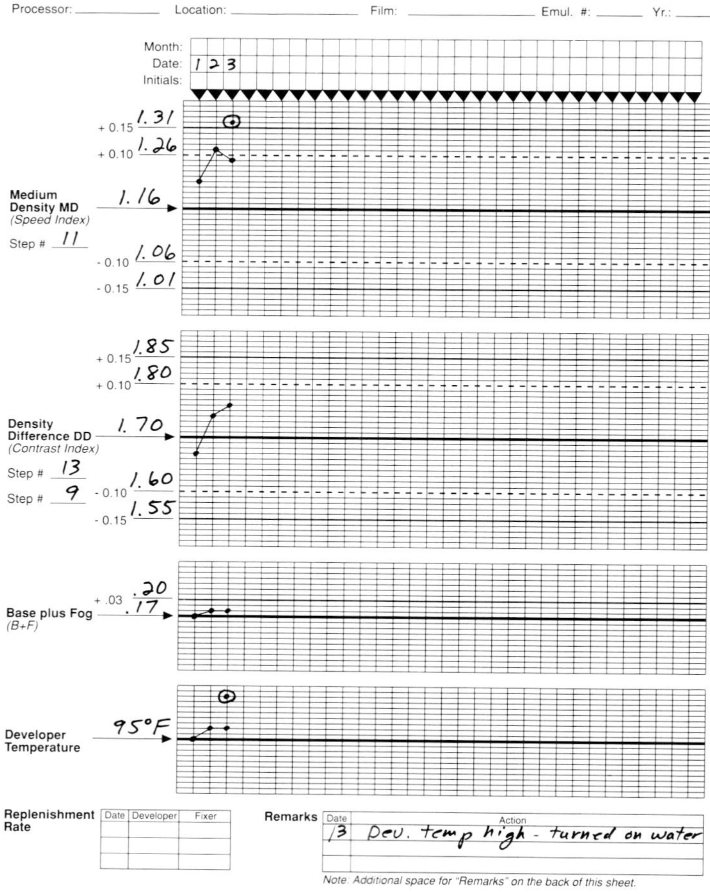

Figure 6. Typical data plotted on a mammography processing control chart.  The out-of-control points have been circled, the in-control points have been replotted and associated actions are noted on chart.

## When to Perform Processor Quality Control

The best time to perform the processor quality control procedure is the first thing in the morning, before processing any mammography films. In addition, doing processor quality control before and after processor cleaning and after adding fresh chemicals to the replenisher holding tanks will help ensure that the proper processing environment is maintained.

## The Crossover Procedure

A crossover procedure must be performed when a new box of mammography film is opened for quality control because the new box will usually have a different emulsion number. This procedure must be done at the same time on the same day and when the chemicals in the processor are in a seasoned, not fresh, state. Following the usual quality control procedure, expose five films from the current box of film and five from the new box. Working only with the steps usually measured for MD and DD, determine the average for MD and DD for the current film and the new film. If the difference in the values between the current film and new film for MD and/or DD is greater than 0.05, then the aims on the control chart should be adjusted to the new values. If the difference is less than or equal to 0.05, no adjustment is necessary; however, making an adjustment is acceptable. The B+F difference should not differ by more than 0.02. A greater difference than this warrants investigation. The emulsion number of the new box of quality control film should be noted on the control chart as well as the date the crossover was performed.

## Summary

Daily processor quality control is not only required in many instances but is absolutely essential for consistent high-quality films. The proper tools and a consistent daily procedure must be used. Before establishing a comprehensive program, the entire darkroom, processor and chemicals must be thoroughly evaluated and any deficiencies corrected. The program should be initiated based on an average of five days. Control charts are used to evaluate whether or not the processor is in control and to note all activity affecting that control. Finally, a crossover procedure should be performed when a new box of film is opened for quality control.

### Reference

Mammography Quality Control for Radiologic Technologists, American College of Radiology, Reston, Virginia, 1992.

# Processor Quality Control: American College of Radiology Mammography Quality Control Manual*

**R. Edward Hendrick**
University of Colarado, Denver, Colorado

**Joel E. Gray**
Mayo Clinic, Rochester, Minnesota

**Arthur G. Haus**
Eastman Kodak Company, Rochester, New York

**E. Lee Kitts**
E.I. du Pont de Nemours & Company, Brevard, North Carolina

**Pamela A. Wilcox**
**Marie D. Zinninger**
American College of Radiology, Reston, Virginia


The American College of Radiology has developed a Mammography Quality Control Manual with separate sections for the radiologist, medical physicist and radiologic technologist. Radiologic technologists are responsible for carrying out tests in the appropriate section on a daily, weekly, monthly, and quarterly basis. Medical physicists are responsible for tests in their section of the manual, on an annual basis. However, the medical physicist must also be familiar with all of the tests and information in the radiologic technologists' section so that the medical physicist can serve as a consultant to the radiologists and radiologic technologists. The following sections, which discuss film processing and film processing quality control tests, are reproduced with the permission of the American College of Radiology from the American College of Radiology Mammography Quality Control for the Radiologic Technologists and Medical Physicists Manuals.

---

*American College of Radiology Committee on Quality Assurance in Mammography. R. E. Hendrick, Chairman, L. Bassett, G. D. Dodd, S. Feig, J. E. Gray, A. G. Haus, M. A. Harvey, R. Heinlein, L. Kitts, R. McLelland, J. McCrohan, R. Rossi, D. Sullivan, P. Wilcox, M. Zinninger.

## Reproduced from the Radiologic Technologists Manual:
- Introduction
- Important Points
- Mammography Quality Control Tests
- Darkroom Cleanliness
- Processor Quality Control
- Analysis of Fixer Retention in Film
- Developer Temperature and Replenishment Rate
- References

## I. Introduction

The American College of Radiology is working with the diagnostic imaging community to help assure that optimum mammographic images are produced consistently, thus providing the best images possible for screening and diagnosis. This effort involves the ACR Mammography Accreditation Program as well as educational programs. These programs are not enough, however, to assure consistent, optimum quality mammograms. It is essential to have an ongoing quality assurance program in place at each mammogarphy site to assure consistent production of quality images.

The ACR Committee on Quality Assurance (QA) in Mammography has developed material to assist the radiologist, medical physicist, and radiologic technologist in establishing and maintaining mammographic equipment quality control programs. This document provides a series of quality control tests which should be carried out by the radiologic technologist with a minimal investment in time and equipment. The purpose and frequency of each test is clearly stated. The equipment and materials required to carry out the test are listed for each test. A step-by-step procedure is provided, followed by a discussion of precautions and caveats. Suggested performance criteria are provided along with suggestions for the types of corrective actions that may be needed to resolve problems. The minimum frequency and the approximate time required to perform each test are summarized in Tables 1 and 2, respectively. Control charts and data forms are provided in this document and may be copied for use in the quality control program.

## Table 1.  Mammographic Quality Control Minimum Test Frequencies

| Test | Minimum Frequency |
|---|---|
| Darkroom Cleanliness | Daily |
| Processor Quality Control | Daily |
| Screen Cleanliness | Weekly |
| Viewboxes and Viewing Conditions | Weekly |

**Table 1 (continued) MinimumTest Frequencies**

| Test | Minimum Frequency |
|---|---|
| Phantom Images | Monthly |
| Visual Check List | Monthly |
| Repeat Analysis | Quarterly |
| Analysis of Fixer Retention in Film | Quarterly |
| Darkroom Fog | Semi-annually |
| Screen-Film Contact | Semi-annually |
| Compression | Semi-annually |

It must be stressed that the frequencies of tests indicated in this document are the minimum frequencies (Table 1). If problems are detected often, or if the equipment is relatively unstable, then it may be necessary to carry out some or all of these tests more frequently, or repair or replace the faulty equipment. If the quality control program is just being initiated, one should carry out the tests more frequently for the first few months. This will provide the QC technologist with more experience in a shorter period of time and will also provide better baseline data regarding the reliability of imaging equipment. For example, it is recommended that the phantom image test be carried out monthly. It would be worthwhile to carry out this test daily for the first few weeks, then weekly for the next few months. At this point the QC technologist will have considerable experience with this test and, more importantly, will have integrated the test into his or her routine.

In addition to performing the Mammographic Quality Control Tests at the minimum frequencies indicated, tests should also be carried out initially (when the quality control program is started), when problems are suspected, or after service or preventive maintenance. For example, the compression test should be carried out initially when a new x-ray system is installed; screen-film contact tests should be carried out whenever new cassettes are placed into service; and the darkroom fog should be checked whenever new safelights or filters are installed in the darkroom or when a new type of film is used. If one suspects a loss of sharpness, then the screen-film contact test should be carried out on every cassette unless the problem can be isolated to a single cassette. Any time the processor is serviced, the Processor Quality Control Test should be performed. In addition, the Phantom Image Test should be carried out to test for processor artifacts.

**Table 2.  Mammographic Quality Control Test Procedure Time**

| Test | Approximate Time to Carry Out Procedure (minutes)* |
|---|---|
| Darkroom Cleanliness | 5-10 |
| Processor Quality Control | 10 |

**Table 2 (continued) Test Procedure Time**

| Test | Appoximate Time to Carry out Procedure (minutes)* |
|---|---|
| Screen Cleanliness | 5 (6 screens) |
| Viewboxes and Viewing Conditions | <5 |
| Phantom Images | 10 |
| Visual Check List | <5 |
| Repeat Analysis | 15-30 |
| Analysis of Fixer Retention in Film | <5 |
| Darkroom Fog | 15 |
| Screen-Film Contact | 5 (6 screens) |
| Compression | <5 |

* It is not possible to add up these times to give the total time required for quality control test since some may be done concurrently.

Due to the importance of quality control in diagnostic imaging in general, and mammography in particular, it is recommended that the medical physicist and radiologist review the control charts, other data, and images with the QC technologist at least quarterly, or more frequently if so desired by the radiologist. This assures that the quality control program is carried out consistently and provides oversight to assure that changes in image quality are not inadvertently overlooked.

The medical physicist has the primary responsibility for performing Quality Control testing on the x-ray equipment itself, including tests such as focal spot size, half value layer, entrance exposure and dose measurements, kVp accuracy and reproducibility. In addition, the medical physicist should be available to answer questions for the QC technologist carrying out the quality control measurements listed in this manual whenever problems are encountered. The medical physicist may serve as the liaison between the QC technologist and service engineer and verify that equipment problems exist before requesting service. This may require the use of more sophisticated tests and test tools as described in the document entitled, "Mammography Quality Control for Medical Physicists." The medical physicist is a resource that both the radiologist and radiologic technologist should rely on for questions and problems regarding mammographic image quality and quality control.

In a facility where more than one technologist does mammography, one technologist should be assigned the responsibilities of quality control. The designated quality control technologist is responsible for insuring standardization of methodology, reviewing all data, overseeing repeat testing before calling the medical physicist, and conferring with the radiologist and medical physicist. The radiologist, medical physicist, and QC technologist, working together as a team, are the key to providing optimum quality mammographic images, which will ultimately provide the best medical care possible to the patient.

There are a number of points which are important to a good, functioning quality control program. These "Important Points" are applicable to most of the tests described in this manual and are presented in Section II. The detailed quality control tests are presented in Section III. Section IV contains some additional, less frequently performed quality control tests. Section V contains an important guide to patient positioning and breast compression, and Section VI contains a glossary of terms used in this manual and elsewhere in mammography quality control.

## II. Important Points
### 1. Time for Quality Assurance Procedures

The approximate times to carry out the quality control procedures described in this manual are listed in Table 2. Only two of the procedures must be carried out daily, darkroom cleaning and processor quality control. Several of the tasks can be carried out at the same time so it is not appropriate to add the times listed in the table. For example, as soon as the processor is turned on, and while waiting for it to warm up, the darkroom can be cleaned, screens can be cleaned, and the viewbox and viewing conditions can be checked. Consequently, only a small amount of time is required for a successful mammographic quality control program.

### 2. Darkroom Cleanliness

The darkroom is a major source of problems in mammography. Any dust or dirt in the darkroom will result in artifacts in the mammographic images. A clean darkroom will result in fewer artifacts and reduce the amount of effort required for cleaning the cassettes and screens. There are a few basic rules regarding darkroom design and cleanliness that will help reduce the amount of dust and dirt and, consequently, the number of dust artifacts in mammographic images.

There should be no smoking, eating, or drinking in the darkroom. In addition, food and drink should not be taken into the darkroom at any time.

There should be nothing on the counter top used for loading and unloading the cassettes. Anything on the counter top makes cleaning more difficult and provides a convenient place for dust and dirt to accumulate.

Although convenient for film storage, there should be no shelves above the counter tops in the darkroom. Such shelves provide another place for dust and dirt to accumulate. Whenever a box of film is removed from the shelves above the counter top, the accumulated dust and dirt are deposited on the area used for loading and unloading cassettes.

The ceiling of the darkroom should be constructed of a solid material such as drywall. Ceiling tiles, often set in metal channels, allow dirt to sift through the ceiling and fall on the surfaces used for handling cassettes. In addition, light can often enter the darkroom through such tiles, resulting in fog on the mammographic films.

The vent for heating and air conditioning should not enter the room over the counter used for handling cassettes. This provides another source for dust and dirt being deposited on the counter.

Ultraviolet lights are available (inexpensive ones at novelty stores) which help demonstrate the dust and dirt in darkrooms. Some dust and dirt particles fluoresce when exposed to ultraviolet light and can readily be seen if all lights are turned off. However, not all dust and dirt particles fluoresce.

Electrostatic air cleaners may prove useful in reducing the amount of dirt and dust in the darkroom. In addition, static electricity can be reduced in several ways. The humidity level in the darkroom must be maintained between 40% and 60% throughout the year. If a new darkroom is being designed, counter top materials which reduce static electricity should be considered. Finally, static discharge systems are available which provide a continuous flow of ionized air to reduce static during the loading and unloading of cassettes.

Other sources of dust and dirt must be controlled. For example, if cassettes are placed on the floor beneath the passbox or in the exposure room they will accumulate dust which will be carried into the darkroom. In addition to other darkroom cleaning tasks, the passbox should be cleaned every day to prevent dust and dirt from being introduced into the darkroom through this route.

### 3. Screen-Cassette Identification

It is important to be able to identify each screen-cassette combination. For example, if the QC technologist or radiologist notices dust artifacts on some mammogarphic images, appropriate identification will allow the QC technologist to quickly locate the dirty cassette and clean the screens.

Each screen should be marked with a unique identification number near the left and right edge of the screen using an opaque, permanent marker. (Note - some markers may damage the screens. The screen manufacturer can provide information regarding appropriate markers.)  The same identification number should also be placed on the outside of the cassette.

### 4. Selecting the Appropriate Film, Processing Chemicals, Processor and Processing Cycle

To obtain the best results, it is necessary to select the appropriate combination of mammographic film, processing chemistry, developer temperature, film processor and processing cycle.

Due to the large number of combinations of film, chemistry, etc., it is extremely important to use the film, developer chemistry, the processor, the developer temperature, and the immersion time recommended by the film manufacturer.

In addition, it is important to use single emulsion film when only a single screen is used and dual emulsion film when a cassette with two screens is utilized

Furthermore, only film designed specifically for mammographic imaging should be used in mammography.

## 5. Film and Chemical Storage

As recommended by NCRP 99, photographic material should be stored at temperature less than 24°C (75°F), preferably in the range of 15° to 21°C (60° to 70°F). Open packages of photographic film should be stored in an area with humidity ranging between 40% and 60%. Photographic materials should not be stored in areas where they can be exposed to chemical fumes or radiation including radioisotopes, radioactive wastes, and direct or scattered x-rays. Photographic materials are also sensitive to pressure damage; consequently, films should be stored standing on edge.

Photographic chemicals should be stored with care. Never allow liquid photochemicals to freeze. If chemicals are frozen and there is any evidence of sedimentation in the container, the chemicals should not be used and should be returned to the vendor.

The emulsion batch that will expire first should be used first. Film should not be allowed to remain in the film bin past that expiration date. New shipments of film should be checked and should not be accepted from the vendor unless they can be used before the expiration date.

## 6. Selecting the Appropriate Thermometer

Only digital thermometers should be used for monitoring mammographic film processors. Glass thermometers are easily broken in the processor and should be avoided. Most importantly, a thermometer containing mercury should never be used in a photographic processor since the mercury is a photographic containment. Even small amounts of mercury, on the order of a few parts per million, will contaminate the processor and cause erratic results.

The thermometer used for monitoring the developer temperature must be accurate to at least ±0.5°F. Many inexpensive digital thermometers are available but they are seldom accurate enough for use in a mammographic quality control program. However, a clinical fever thermometer is inexpensive (less than $10) and usually has an accuracy of better than ± 0.5°F over a range from 90° to 100°F. Fever thermometers must be reset after each reading since they are designed to take a peak reading and hold that reading, i.e., they are continuous reading thermometers. In addition, most fever thermometers do not function properly, or at all, below 90°F.

## 7. Selecting the Appropriate Sensitometer

It is essential to select a sensitometer for the quality control program which exposes the film in a manner similar to the exposure received by the film in clinical use. Matching of the sensitometer to the clinical exposure conditions is important since some films may respond differently to changes in the processing chemicals, depending on the type of exposure received. If a single-sided film is used, then the sensitometer should be a single-sided device. If dual- emulsion film is used with dual screens, then the sensitometer should be a dual-sided device. In either case the spectrum of the light from the sensitometer should be similar to that of the intensifying screens used. For example, most mammographic films are exposed to green emitting screens so a sensitometer which produces a green output should be selected, as opposed to one with a blue output spectrum or a sensitometer with an unfiltered tungsten light source.

## 8. <u>Processing and Reading of Sensitometric Control Strips</u>

The purpose of processing a sensitometric control strip to determine the developer activity level of the processor before processing clinical films. Consequently, it is essential that the sensitometric strip be exposed, processed, and read with a densitometer, and the data plotted to determine whether the processor is operating properly first thing in the morning before processing any mammograms. Sensitometric strips that are pre-exposed (hours or days in advance) will suffer from latent image changes and will not be as sensitive as freshly exposed strrips to changes in the processor. In addition, changes in the film density may result over time due to latent image decay, so it will be difficult to determine whether the processor is operating properly. Likewise, the densities of the strips must be read and plotted immediately to determine whether any processor changes have occured. It is inappropriate to process clinical films and then determine hours or days later that the film processor was not operating optimally. Likewise, the processed sensitometric strips must be read with a densitometer, i.e., it is inappropriate to only visually compare sensitometric control strips.

## 9. <u>Control Charts</u>

For reliable monitoring of the measurements in a quality control program, it is essential to immediately plot data on control charts. For example, the film density, density difference, exposure time or mAs, and the number of visible objects seen on the phantom image should be plotted on a control chart (see Figures 1a and 1b). The date should be indicated, along with the initials of the individual performing the test. Notes regarding changes in operating conditions, e.g., a change in the developer temperature or replenishment rate, should be recorded on the control chart.

Control charts provide an easy means of reviewing related data. Whenever a data point reaches or exceeds the control limits, the test should be repeated immediately. If the repeated measurement data still reach or exceed the control limits, then immediate corrective action is required. In this case, the out-of-control data point should be circled, the cause of the problem noted, and in-control data point plotted (see Figure 1b).

Control charts also allow for the detection of trends which indicate an unstable process. A trend is an upward or downward change in the measured data when three data points move in the same direction. The cause of trends should be investigated.

For example, a trend is evident in Figure 1b, from May 4 through May 6 where the density of the films was steadily before the control limits are reached or exceeded. increasing as a result of overreplenishment.

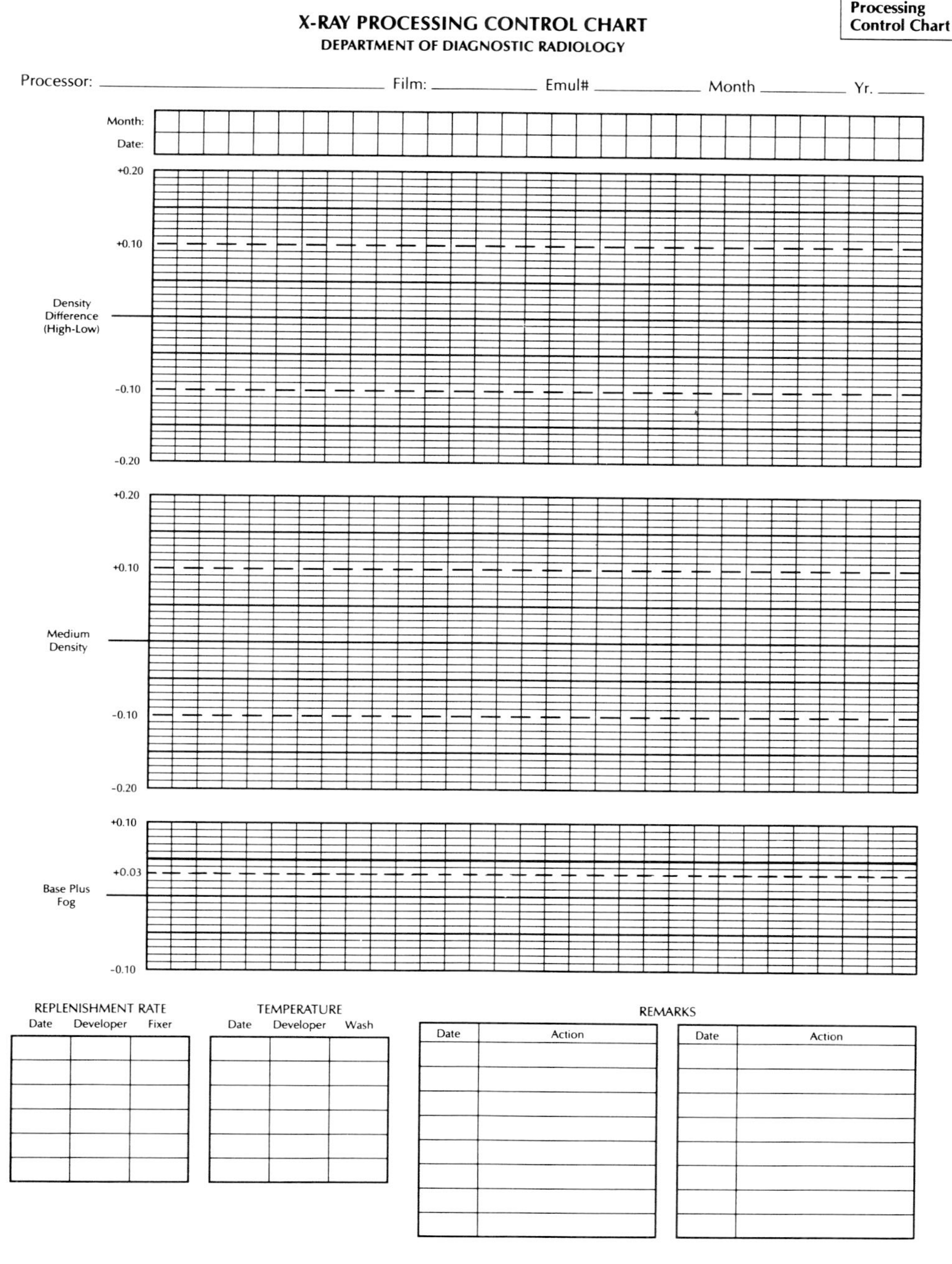


**Figure 1a. Daily processor quality control charts.**

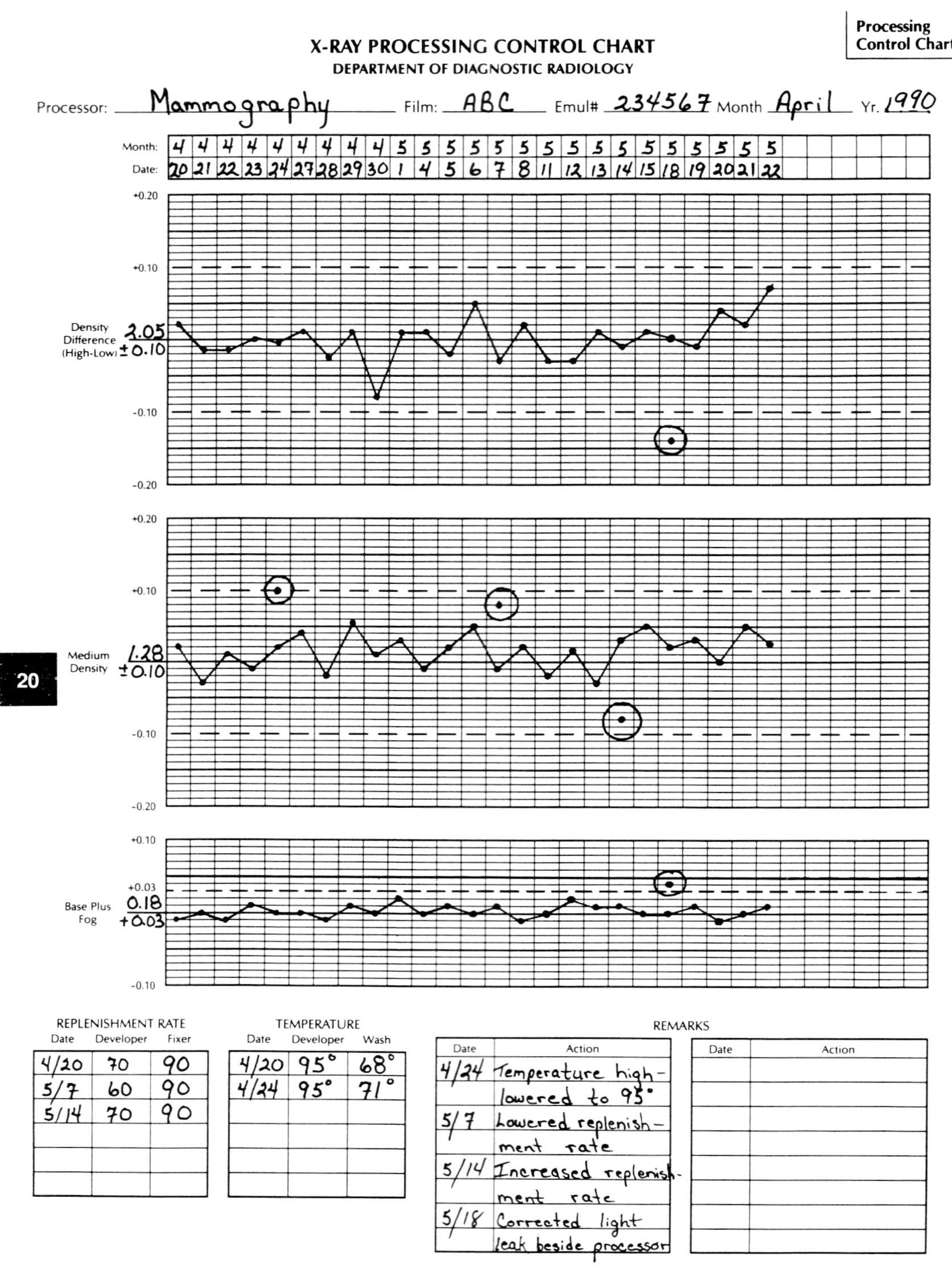



Figure 1b. Processor control chart showing typical data with trends on May 4-6.

10. <u>Establishment of Operating Levels and Control Limits</u>

When a quality control program is started it is necessary to establish operating levels and control limits. The operating level is that level which is normally expected. For example, the density measured on a film would be expected to be at, or close to, some particular value which is the operating level. The operating level for the kVp should be the kVp normally set on the x-ray generator. The control limits are those measured values which, if reached or exceeded, require additional action. Normally if the control limits are reached or exceeded the test is repeated immediately to confirm the problem. If a repeat of the test gives the same measurement, then corrective action is required. Corrective action may include contacting the medical physicist to investigate the problem or contacting a service engineer to correct a confirmed problem.

If the suggested performance criteria, or control limits, from this manual are consistently exceeded, then it will be necessary to determine the cause of the problem. This may be due to the measurement technique. For example, if the sensitometric control strip is processed on the left side of the processor one time and the right the next, with the emulsion up one time and down the next, or immediately after exposure one time and after a delay the next, then one may suspect such variations. All of these "human variables" should be eliminated and data collected for another period of time before making a decision. If the control limits are still consistently exceeded then the measurement equipment, e.g., the sensitometer and densitometer, should be evaluated. If the measurement equipment is found to be functioning properly and all "human variables" have been eliminated, then it is probably time to replace the equipment being monitored. All of the problem data should be reviewed by the medical physicist, and recommendations regarding modifications to the qualify control program, the repair or renovation of present equipment, or the purchase of new equipment should be discussed with the radiologist.

If it is apparent that the "Suggested Performance Criteria" are too wide, then one can consider narrowing the control limits. This should be done in consultation with the medical physicist and radiologist.

For example, the "Suggested Performance Criteria" for the Processor Sensitometric Evaluation indicate a retest if the measured density varies from the operating level by $\pm 0.10$ and immediately corrective action if it exceeds $\pm 0.15$. However, if the data seldom exceed $\pm 0.10$, then one may wish to make this the control limit, the limit which requires immediate corrective action. In this case one is assured of even better, more consistent quality.

One caveat must be stressed:

If the control limits are consistently exceeded, then it is necessary to improve the quality control procedures, or repair or replace the appropriate equipment. DO NOT widen the control limits since the data are indicating that the process is "out of control" and corrective action is essential.

## 11. Viewing Conditions

Viewing conditions are extremely critical in mammography. The information for the procedure entitled "Viewboxes and Viewing Conditions" should be read and followed with great care. High-luminance viewboxes with proper masking of each film are essential for good mammography.

Whenever mammograms or phantom images are viewed, they should be viewed under identical conditions. For example, phantom images should be viewed on the same viewbox, with the same lighting conditions, and using the sme magnifier as is used for viewing clinical mammographic images and at the same time of day, for example, first thing in the morning. In addition, the same viewbox masking should be used for both clinical and phantom images.

Whenever it is necessary to make subjective judgements about phantom images, e.g., determining the number of objects in the phantom image, the evaluation should be carried out by the same person using conditions identical to those used for previous evaluations.

## 12. Frequency of Tests

The frequency of tests specified in this manual (Table 1) is the minimum frequency. The frequency of quality control tests can vary considerably depending on many factors including the age and stability of the imaging equipment, and the number of problems being encountered, to name just a few. The baseline operating levels should be determined just after calibration of x-ray equipment and with fresh chemistry in the processor.

After the operating levels have been determined, the tests should be run more frequently than specified in this document for ten to twenty test periods. For example, if the recommended frequency is weekly, then the test should be performed daily for a few weeks. This provides a large amount of data quickly to determine if rapid changes are occurring and allows for an accurate determination of operating levels, where appropriate. It also provides the individual performing the tests with more experience in a short period of time.

The frequency of the tests may be modified in consultation with th radiologist responsible for the facility and the consulting medical physicist after significant experience has been gained. It may be necessary to increase the frequency of the tests if problems are frequently detected. It may also be possible to decrease the frequency of some tests if only a few problems have been detected. In this latter case one may wish to decrease the control limits, while maintaining the frequency of the test, and operate with tighter controls and more consistent image quality.

One caveat must be stressed:

If problems are seldom detected, DO NOT discontinue the quality control program! The lack of problems indicates that the process is "in control" at the present time, but does not predict the stability of the process in the future.

As noted in "Establishment of Operating Levels and Control Limits," the control limits should not be increased. If the equipment produces results which are consistently outside of the control limits suggested in this manual, then it will be necessary to have the appropriate repairs made or the equipment replaced.

### 13. Mammography Quality Control Checklists

In order to assist in the oversight of the quality control tests, two mammography quality control checklists are provided (Figure 1). These checklists provide a quick reminder as to when quality control tasks are due and also provide a record indicating that the appropriate tasks have been completed in a timely manner. All dates should be filled in prior to use of the checklist. Each time a task is completed, the individual carrying out the task should initial the appropriate area on the checklist.

### 14. Screening Mammography Phototimer Technique Chart

Many phototimers do not produce the correct densities for all thicknesses of breasts nor for all kVps. This problem may be reduced by the use of a phototimer technique chart (following page). The necessary changes in kVp and the density setting to produce consistent density mammograms can be determined with the help of the medical physicist.

It may be necessary to use manual techniques to obtain appropriate films of breasts containing implants. This information can be recorded in the manual technique chart.

Once these technique charts have been filled out, they should be posted on the mammographic unit adjacent to the control panel.

## III. Mammography Quality Control Tests

## 1. Procedure: Darkroom Cleanliness

Objective: To minimize artifacts on film images by maintaining the cleanest practicable conditions in the darkroom.

Artifacts due to bits of dirt and dust between the screen and film are particularly troublesome with single emulsion imaging in mammography, not only because they are much more prominent than on double emulsion films, but also because they may mimic microcalcifications and lead to misdiagnosis.

Frequency
This procedure should be carried out daily at the beginning of the work day before

processing or handling any films in the darkroom.

<u>Required Equipment</u>
Wet mop and pail
Lint-free towels
Liquid hand soap

<u>Procedure Steps</u>
1.   Turn the processor water and power on so that the developer temperature can stabilize during this procedure.
2.   Damp mop the darkroom floor.
3.   Remove all unnecessary items from counter tops and work surfaces.
4.   Use a clean, damp towel to wipe off the processor feed tray and then the counter tops and other surfaces in the darkroom.
5.   Keep hands clean to minimize fingerprints and handling artifacts.
6.   Wipe or vacuum overhead air vents and safelights weekly before cleaning the feed tray and counter tops.

<u>Precautions and Caveats</u>
Smoking and eating in the darkroom should be prohibited. Adequate closed storage space is required to minimize dirt-collecting clutter.

<u>Suggested Performance Criteria and Corrective Action</u>
Darkroom cleanliness may be evaluated best in terms of screen cleanliness, i.e., the number of dust artifacts appearing on the mammographic images.


## 2. Procedure: Processor Quality Control

<u>Objective:</u> To confirm and verify that the film processor-chemical system is working in a consistent manner according to pre-established specifications (manufacturer's specifications).


<u>Frequency</u>
Procedure 2B should be carried out daily at the beginning of the work day before processing any films. For mobile mammographic equipment, Procedure 2B must be carried out for the processor used for processing the clinical films before processing any mammogram. This is essential if the processor is located near the mobile equipment site or if the films are processed later at the home location of the mobile equipment.

<u>Required Equipment</u>
Sensitometer – a sensitometer that exposes one side of the film should be used for single-emulsion film, while a sensitometer that exposes both sides of the film simultaneously should be used for double- emulsion films. The spectral characteristics of the light source of the sensitometer must be similar to the light source used for exposing the film in clinical use, e.g., it should be green if green emitting screens are used. The sensitometer must have a 21-step optical attenuator with densities ranging from approximately 0.00 to 3.00 in steps of 0.15.

Densitometer
Fresh box of control film (of the same type of film used in mammography)
Control chart
Clinical digital fever thermometer accurate to at least $\pm 0.5^\mathrm{O}$F.

<u>Procedure Steps</u>
Two distinct procedures are described in this section. The first procedure describes the steps necessary to establish the correct operating levels of the processor. This procedure will be carried out when the quality control program is initiated or when a different type of film or developer is to be used. The second procedure is carried out daily at the beginning of the work day before processing any patient films, but after processor warm-up. This procedure assures consistent film quality through consistent film processing.

**Procedure 2A: Establishment of Processor Quality Control Operating Levels**

1.  Select a fresh box of film, of the same type used for mammography, and reserve this box for quality control purposes only. (Note the emulsion number of the box of film on the control chart.)
2.  Drain the chemicals from the processor and thoroughly flush the racks and tanks with water.
3.  Drain the replenisher tanks and refill with fresh replenisher.
4.  Fill the fixer tank with fixer solution.
5.  Once again flush the developer tank with water.
6.  Fill the developer tank about one-half full with developer solution and add the specified amount of developer starter solution. Add sufficient developer solution to fill developer tank.
7.  Set the developer temperature control at the temperature specified in the film manufacturer's written literature.
8.  Set the developer and fixer replenishment rates as specified by the film manufacturer.

9.  After the developer temperature has stabilized, check the temperature of the developer solution with a clinical fever thermometer and assure that the processor is operating at the temperature specified by the film manufacturer. Clean the thermometer stem of developer solution after each use.

NOTE: A thermometer containing mercury should never be used in a photographic processor. If the thermometer were to break, minute amounts of mercury could contaminate the processor and cause inconsistent processing results.

10.  Using a sensitometer, expose and process a sensitometric strip. Repeat this exposure and processing once each day for five consecutive days.

Before processing sensitometric strips be sure that the:
- developer temperature is correct
- sensitometric strip is processed with the less-exposed end being fed into the processor first
- sensitometric strip is processed on the same side of the processor, i.e., it is inserted on the same side of the processor feed tray each time
- sensitometric strip is processed with the emulsion in the same orien tation (for single-emulsion films), for example, with the emulsion side down
- delay between exposure and processing is similar each day to avoid any latent image changes that may occur with time.

11.  Read and record the densities of each step of the sensitometric strip using the densitometer, including an area of processed film which has not been exposed. Note, the densities of the steps should be measured in the center of each step.

12.  Determine the average of the densities for each step using the densities for that step from the five strips.

13.  Determine which step has an average density closest to 1.20. Put a small mark on the corresponding step of the step wedge on the sensitometer and designate this step the mid-density (MD) step. (This step is often referred to as the speed point, speed index, or speed step.)

14.  Determine which step has a density closest to 2.20 and which step has a density closest to but not less than 0.45. Put a small mark on the corresponding steps of the step wedge on the sensitometer. The difference in densities between these two steps should be designated as the density difference (DD).

NOTE: The density difference determined by this method is to be used only to assess consistency of film and processing. It is not appropriate for comparing different film types nor for comparing film types processed at different facilities.

15.  Determine the average of the densities from the unexposed area of the five

strips. This density will be designated as the base-plus-fog level (B+F) of the film.

16. Record the average numerical values of the MD, DD, and B+F on the center line of the appropriate areas of the control chart (Figures 1A and 1B).

17. Record the upper and lower control limits for each value on the control chart. See Figures 1A and 1B and the following section entitled "Suggested Performance Criteria" for examples and further information.

## Procedure 2B: Daily Processor Quality Control

1. Expose and immediately process a sensitometric strip before processing clinical mammograms.

Before processing sensitometric strips be sure that the:
- developer temperature is correct
- sensitometric strip is processed with the less-exposed end fed into the processor first.
- sensitometric strip is processed on the same side of the processor, i.e., it is inserted on the same side of the processor feed tray each time
- sensitometric strip is processed with the emulsion in the same orien tation (for single-emulsion films), for example, with the emulsion side down
- delay between exposure and processing is similar each day to avoid any latent changes that may occur with time

2. Read the densities of the three indicated steps and the base-plus-fog.

3. Plot the mid-density (MD), the density difference (DD), and the base-plus-fog level (B+F) on the control chart.

4. Determine if any of the data points exceed the control limits.

5. Circle the out-of-control data points, correct the cause of the problem and repeat the test, note the cause of the problem in the "Remarks" section of the control chart, and plot the in control data point.

6. Determine if there are any trends, i.e., three or more data points moving in one direction (either upwards or downwards), in the MD, DD, or B+F. If trends are present but the data points have not, as yet, exceeded the control limits clinical mammograms can be processed. However, it will be necessary to determine the cause of the trend and to monitor the processor closely to assure that the control limits are not exceeded.

Precautions and Caveats

It is essential that sensitometric strips be exposed, processed, and the data evaluated before clinical films are processed each day. If problems are detected, corrective action can then be taken before clinical films are processed under less than optimal conditions.

The use of sensitometric strips exposed more than an hour or two before use is not acceptable since these strips may be less sensitive to changes in the processor than freshly exposed strips. In addition, as noted before, the sensitometric strip must be evaluated before clinical films are processed. Reading of the sensitometric strips and evaluation of the results hours or days after the strip has been processed does not provide adequate quality control. Many clinical films may be improperly processed before the results are available. In order to maintain good quality control of the photographic processor, it is essential to read the densities of the sensitometric control strips with a calibrated densitometer. Visual comparison of the steps of the control strips is not adequate.

As indicated above, each sensitometric strip must be processed on the same side of the processor and fed into the processor with the less-exposed (lower density) end of the strip leading. This reduces variation in the results and avoids development artifacts.

Radiographic film is produced in batches. Consequently, there may be slight variations in the characteristics of film between batches. In addition, film aging and storage conditions can also affect the sensitometric characteristics of the film. Whenever a new box of film is opened for quality control purposes it is necessary to perform a "cross-over" with the old film. The "cross-over" should be carried out only with a processor with seasoned chemistry. Expose and process, at the same time, five sensitometric strips each from the old and new boxes of film. Determine the average of each of the three indicated steps and of the base-plus-fog for the old film and for the new film. If the difference in the MD or DD between the old and new film is greater than 0.05, then the operating level on the control chart should be adjusted to this new level. If the B+F of the new film exceeds the B+F of the old film by more than 0.02, the cause for this increase should be investigated.

Quality control must also be performed on the densitometer, sensitometer, and thermometer themselves, to ensure their proper calibration. Manufacturer recommendations for quality control on these instruments should be followed, where available.


<u>Suggested Performance Criteria and Corrective Action</u>
If the MD and DD are within ± 0.10 of their respective operating levels, and the B+F is within +0.03 of its operatinglevel, the processor is in control and no further action is required. If the MD or DD falls outside of the ± 0.10 control limits but within ± 0.15 the test should be repeated immediately. If the same result is obtained it is acceptable to process clinical films, but the processor should be monitored closely. If the MD or DD exceeds the control limits of ± 0.15, the source of the problem must be determined and corrected before clinical mammograms are processed. Likewise,

if the B+F exceeds +0.03, immediate corrective action must be taken before clinical mammograms are processed.

If a change in the mid-density, density difference, or base-plus-fog exceeds the suggested performance criterion then it will be necessary to determine the source or sources of this change (temperature, chemistry, replenishment, etc.) and the problem(s) should be corrected immediately. In addition, the out-of-control data point should be circled, the cause of the problem noted in the "Remarks" section of the control chart, and the in control data point plotted (see Figure 1b).

## Procedure: Analysis of Fixer Retention in Film

<u>Objective</u>: To determine the quantity of residual fixer (or hypo) in processed film as an indicator of keeping quality.

Residual hypo indicates insufficient washing and considerably degrades image stability.

<u>Frequency</u>

This test should be carried out quarterly.

<u>Required</u>

Hypo estimator (e.g., Kodak hypo estimator, publication no. N-405, or equivalent)

Residual hypo test solution (commercially available or see Note at the end of this section)

<u>Procedure Steps</u>

1. Process one sheet of unexposed film in the photographic processor.
2. Place one drop of the residual hypo test solution on the film.
3. Allow the solution to stand for two minutes.
4. Blot off the excess solution.
5. Compare the stain with the hypo estimator (Figure 2) by placing the radiographic film on a sheet of white paper. The comparison should be made with the estimator over the film sample to help compensate for differences in the color of the base of the film and with the hypo estimator in its sleeve (for protection).
6. For dual-emulsion films repeat steps 2 through 5 for the other emulsion selecting a different area so that the spots will not overlap.

<u>Precautions and Caveats</u>

The comparison should be made immediately after the excess test solution has been removed from the film. Direct sunlight will cause the spot to darken rapidly, and a prolonged delay between the blotting of the solution and comparison will also allow the spot to darken.

The test solution should have a shelf life of about two years provided that it is stored in a dark, airtight bottle and away from light.

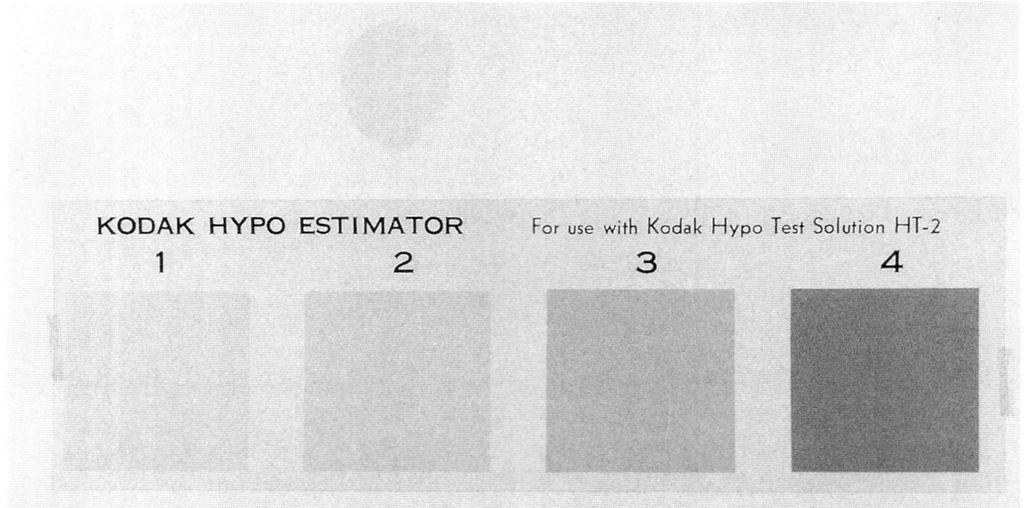


Figure 2. Hypo estimator and test film, showing a match with step 2. This indicates a lower amount of retained fixer than the suggested performance criteria.

Suggested Performance Criteria and Corrective Action

The hypo estimator provides estimates of the amount of residual hypo in the film in units of grams per square meter. The estimated amount of residual hypo should be 0.05 grams per square meter (5 micrograms per square centimeter) or less.

If the stain indicates that there is more than 5 micrograms per square centimeter residual hypo in the film, the test should be repeated. If the same result is obtained, then corrective action is necessary.

The processor wash water tank should be checked to assure that it is full of water, if appropriate. The wash water flow rate should be verified to determine if it meets the specifications of the processor manufacturer. Also, the fixer replenishment rate should be checked to determine if it is close to the recommended rate, since the efficiency of the wash water in removing fixer from the film is dependent upon the correct fixing of the film. If these items appear to be correct, a technical representative of the film manufacturer should be consulted to assist in resolving the problem.

NOTE: If the residual hypo test solution is not available commercially, it can be prepared easily. Place 75 ml of distilled water in a container. Add 12.5 ml of 28% acetic acid and stir. While continuing to stir, add 0.75 gram of silver nitrate. (Acetic acid and silver nitrate should be available from a photographic supply store. to make approximately 28% acetic acid from glacial acetic acid, with caution, add 3 parts of glacial acetic acid to 8 parts of distilled water.) Stir until all of the solid material has dissolved. Add sufficient distilled water to make 100 ml of solution. Place the solution in a dark container and store in a cool, dark area.

Both acetic acid and silver nitrate are dangerous and must be handled with caution. If either of these chemicals comes in contact with your skin, wash the area with cold water immediately and seek medical assistance.

## IV. Developer Temperature and Replenishment Rate

### Procedure: Monitoring Developer Temperature and Replenishment Rate in Photographic Processors

Although these procedures are not as frequently performed as quality control tests, they will be useful to the QC technologist in troubleshooting photographic processor problems.

### A. Developer Temperature
<u>Objective</u>
To confirm and ensure that developer and fixer temperatures are within the manufacturers' recommendations for a particular processor and processing cycle. Low developer temperature can result in underdevelopment which results in reduced image contrast and is often compensated for by increased patient exposure. Fluctuating developer temperature can result in fluctuating image quality.

<u>Required Equipment</u>
Alcohol, dial, or digital (electronic) thermometer
Built-in thermometer

<u>Procedure Steps</u>
1. Read the temperature of developer and fixer solutions and record on the control chart. Clean the thermometer stem of any chemical traces between measurements of developer and fixer and before storage.
2. Compare the measured developer temperature with the temperature reading from the built-in thermometer. If there is a significant discrepancy, e.g., greater than $0.5°$ F, the calibration of both thermometers should be verified, with appropriate corrections (i.e., calibrations) being made by a qualified service engineer.

<u>Precautions and Caveats</u>
Mercury-filled thermometers should never be used to monitor temperatures in a photographic processor. Mercury is a sensitizing agent for photographic films and minute amounts in the processor or darkroom can cause serious problems.

<u>Suggested Performance Criteria and Corrective Action</u>

The developer temperature should be within $\pm 0.5^\circ F$ ($\pm 0.3^\circ C$) of that recommended by the manufacturer for the specific film-developer combination being used. Fixer temperature is not as critical and should be maintained within $\pm 5^\circ F$ ($\pm 3^\circ C$) of the developer temperature.

If developer or fixer temperature is not within specifications it should be adjusted appropriately.

## B. Replenishment Rate

<u>Objective</u>: To verify the replenishment rate based on daily film usage (milliliter / sheet of film). This insures 1) proper film speed and film contrast, and 2) appropriate solution tank operating levels.

<u>Required Equipment</u>

Consult the manufacturer's processor service manual for obtaining this information.

<u>Procedure Steps</u>

1. Consult the manufacturer's processor service manual for obtaining this information.

2. The personnel performing the replenishment rate check must have proper training from the manufacturer or a local service representative (dealer, vendor, etc.).

3. Replenishment rates should be compared to the chemistry manufacturer's pre-established rate per sheet of film based on the daily volume of processed film.

<u>Precautions and Caveats</u>

Replenishment rate checks vary from direct visual readings on some processors to invasive, more labor intensive procedures.

Replenishment rate recommendations are available from most film and chemical manufacturers. However, there are no readily available tables or charts that provide replenishment rate information in a concise and standardization format.

## References


1. AAPM Report #29. Performance Specifications and Equipment Requirements for Mammography, Report of Diagnostic X-ray Imaging Task Group #7, 1991.

2. Gray JE, Winkler NT, Stears J, Frank ED. *Quality Control in Diagnostic Radiology*. Rockville, MD: Aspen Publisher, 1983.

3. Haus AG, Feig SA, Ehrlich S, Hendrick RE, Tabar L. Mammography Screening: Technology, Radiation Dose, Quality Control, and Benefits to Society.

Radiology 174:627;1990.

4. Medicare Program: Medicare Coverage of Screening Mammography. *United States Federal Register*, Washington, DC. Volume 55, No. 251, December 31, 1990, pp. 53510-53525.

5. NCRP, Mammography – A User's Guide. NCRP Report #85, National Council on Radiation Protection and Measurements, Bethesda, MD, 1986.

6. NCRP, Quality Assurance for Diagnostic Imaging. NCRP Report #99, National Council on Radiation Protection and Measurements, Bethesda, MD, 1988.

7. Vyborny CJ, Schmidt RA. Mammography as a Radiographic Examination: An overview. *RadioGraphics* 9:723-764, 1989.

**Reproduced from the ACR Medical Physicists Manual:**
- Introduction
- Mammography Quality Control Tests
- Image Quality Evaluation
- Artifact Evaluation

## Introduction

The success of mammography, whether for screening or diagnosis, depends on the production of high-quality, low-dose images. Production of such images is a complex and difficult task. Poor quality mammograms will lower the detection rate of early breast cancer, reducing the patient's chances of survival and undermining the public's confidence in the value of mammography. Furthermore, substandard mammography will generate unnecessary equivocal examinations leading to increased costs and anxiety to the patient. Achieving high-quality studies at low dose requires vigilant attention to quality control, not only on the part of radiologists and technologists, but also on the part of medical physicists.

This section of the Mammography Quality Control Manuals provides detailed procedures for a number of tests designed to be conducted at least annually by a medical physicist and intended to assess the continuing performance of mammography equipment . Similar sections are included for technologists that detail the procedures appropriate for routine quality control (QC) testing. The tests presented in the Medical Physicist's Manual were selected as the minimum set of tests that should be conducted on an annual basis to help assure proper mammographic system performance. It is assumed that mammographic equipment will have been subjected to extensive acceptance testing or a thorough performance evaluation prior to the initiation of quality control testing.

It is the responsibility of the medical physicist conducting these tests to accurately convey test results in a written report, to make recommendations for corrective actions according to the test results, and to review the results with the radiologist and QC technologist. Communicating test results and recommending corrective actions are areas that can be improved in the practices of most medical physicists. Corrective actions should not be limited to repair of x-ray equipment by a qualified service-person, but should include recommendations that might improve image quality, including recommendations concerning image receptors, technique factors, processing, viewing conditions, and quality control. The medical physicist should periodically review the results of the routine quality control tests conducted by the QC technologist and make recommendations regarding these tests, if appropriate. Furthermore, the medical physicist should participate in periodic reviews of the mammography quality control program as a whole in order to assure that the program is meeting its objectives.

## Medical Physicist's Responsibilities

The medical physicist's responsibilities relate to equipment performance, including image quality, and patient doses, and operator safety. Specific tests include:

Annually:
Mammographic Unit Assembly Evaluation
Collimation Assessment
Focal Spot Size Measurement
kVp Accuracy / Reproducibility
Beam Quality Assessment (Half-Value Layer Measurement)
Automatic Exposure Control (AEC) System Performance Assessment
Uniformity of Screen Speed
Breast Entrance Exposure and Average Glandular Dose
Phantom Evaluation of Image Quality
Artifact Assessment

## Procedure: Image Quality Evaluation

Objective: To assess mammographic image quality and to detect temporal changes in image quality.
Required Test Equipment
Mammographic phantom (approximately 4.5-cm-thick 50/50 tissue equivalent breast phantom) containing appropriate details ranging from visible to invisible on

the mammographic image, e.g., the RMI-156 Mammographic Phantom used for the ACR Mammography Accreditation Program (MAP) or a similar phantom.

Acrylic disc, approximately 4 mm thick and 1 cm in diameter, attached to the top of the phantom in the image area, but not superimposed over details within the phantom.

Cassette and film of the types used clinically for mammography.

A film mask to eliminate light reaching the viewer's eye from beyond the borders of the exposed phantom image. Images should be viewed on the same viewbox(es) used clinically. If a 14" x 17" box is used, a film mask for a 14" by 17" viewbox can be made by exposing a 14" by 17" film to light, processing it, and cutting a hole just the size and shape of the phantom being used.

Original phantom image and the previous phantom image acquired on this unit.

Magnifying lens of the same type used clinically.

Densitometer


<u>Test Procedure Steps</u>
1.   Load the film in the cassette.
2.   Place the cassette in the cassette holder assembly of the x-ray unit.
3.   Place the phantom on the cassette holder, positioning the phantom so that the chest wall edge of the phantom is aligned with the chest wall side of the image receptor.
4.   Lower the compression paddle so that it is just in contact with the top of the phantom. Do not exert excessive compression force on the phantom, as this may damage the compression paddle.
5.   a. For sites using phototimed techniques, verify that the phototimer detector is located beneath the center of the phantom and in the same location as used for previously acquired phantom images.

b. For sites using manual techniques, select the appropriate exposure time and mA setting (or mAs setting) for the phantom thickness, matching technique factors used for previously acquired phantom images.
6.   Select the kVp and density control settings used clinically for a breast of thickness and density corresponding to the phantom. Make sure that these agree with previously acquired phantom image techniques.
7.   Make an exposure, recording all technique factors on the image quality evaluation form.
8.   Process the film in the processor normally used for mammography films.
9.   Measure the central background optical density on the film (usually measured in the center of the phantom insert, away from any test objects), recording this density as the background optical density on the data sheet. Be sure to measure this density at the same location each time.

10. Measure the optical density of the film in the area of the disc (if present) and just outside the disc to the left or right (perpendicular to the anode-cathode axis), recording the difference as the density difference on the image quality evaluation form.

11. Using the mask to give good viewing conditions (see Note below), determine the number of test objects of each type that is visible in the phantom image.

a. If an alternative phantom is used, use the scoring methodology recommended by the phantom manufacturer.

b. If the ACR Mammography Accreditation Phantom is used, and you want your scoring system to match that of the ACR MAP Phantom Reviewers, then use the following criteria. Always count the number of visible objects from the largest object of a given type (fiber, speck group, or mass) downward, until a score of 0 or 0.5 is reached, then stop counting for that object type.

(i) Count each fiber as one point if the full length of the fiber is visible and the location and orientation of the fiber are correct. Count a fiber as 0.5 point if not all, but more than half, of the fiber is visible, and its location and orientation is correct. If a fiber-like artifact appears anywhere in the insert area of the image, but is not in an appropriate location or orientation, deduct the "artifactual" fiber from the last "real" fiber scored if the artifactual fiber is equally or more apparent.

(ii) Use a large field of view magnifying lens (approximately 2x) to assist in the visualization of specks. Count each speck group as 1 point. A full speck group is counted if 4 or more specks are visible in the group in the proper locations. Count a speck group as 0.5 if two or three specks of the group are visible. If noise or speck-like artifacts are visible in the wrong locations in the phantom insert but are as apparent as the "real" specks you are counting, deduct them one for one from the individual specks that you are counting. Artifactual specks should only be deducted from "real" specks in the last group counted.

(iii) Count each mass as 1 point if a density difference is visible in the correct location and the full circular edge of the mass is visible against the background. Count each mass as 0.5 point if a density difference is visible in the correct location, but the full circular edge of the mass is not visible, so the mass does not have a circular appearance. If there is a mass-like artifact appearing in the wrong location anywhere in the phantom insert, deduct the "artifactual" mass from the last "real" mass scored if the artifactual mass is equally or more apparent.

(iv) Enter the results in each category (fibers, specks, and masses) on the image quality evaluation form.

12. Examine the phantom images carefully for artifacts, including dust or dirt, film handling artifacts, processing artifacts, grid lines, and other equipment-induced artifacts. If artifacts are present in the phantom image, be sure to conduct the Artifact Evaluation Test.

NOTE: Mammography phantom images, like mammograms, should always be viewed under good viewing conditions, consisting of:

1. Masking of the viewbox so that extraneous light does not come from the viewbox to the viewer's eye without passing through the exposed portion of the phantom image. A mask is essential for appropriate viewing of phantom images.

2. No backlighting; ambient room lighting reflecting off the film should be minimized.

3. Use of a large field of view magnifying lens (2x is recommended), preferably the same type of magnifying lens used for reading clinical mammograms.

## Precautions and Caveats

This test measures all components of the imaging chain, other than breast positioning by the technologist, patient-induced errors such as motion, and image interpretation by the radiologist. Observed changes in phantom image quality may be due to any component of the imaging chain, from x-ray tube to processor. As a result, other tests will be needed to determine the component(s) of the imaging chain that are at fault and in need of corrective action.

Since the medical physicist may not have the opportunity to measure phantom image quality as frequently as the QC technologist, it is important to review the phantom images acquired by the technologist since the previous visit, comparing results with your own assessment of image quality.

## Suggested Performance Criteria and Corrective Action

The optical density of the film in the center of the phantom image should be about 1.25 (between 1.10 and 1.50), while the density difference should be about $0.40\pm0.05$ for a 4-mm-thick disc and films exposed at 28 kVp. Some discs available commercially have thicknesses different than 4 mm, so optical density differences will be different than 0.40. Constancy from phantom image to phantom image is the crucial factor. If the exposure is made identically to previous phantom images, the optical density in the center of the phantom should not change by more than $\pm0.20$ and the density difference should not change by more than 0.05. The exposure time or mAs noted on the generator read-out should not change by more than $\pm15\%$ from one phantom image exposure to another.

The number of objects detected in each group (fibers, specks, and masses) should not change by more than 0.5 if viewed under ideal conditions by the same observer. If the observed number of test objects in one or more groups changes by more than 0.5, then further comparison with the original or previous phantom image and previously acquired phantom images should be made to determine whether the change is real.

Any change between the current phantom image and the original or previous phantom image in density, density difference, or number of test objects that exceeds the suggested performance criteria should be investigated to determine the source or sources for the change. Once the source has been identified, the problem or problems should be corrected immediately.

## Procedure: Artifact Assessment

Objective: To assess the degree and source of artifacts visualized in mammograms or phantom images. This procedure allows the source of artifacts to be isolated to x-ray equipment or film processor so that appropriate measures for elimination of artifacts can be taken.

Required Test Equipment
A 1-inch-thick uniform sheet of acrylic or 1-2 cm thick sheet of high-grade, uniform BR-12 free from defects that covers the mammographic cassette.
Mammographic cassette and film. The same cassette should be used for all tests.
A mask appropriate for full-field mammographic films.
A densitometer.

Test Procedure Steps
1.   Use technique factors normally used clinically, choosing the lowest kVp setting used clinically (to be most sensitive to artifacts). If phototiming is normally used, use it in this test, choosing the density adjustment on the unit to produce an optical density in the range of 1.10 to 1.50. Use the most commonly used image receptor size (usually 18 x 24 cm). If a grid is normally used, make sure the same grid is used in this testing. Record these technique factors on the data form.
2.   Place a uniform sheet of acrylic or BR-12 that is large enough to cover the mammographic cassette and thick enough to have an exposure time of 0.5 second or greater on the image receptor holder assembly. Use a collimator that permits irradiation of the entire cassette.
3.   Use a single mammographic cassette that is known to have good screen-film contact. Load the cassette with the appropriate type of mammographic film used clinically.
4.   Position a lead marker such as number 1 or an arrow on the acrylic sheet in a corner of the radiation field, preferably outside the normal location of the breast, and pointing along the long axis of the film and cassette.
5.   Make an exposure.
6.   Process the film, taking care to insert the film lengthwise into the processor as shown in the upper part of Figure 3 (so that the film travels parallel to the direction of the arrow on the latent image). Measure the optical density in the center of the film,

verifying that it is in the range of 1.1 to 1.5, and record this on the data form for this test.

7. Reload the same cassette with film, place it in the image receptor holder assembly under the same sheet of acrylic. Orient the lead marker at 90° to its original direction so that the marker runs parallel to the short axis of the film. Repeat the exposure using exposure factors identical to the previous image.

8. Process this film, taking care to insert the film widthwise into the processor as illustrated in the lower part of Figure 3 (at right angles to the previous film) so that the film travels through the processor parallel to the direction of the arrow on the latent image.

9. Repeat this process for other image receptor sizes, using a grid for the other image receptor sizes, if available. Also repeat for all available focal spot sizes and filters used clinically.

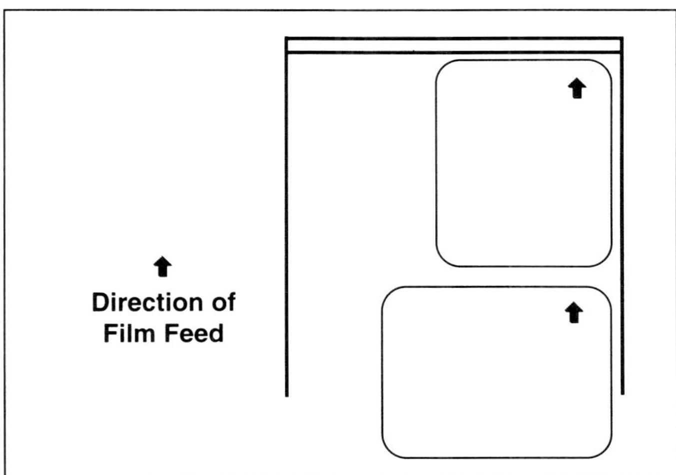


Figure 3. Direction of insertion of film into the film processor. The first exposed fim should be inserted lengthwise, parallel to the direction of the arrow on the latent image. The second film should be inserted widthwise, again parallel to the direction of the arrow on the latent image.

<u>Suggested Performance Criteria and Corrective Action</u>
1. Using appropriate masking, examine the two processed images acquired for each image receptor size for density variations, especially those that might simulate breast structure or breast pathology. Orient the two films for viewing at right angles to one another so that the arrows indicating the direction that they were run through the processor are parallel, as shown in Figures 4 and 5.

2. Any artifacts that are parallel in the two films, as illustrated in Figure 4, are localized to the processor. This is true whether the artifacts run parallel to or perpendicular to the direction of film travel. For example, film processor artifacts due to dirty or defective rollers can produce plus or minus density streaks running parallel to the direction of film travel or plus density bands running perpendicular to the direction of film travel. If film processor artifacts are detected, contact the person maintaining the processor or the film processor service organization or dealer.

3. Any artifacts that are oriented perpendicular between the two films, as illustrated in Figure 5, are localized to the x-ray equipment. Artifacts localized to the x-ray equipment can be due to several sources, including the grid, the image receptor holder, the collimator, the filter, or the x-ray tube itself. Further testing will be required to determine the specific source within the x-ray equipment that is causing the artifact. Contact the x-ray equipment service person for suggestions on additional testing procedures and for help correcting x-ray equipment artifacts.

4. Other artifacts may appear sporadically in mammography images, having no consistent appearance in artifact evaluation images. These artifacts may be due to other sources, such as the patient, film handling, a defective cassette screen (that was not used in these tests), or moving grid artifacts that show up only under certain patient or timing conditions. Additional testing under specific conditions may be necessary to isolate the causes of sporadically occuring artifacts.

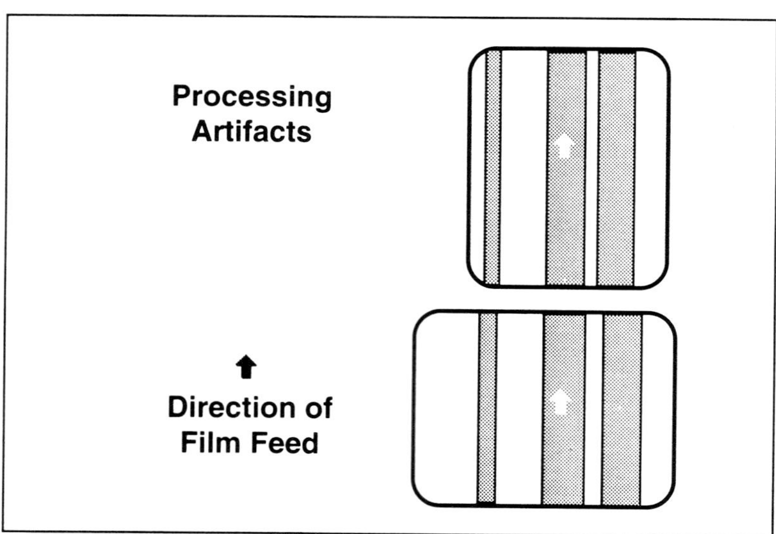


Figure 4. Orient the films for viewing at right angles to one another, so that the arrows or markers indicating the direction of film travel through the processor are parallel. Any artifacts running parallel in the two films are due to the processor.

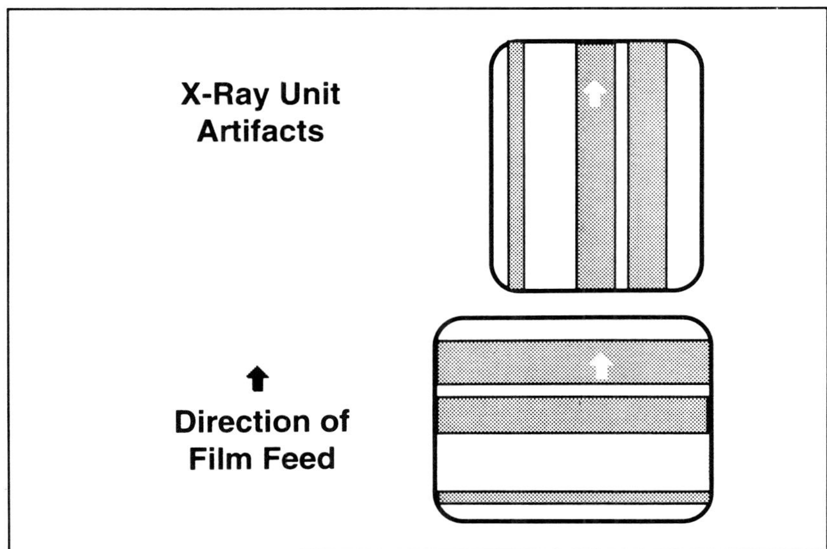


**Figure 5.** Orient the two films at right angles to one another, as in Figures 3 and 4. Any artifacts running perpendicular in the two films are due to x-ray equipment.

## References

1. AAPM Report No.29. Equipment requirements and quality control for mammography. Report of Task Group No. 7: Diagnostic x-ray imaging, Martin J. Yaffe, chairman. New York: Am Assoc Physicists Med; August 1990

2. Barnes GT, Brezovich IA. The intensity of scattered radiation in mammography. *Radiology* 126:243-247, 1978

3. Barnes GT, Frey GD (eds). Screen-film mammography: imaging considerations and medical physics responsibilities. Madison, WI: Medical Physics Publishing, 1991

4. Bunch PC. Detective quantum efficiency of selected mammographic screen-film combinations. *Proc SPIE*, Medical Imaging III, vol. 1090, 1988

5. Bunch PC, Huff KE, Van Metter RL: Analysis of the detective quantum efficiency of a radiographic screen-film combination. *J Opt Soc Am A* 4:902, 1987

6. Burgess A. A mammography quality assurance test program. *Radiology* 133:491-495, 1979

7. Dance DR. Montecarlo calculation of conversion factors for the estimation of mean glandular breast dose. *Phys Med Biol* 35:1211-1219, 1990

8. deParedes ES, Frazier AB, Hartwell GD, Strash AM, Sheer C, Smith DC, Barnette PA, Noel W, Kenneweg D. Development and implementation of a quality assurance program for mammography. *Radiology* 163:83-85, 1987

9. Dershaw DD, Malik S. Stationary and moving mammography grids: comparative radiation dose. *AJR* 147:491-492, 1986

10. Galkin BM, Feig SA, Muir HD. The technical quality of mammography in centers participating in a regional breast cancer awareness program. *RadioGraphics* 8:133-145, 1988

11. Gray JE, Winkler NT, Stears J, Frank ED. Quality control in diagnostic radiology. Rockville, MD: Aspen Publishers; 1983

12. Haus AG, Gray JE, Daln T. Evaluation of mammographic viewbox luminanceilluminance and color. *Medical Physics,* 1993 (in press)

13. Haus AG. Evaluation of image blur (unsharpness) in medical imaging. *Med Radiogr Photog* 61:42-53, 1985

14. Haus AG. Recent advances in screen-film mammography. *Radiol Clin North Am* 25:913-928, 1987

15. Haus AG. State-of-the-art screen-film mammography: a technical overview. In Barnes GT, Frey DG (eds), Screen-film mammography imaging considerations and medical physics responsibilities. Madison, WI: Medical Physics Publishing Corporation, 1990

16. Haus AG. Technologic improvements in screen-film mammography. *Radiology* 174:628-637, 1990

17. Haus AG, Cullinan JE. Screen-film processing systems for medical radiography: a historical review. *RadioGraphics* 1203-1224, 1989

18. Hendrick RE. Quality assurance in mammography: accreditation, legislation, and compliance with quality assurance standards. In: Bassett LW (ed.), Breast imaging: current status and future directions. *Radiol Clin North Am* 30:243-255, 1992

19. Hendrick RE. Standardization of image quality and radiation dose in mammography. *Radiology* 174:648-654, 1990

20. Hessler C, Depeursinge C, Grecescu M, Pochon Y, Raimondi S, Valley JF. Objective assessment of mammography systems, part 1: Method. *Radiology* 156:215-220, 1985

21. Hessler C, Depeursinge C, Grecescu M, Pochon Y, Raimondi S, Valley JF. Objective assessment of mammography systems, part 2: Implementation. *Radiology* 156:221-225, 1985

22. Hubbard LB. Mammography as a radiographic system. *RadioGraphics* 10:103-113,1990

23. Karila KTK. Image quality of mammographic system. *Eur J Radiol* 7:194, 1987

24. Kimme-Smith C, Bassett LW, Gold RH. Focal spot measurements with pinhole and slit for microfocus mammogarphy units. *Med Phys* 15:293-298, 1988

25. Kimme-Smith C, Bassett LW, gold RH, Roe D, Orr J. Mammographic dual screen, dual emulsion film combination: visibility of simulated microcalcifications and effect on image contrast. *Radiology* 165:313-318, 1987

26. Kimme-Smith C, Rothchild PA, Bassett LW, Gold RH, Moler C. Mammographic film-processor temperature, development time, and chemistry: effect on dose, contrast, and noise. *AJR* 152:35-40, 1989

27. LaFrance R, Gelskey DT, Barnes GT. A circuit modification that improves mammographic phototimer performance. *Radiology* 166:773-776, 1988

28. McLelland R, Hendrick RE, Zinninger MD, Wilcox PA. The American College of Radiology Mammography Accreditation Proram. *AJR* 157:473-479, 1991

29. Mount CJ, Gray JE. Mammography screen-film contact: problems with conventional screen-film contact setting. *RadioGraphics* 10:1049-1054, 1990

30. NCRP Report No. 85. Mammography - a user's guide. Rothenberg LN (ed), National Council on Radiation Protection and Measurement. Bethesda, MD: March 1, 1986 (see references therein to mammography literature prior to 1986)

31. Niklason LT, Barnes GT, Rubin E. Mammography phototimer technique chart. *Radiology* 157:539-540, 1985

32. Nishikawa RM, Yaffe MJ. Signal-to-noise properties of mammographic film-screen systems. *Med Physics* 12:32-39, 1985

33. Prado KL, Rakowski JT, Barragan F, Vanek KN. Breast radiation dose in film/screen mammography. *Health Physics* 55:81-84, 1988

34. Rothenberg LN. Patient dose in mammography. *RadioGraphics* 10:739-746, 1990

35. Sickles EA, Weber WN, High-contrast mammography with a moving grid: assessment of clinical utility. *AJR* 146:1137-1139, 1986

36. Skubic SE, Fatourros PP. Absorbed breast dose: dependence on radiographic modality and technique, and breast thickness. *Radiology* 161:263-270, 1986

37. Stanton L, Viillafana T, Day JL, Lightfoot DA. Dosage evaluation in mammography. *Radiology* 150:577-584, 1984

38. Tabar L, Dean PB. Optimum mammography technique: the annotated cookbook approach. *Admin Radiology* 8:54-56, 1989

39. Tabar L, Haus AG. Processing mammographic films: technical and clinical considerations. *Radiology* 173:65-69, 1989

40. Villfana T. Generators, x-ray tubes, and exposure geometry in mammography. *RadioGraphics* 10:539-554, 1990

41. Wu X, Barnes GT, Tucker DM. Spectral dependence of glandular tissue dose in screen-film mammography. *Radiology* 179:143-148, 1991

42. Yaffe MJ. Physics of mammography: image recording process. *RadioGraphics* 10:341-363, 199010:103-113, 1990